Leadership for Public Health

Leadership for
Public Health

Theory and Practice

JAMES W. HOLSINGER JR. | ERIK L. CARLTON

Health Administration Press, Chicago, Illinois

Your board, staff, or clients may also benefit from this book's insight. For more information on quantity discounts, contact the Health Administration Press Marketing Manager at (312) 424-9450.

22 21 20 19 18   5 4 3 2 1

Library of Congress Cataloging-in-Publication Data

Names: Holsinger, James W., author. | Carlton, Erik L., author.
Title: Leadership for public health : theory and practice / James W. Holsinger, Jr., Erik L. Carlton.
Description: Chicago, Illinois : Health Administration Press, [2018] | Includes bibliographical references and index.
Identifiers: LCCN 2017041130 (print) | LCCN 2017035208 (ebook) | ISBN 9781567939361 (eBook 13) | ISBN 9781567939378 (Xml) | ISBN 9781567939385 (Epub) | ISBN 9781567939392 (Mobi) | ISBN 9781567939354 (print : alk. paper)
Subjects: LCSH: Health services administration. | Leadership.
Classification: LCC RA971 (print) | LCC RA971 .H573 2018 (ebook) | DDC 362.1068—dc23
LC record available at https://lccn.loc.gov/2017041130

Acquisitions editor: Janet Davis; Project manager: Michael Noren; Cover designer: James Slate; Layout: Cepheus Edmondson

Found an error or a typo? We want to know! Please e-mail it to hapbooks@ache.org, mentioning the book's title and putting "Book Error" in the subject line.

Health Administration Press
A division of the Foundation of the American
   College of Healthcare Executives
One North Franklin Street, Suite 1700
Chicago, IL 60606-3529
(312) 424-2800

BRIEF CONTENTS

DETAILED CONTENTS

PREFACE

As the twenty-first century unfolds, the effective practice of public health leadership is critical. The popular press is replete with stories of failed leadership in otherwise well-run for-profit corporations, public not-for-profit entities, and governmental agencies. As the health of the public rapidly evolves and the discipline of public health continues to develop, new demands are placed on leaders in the field. In this rapidly changing landscape, a thorough understanding of the principles, attributes, and skills of leadership is essential for all current and prospective practitioners.

In both a letter[1] and a concept paper, leaders of several organizations—specifically, the National Public Health Leadership Development Network, the Public Health Leadership Society, the Association for State and Territorial Health Officials, the National Association for County and City Health Officials, the National Public Health Leadership Institute, the National Network of Public Health Institutes, and the American Public Health Association[2]—argued for leadership development as an integral part of public health workforce development. The organizations addressed their argument to senior leaders at the Centers for Disease Control and Prevention (CDC) and the Health Resources and Services Administration (HRSA). The CDC has been the principal funding source of national, regional, state, local, tribal, and territorial leadership institutes, and HRSA has supported a national network of public health training centers (PHTCs). The authors of the letter argued for closer collaboration between existing public health leadership development efforts. They suggested affiliation of each leadership institute with a federally funded PHTC, continued support for the development of the National Alliance for Workforce and Leadership Development (a partnership among the aforementioned organizations), the development and adaptation of new models for training public health partners, the provision of leadership development opportunities to a wider array of public health professionals, an effort to maximize the use of distance-learning technologies, and support for the development of citizen leaders.

A major impetus behind the letter and concept paper, aside from the need for continued funding, was the aim of creating a unified voice among these organizations and their leadership development efforts. Such a voice could merge the unique efforts and processes of each organization across shared values, objectives, and activities. The future of public health leadership development will grow from this collaborative effort, with a focus that includes preparation, crisis and disaster management, and greater leadership both within and outside of public health organizations. Instead of *public health leadership*, the emphasis will be on *leadership for the public's health*—in particular, leadership that not only rises to the challenges presented by public health agencies but also transforms public health practitioners, public health agencies, and, therefore, the health of the public.

These organizations have developed several frameworks for ensuring a competent and professional public health workforce, and the models incorporate themes of communication, collaboration, cultural and community awareness, ethics and professionalism, and policy and program assessment and analytics. Clearly, the overarching theme of public health leadership development is the need for well-skilled and well-educated leaders capable of galvanizing organizations and communities in transformational change processes that can ensure and improve the health and well-being of communities and the population at large. This is the essence of effective public health leadership.

Today's practitioners must have the managerial skills necessary to ensure effectiveness across the various public health professional disciplines at a time when these fields have become increasingly demanding and complex. At the same time, today's practitioners must also have the ability to lead people regardless of professional discipline. Although leadership is one of the cornerstones of effective management, not all great managers are great leaders—and vice versa. Current and prospective practitioners must therefore study the principles of leadership so that they become qualified to lead as well as manage their organizations.[3]

The word *leadership* has more than 100 definitions[4]; thus, the topic can be approached in a variety of ways. For our purposes, leadership is "a process that occurs whenever an individual intentionally attempts to influence another individual or group, regardless of the reason, in an effort to achieve a common goal which may or may not contribute to the success of the organization."[3(p3)] The nature of leadership itself—as a process involving two or more people—is an important concept in leading an organization, group, or team. Whereas some leaders may be born with the inherent traits to lead, most effective public health leaders develop the required knowledge, skills, and abilities through education, training, and practice.

The aim of this book is to focus the attention of public health practitioners on the importance of effectively leading their organizations. Skilled public health managers recognize that the people they lead are their organizations' most valuable resource, and they understand that leadership can be applied in a variety of ways, depending on the person and the situation. As we consider the various models and theories of leadership, we strongly recommend that the reader test the various approaches. No single leadership model or theory fits everyone, and effective public health leaders often use more than one. We challenge our readers to try the various leadership models and theories presented in this book, determine which are the best fit for their public health practice, and utilize those approaches in day-to-day practice.

The chapters of this book are arranged in three parts: part I, titled "The Basis for Effective Public Health Practice"; part II, "Leadership Theories and Concepts"; and part III, "The Effective Practice of Public Health Leadership." The book also contains a leadership application case that describes a series of events at the Missouri City Metropolitan Health Department and provides realistic scenarios corresponding with the book's chapters.

Part I comprises two chapters. Chapter 1, "The Nature of Effective Public Health Leadership," provides an overview of the concept of leadership and develops the definition of *leadership* that will serve as the basis of our study. Although leadership is often considered one of the core functions of management (i.e., planning, organizing, leading, controlling), we consider leadership and management separately. We define *management* as "working with and through people in order to complete the work at hand in an effective and efficient manner." Leadership, on the other hand, occurs whenever an individual attempts to influence another individual or group, regardless of the reason, in an effort to achieve a common goal that may or may not contribute to the success of the organization.

Chapter 2, "Professionalism for the Effective Public Health Leader," establishes that public health is a profession staffed by practitioners from a variety of disciplines. As such, it has an educational basis with core competencies that enable practitioners to perform their duties in an appropriately professional manner. The chapter uses Reinhard Priester's framework of healthcare values as the basis for a professional framework for the effective practice of public health leadership.

Part II of the book explores the models and theories of leadership likely to be most helpful to aspiring public health leaders. Chapter 3, "Traits, Skills, and Styles of Leadership," examines the importance of traits (e.g., self-confidence), skills (e.g., interpersonal and human skills), and personality factors (e.g., conscientiousness) to the effective practice of leadership. It discusses the Myers-Briggs Type Indicator, which can help identify one's cognitive style, and the concept of emotional intelligence, which can serve as a means for self-understanding.

Chapter 4, "The Contingency Model and Situational Leadership," emphasizes the situation or context within which leadership transpires—an important aspect of leadership regardless of the specific approach being used. Situational leadership is a contingency model based on the premise that the needs of the follower come before the ego needs of the leader. To effectively apply this theory, practitioners must match their leadership style to the developmental level of their followers. They must constantly be aware of the developmental level of each follower, recognizing that each follower's level is individualized and can change rapidly, requiring a quick response by the leader.

Chapter 5, "Path–Goal Theory and the Vroom-Jago Model of Leadership," builds on chapter 4 and focuses on understanding the influence of the leader's behaviors on the performance and satisfaction of the followers. The path–goal theory may be the most comprehensive and sophisticated of the contingency models. Unlike situational leadership, in which the leader adapts to the needs of the follower, the path–goal theory emphasizes the interaction between three elements: the leader's style, the follower's characteristics, and the work setting in which the leader and follower interact. The theory specifies four leadership behaviors that, when matched to situational contingencies, provide a useful means of motivating followers.

Chapter 6, "The Leader–Member Exchange Theory," focuses on the development of leader and follower roles and the exchange relationship that occurs over time between them. A key element of the leader–member exchange theory, or LMX theory, is the trust that develops between pairs of individuals. The dyadic pair of the leader and follower is the basic unit of analysis of that trust, and the trust can be assessed via the Conditions of Trust Inventory, a validated trust inventory. The LMX theory is similar to situational leadership, in that it deals with the relationship between two individuals, the leader and the follower. The LMX theory differs, however, in its expectation that each follower will have a different and unique relationship with the leader.

Chapter 7, "Transformational Leadership," furthers the idea that leadership occurs within the context of relationships, and it distinguishes transformational leadership from transactional leadership. Transformational leadership emphasizes risk taking, change, and motivation in a way that transactional leadership does not. Although it does include certain elements of transactional leadership (e.g., contingent rewards, management by exception), transformational leadership relies heavily on such concepts as idealized rewards, intellectual stimulation, inspirational motivation, and individualized consideration. Several studies have linked transformational leadership to improved quality, employee satisfaction, productivity, and leadership efficacy.

Part III of the book explores key leadership concepts that expand on the theories and models presented in part II. Chapter 8, "The Ethical Basis of Public Health Leadership," develops the ethical and moral basis for the effective practice of public health leadership. To be effective, public health leaders must have an understanding of moral reasoning and ethical decision making, and they must understand how to apply utilitarian analysis to their community's needs while recognizing that resources are limited. Leaders also must discern the right and wrong of certain behaviors. They must understand that having a positive impact on the community they serve depends on their character and on the character of those they lead.

Chapter 9, "The Cultural Basis of Public Health Leadership," examines the cultural processes that exist in every organization, public health or otherwise. Every organization has its own identifiable culture based on the information exchanged in speech, actions, and rituals; the organization's artifacts; and the organization's social structure. In addition, organizations, like society at large, have subcultures within the wider culture. All public health practitioners function within a set of cultures ranging from the nation as a whole, to a state or jurisdiction, to a local community, to the specific public health organization. Each of these cultures has practices guided by values and beliefs.

Chapter 10, "Followership," examines the concept of followership and explores its relationship to leadership. Followership has traditionally been deemed secondary to leadership, but its importance has become more widely recognized in recent years. Leadership cannot exist without followers, and leaders must be closely engaged with the people they lead. Leaders who are far out in front of their followers are no longer leading. Followers share a common purpose with their leaders. They believe in what their organizations are trying to accomplish, and they work closely with their leaders to make it happen. In addition, public health leaders may serve as followers in several contexts in which they function, just as followers in one context may be leaders in another.

Chapter 11, "Team Leadership for Public Health," explores the ways that effective public health leaders engage their followers in teams or groups. Teams are small organizational units (typically ranging from 3 to 20 members) that work together on a regular basis and share a common goal or goals. Teams in the public health setting may include employees, colleagues, collaborators, constituents, or other public health leaders. To lead these organizational elements effectively, public health practitioners must possess team-oriented leadership skills that are built from the skills associated with leading individuals. Among the team leadership approaches described in the chapter are the Hersey, Blanchard, and Johnson application of situational leadership and Hill's team leadership model, which is based on diagnosing team problems. Teams can be highly effective, but they can also be plagued by five common dysfunctions: absence of trust, fear of conflict, lack of commitment, avoidance of accountability, and inattention to results.

Chapter 12, "Power and Public Health Leadership," considers the relationship between leadership and power. As Lord Acton famously stated, "power tends to corrupt," and public health practitioners must be constantly aware of the possibility of such corruption in their practice of leadership. Power is the capacity or potential for leaders to influence one or more followers to achieve the goals or outcomes desired by the leader. Power can be based on the leader's position within the organization (i.e., hard power), or it can come from the leader's personal attributes and relationships with followers (i.e., soft power). The chapter presents an expanded French-Raven taxonomy of power, which can be a useful tool for public health leaders.

Chapter 13, "Mentoring and Coaching Leaders in Public Health," examines the nature of mentoring and coaching and differentiates between the two concepts. Mentoring is based on concern for an individual's professional success, and it is personal in nature, relying on face-to-face interaction. In mentoring relationships, mentors who have extensive knowledge and wisdom share their experiences with mentees, with the aim of developing the mentees' abilities and helping them reach their full potential. Coaching, meanwhile, involves instructing, training, and directing one or more people so that they learn specific skills or achieve a goal. Coaching can help individuals complete their work and enhance their careers, and it is effective in addressing performance issues. Effective public health leaders must develop the skills to both mentor and coach their followers.

Public health practitioners, like most of the workforce, spend the bulk of their time working for organizations. Because they rarely engage in their practice alone, their ability to work effectively with others is of paramount importance. The theories, models, and practices in this book offer a framework for effective public health leadership that can be applied at all public health organizations, regardless of the size or type of organization, or the position of the leader in the organization's hierarchy. Public health in the twenty-first century demands leadership that is intelligent, purposeful, caring, competent, and ethical, with a commitment to making a difference in the lives of the people served.

James W. Holsinger Jr., MD, PhD
Erik L. Carlton, DrPH

References

1. Peck, M., K. Wright, D. Williams, et al. 2010. Letter to Dr. Judith A. Monroe, director, Office for State, Tribal, Local, and Territorial Support (OSTLTS), Centers for Disease Control and Prevention, and Dr. Kyu Rhee, chief public health officer, Health Resources and Services Administration. July.

2. National Public Health Leadership Development Network, the Public Health Leadership Society, the Association for State and Territorial Health Officials, the National Association for County and City Health Officials, the National Public Health Leadership Institute, the National Network of Public Health Institutes, and the American Public Health Association. 2010. *Public Health Leadership: A Vital Component of Workforce Development*. Concept paper.

3. Holsinger, J. W., Jr., E. L. Carlton, and E. D. Jadhav. 2015. "Leading People—Managing Organizations: Contemporary Public Health Leadership." *Frontiers in Public Health* 3: 268.

4. Rost, J. C. 1991. *Leadership for the Twenty-First Century.* Westport, CT: Greenwood.

Instructor Resources

This book's Instructor Resources include a test bank, PowerPoint slides, and answer guides to the in-book discussion questions.

For the most up-to-date information about this book and its Instructor Resources, go to ache.org/HAP and browse for the book's title or author name.

This book's Instructor Resources are available to instructors who adopt this book for use in their course. For access information, please e-mail hapbooks@ache.org.

ACKNOWLEDGMENTS

We would like to take this opportunity to express our appreciation to our colleagues and friends who have contributed to this book: Dr. Emmanuel Jadhav, Dr. Jennifer Redmond Knight, Dr. William Mase, Dr. Donna Schmutzler, and Dr. James Thobaben. We greatly appreciate the assistance of Dr. Quan Chen and Dr. Andrea Durst, who, while serving as graduate assistants, developed many of the exhibits. Without the support, encouragement, and professionalism of our editors, Janet Davis and Michael Noren, this book would not have seen the light of day. We are deeply grateful to them and to Health Administration Press.

JWH

I am grateful for the forbearance of my spouse, Dr. Barbara Holsinger, during the long hours required to bring this book into existence. She is a pearl of great price! I appreciate the years of assistance provided to me by Rebecca Friend, who gave 20 years of her life to keeping me straight at the University of Kentucky. I treasure her friendship.

ELC

Jim, my coauthor and friend, from hiking together the Great Wall to writing this book, working with you has been a singular professional pleasure. You have been the mentor of mentors, a confidant, a cheerleader, and a voice of reason and wisdom. I am forever in your debt. Scutch, on each step of my professional public health journey, you have been one of my greatest champions. You have set me straight and lifted me up, have lighted the path and allowed me to learn and grow. One could reasonably say this is all your fault! Ann Vail, your encouragement to walk across the street and talk to Scutch opened a door that I could not have foreseen. You trusted and supported me as I led projects under your wonderful leadership, and you have continued to be one of my biggest supporters. Your overt belief in me has helped me believe in myself. Jason Whiting, Kay Bradford, and Leigh Ann Simmons, you brought me on as a young graduate student and gave me the experiences that planted within me the seeds of scholarship. May this book be just one of its many fruits. Finally, and most importantly, I am forever indebted to my best friend and wife, Tamara, whose loving patience with my professional pursuits has been a blessing beyond measure.

LEADERSHIP APPLICATION CASE: MISSOURI CITY METROPOLITAN HEALTH DEPARTMENT

Emmanuel D. Jadhav and James W. Holsinger Jr.

The following case provides realistic scenarios for the application of the leadership principles presented in this book. The sections of the case—and the questions at the end of each section—correspond with the chapters of the book, and they should be completed sequentially as the reader advances through the book.

The Setting

Dr. John Marshall recently completed a residency in preventive medicine. As part of his training, he earned a master's degree in public health, with a concentration in epidemiology, from the state university. He has now received an appointment as the director of the epidemiology division of the Missouri City Metropolitan Health Department (MCMHD).

Previously, John had completed a residency in internal medicine, and prior to entering the preventive medicine program, he had served for two years as an assistant professor of internal medicine at the same university. He had also served as a research associate at the local Department of Veterans Affairs Medical Center, which was affiliated with the state university's medical school. John's interest in the practice of public health began during his internal medicine residency and steadily progressed through his preventive medicine program. He has developed a keen interest in demystifying the healthcare delivery system, which has led to his involvement with a variety of settings, including government and private healthcare systems, academic institutions, and service organizations. At age 35, John is eager to begin working in public health and keenly interested in developing a career in public health leadership. Throughout his medical training, John has studied the art and science of leading, and he possesses a good understanding of the responsibility and authority associated with leadership. However, the position at MCMHD represents John's first experience as an independent leader.

MCMHD serves the residents of Missouri City and the immediate surrounding area of the state of Transylvania. It is one of two health departments serving residents of Jefferson County, and it is staffed by 522 employees. Employees of the department are for the most part members of a collective bargaining unit or union, which is not typical of local public health organizations in Transylvania. In fact, the other six health departments in the state are nonunionized. The unionization of MCMHD employees has a real and significant impact on the work culture and the conduct of employees and their supervisors. In general, the department has a fairly rigid, nonflexible approach toward work and work-related activities, with strict adherence to union policy. The department must pay explicit attention to the Institutional Review Board processes by the commissioner of health, and it must monitor staff work schedules to ensure that lunch breaks and regular staff breaks are honored.

MCMHD is truly a "large city" health department addressing "large city" public health issues. It has a substantial workforce in place to provide clinical services that are unmet by traditional points of service. The department operates six health centers throughout the city and an additional six dental clinics, a service often not addressed by local public health programs. In addition to these 12 direct service facilities, the department has a designated women, infants, and children (WIC) facility to support qualified/eligible residents and a sexually transmitted disease (STD) clinic that offers such programs as reproductive health education, HIV/AIDS testing, and supportive counseling. The Health Department organization includes divisions addressing such areas as community health, epidemiology, and environmental services; the office of the medical director; the office of community outreach advocacy and affairs; the bureau of nursing; and a center for public health preparedness. Missouri City is one of the few cities in the United States that has an operational syndrome surveillance system in place to detect disease outbreaks at the earliest possible point in time.

Missouri City's service delivery design is truly diverse. Each of six divisions—central administration, epidemiology, environmental health and safety, community health development, clinical services, and administration and accounting—is charged with developing, ensuring, and providing public health services to all residents of a large metropolitan region. Given the variability within the communities served, developing policy and providing appropriate and effective services can be challenging.

Chapter 1 Application: Getting Started

As John begins his new assignment, he considers his current status as a leader. The son of a naval officer, John has regarded leadership as a significant concept since his formative years. Thinking back over his life, he remembers being nine years old and attending camp with his cousin, who was the same age. They attended two one-month sessions at the camp, and each session concluded with an awards presentation in front of a campfire. At each event, he received seven awards, one for each area of camp life at which he excelled. Meanwhile, his cousin received only one award, for leadership. As he reflects on these events, John ponders several questions:

1. Was leadership a trait that his cousin was born with?
2. If leadership was an inborn trait and John, at age nine, did not seem to be a born leader, would he be able to become a leader?
3. Could John, as an adult, analyze the skills necessary to be a truly effective public health leader and apply those skills in his public health career?
4. If so, how could he formulate a plan to develop such skills?
5. Analyze the skills John will need to develop in order to become an effective public health leader.

Chapter 2 Application: The Other Side of the Story

In his new position, John is responsible for providing epidemiological services at the six health centers managed by MCMHD. The health centers serve the residents of Jefferson County, as well as the cities of Wilmore, Bracken, Nicholasville, Norfolk, and Anderson. Each health center has an epidemiology section staffed with a section chief and a number of epidemiologists and other staff members; these individuals are responsible for the epidemiological services for their city and the surrounding area. The six section chiefs report directly to John, the epidemiology division director.

Into his second week as the division director, John receives an urgent meeting request from Jack Snow, the section chief of Wilmore. In their meeting, Jack elaborately tells John that the Bracken City section chief, Dr. Jacob Chadwick, has been abusing power and mismanaging the contract protocol for vehicle maintenance. Vehicle maintenance is a major cost center for the six health centers and is at the top of John's agenda. John asks his administrative assistant to contact Jacob, tell Jacob to stop whatever work he is doing, and arrange for Jacob to meet with John immediately. Jacob is in the middle of an epidemiological survey in his city when he receives the call, but he stops his work and arrives at John's office. During the meeting, John allows his temper to get the better of him and explodes with a verbal barrage that conveys his anger and disappointment. After a nearly 15-minute tirade, John stops, takes a breath, and gives Jacob a questioning look. Jacob, in a controlled and polite voice, asks, "Would you like to hear my side of the story?"

1. Has John acted professionally?
2. How should John have acted in this situation?
3. Apply the medical model and Priester's framework to explain how the situation could have been handled differently.
4. After appraising the situation, how would you deal with it?
5. Create your own professional approach to dealing with conflict situations.

Chapter 3 Application: To Change or Not to Change

Having survived two financial quarters and having learned a few lessons about leading people and the department, John reflects on ways he might improve his leadership skills and strengthen his management of the epidemiology division. While reflecting, he receives an e-mail from the human relations department. The e-mail announces a program by the Transylvania Public Health Leadership Institute (TPHLI) that seeks to develop emerging leaders. A one-day orientation workshop will be held at the local university, and, from the people attending that session, a smaller group will be selected to complete yearlong training in the areas of leadership, systems thinking, and change. John is not sure he can find the time, but he is excited about the program and decides to explore the opportunity.

One of the program's requirements is that John complete the Myers-Briggs Type Indicator. Upon taking the test, John determines that his type is ISTJ (introversion, sensing, thinking, judging), reflecting his practical, orderly, logical, realistic, and dependable attitude toward work—an attitude that persists especially once he has made decisions, regardless of protests or distractions. His personality undoubtedly helped him as a resident and assistant professor of preventive medicine.

At the leadership program orientation, John learns the importance of understanding his growth areas, which are found among the traits in the Myers-Briggs type directly opposite one's own. Since he cannot grow by focusing only on his own type, John must engage the traits found in the ENFP (extraversion, intuition, feeling, perceiving) type. Among other growth areas, John will need to work on being warmly enthusiastic and high-spirited, even though he feels more naturally inclined toward seriousness and quiet. John also must address his tendency to do things himself rather than delegate responsibility to others. John is not sure he is ready to make such changes in the way he conducts himself, nor is he certain of a good starting point for initiating them.

1. Identify an appropriate starting point for John to initiate his development of new leadership traits.

2. Review the traits associated with John's personality type (ISTJ) and its opposite (ENFP). Which elements do you think will be easier to implement than others as John goes about finding a balance between them?

3. Assess the amount of influence a leader's personality and behavior have on follower performance.

4. Describe the possible effects of leader characteristics on the outcomes of a public health agency—for instance, the number of epidemiological services offered by MCMHD.

Chapter 4 Application: A New Leadership Model

Eight months into John's appointment as division director, a continuing medical education (CME) opportunity has become available—the Leadership for Physician Executives seminar developed by the Blankenship Institute in association with a major medical school. This opportunity will bring John into contact with new physician executives who come from other states and who have different management portfolios, thus expanding his awareness across a variety of work environments. John realizes that every work environment is a unique, dynamic, and complex living system determined by the sum of the organization's individual members. At the seminar, he learns about human motivation and its tangible application to the work environment, and he gains a better understanding of individual motivators, the concept of responsibility versus accountability, psychological contracts, leading under stress, and management of change. As he progresses through the seminar, he studies contingency theories of leadership and is especially interested in situational leadership.

Over the course of his daily work, John has become more familiar with his section chiefs. Jane Jenner, the Norfolk section chief, is young and enthusiastic about her job, and she wants to progress in the organizational hierarchy. However, John has noticed that she is not consistently following through with assigned tasks. In addition, for the last three months, John has been working closely with the other section chiefs on an important new project, and he has carefully explained their roles and their expected levels of performance and responsibility. Yet, owing to setbacks in funding and budget restrictions, the chiefs are somewhat disheartened. Their confidence has dropped, and so has their operational functioning.

1. Assess the usefulness of the situational leadership model for John as he gains additional leadership experience.

2. Would a contingency model of leadership be appropriate for John to use with his section chiefs?

3. Specify Jane's situational leadership developmental level, and describe the leadership style that would be most appropriate for her.
4. What is the developmental level of the section chiefs as a group?
5. Describe the conditions, if any, in which the situational leadership model might not be appropriate.

Chapter 5 Application: Making a Decision

John is enthusiastic about everything he learned at the Transylvania Public Health Leadership Institute orientation workshop and the Blankenship Institute's Leadership for Physician Executives seminar. Weighing the time requirements of his job and his need to further improve his leadership skills, he accepts the invitation to undertake the yearlong training program at TPHLI. He is eager to begin the program's first phase.

Meanwhile, the division directors at MCMHD are in the midst of deciding whether they should apply for Public Health Accreditation Board (PHAB) accreditation. The issue centers on the department's ability to undertake the accreditation process, as well as its resource limitations. Polling of leadership suggests a significant division within MCMHD, with two-thirds of the staff in favor of accreditation and one-third opposed. Unsure of making the decision by himself, the MCMHD commissioner has engaged the directors in a brainstorming session on the issue. At the session, the group collectively decides that the directors will make recommendations for their divisions, and then a majority vote will decide MCMHD's course of action.

As leader of the epidemiology division, John knows he has a responsibility to ensure that the PHAB decision reflects the division's and the department's best interest. He decides to apply the Vroom-Jago model of decision making, which he learned at the TPHLI orientation workshop. He applies the model's seven questions to determine which leader participation style will effectively engage the members of his division in the decision-making process and will best meet the needs of the situation.

1. Apply the Vroom-Jago decision tree, and answer the seven questions. Which of the five leader participation styles should John employ to effectively engage the section chiefs in the decision making?
2. Assess the applicability of the Vroom-Jago model in this situation.
3. How could the expectancy model of motivation be used to explain accreditation to the section chiefs?
4. Apply the path–goal leadership theory to identify the employee and environmental characteristics John should take into consideration as he makes the accreditation decision.

5. Assess the applicability of the Vroom-Jago model in your own professional and personal life.

Chapter 6 Application: A Leadership Study

John recently attended a TPHLI session that focused on the leader–member exchange (LMX) theory of leadership, including the Conditions of Trust Inventory (CTI). He is intrigued by the 11 dimensions considered by the CTI: supervisor availability, competence, consistency, discreetness, fairness, integrity, loyalty, openness, promise fulfillment, receptivity, and overall trust. Having long known that trust is a key component of leadership, John, in follow-up to the TPHLI session, suggests to the MCMHD commissioner that the department undertake a study of trust throughout the organization. He recommends using the CTI while at the same time collecting demographic data on the individuals participating in the study. After hearing John's persuasive case about the study and its potential usefulness for improving vertical dyad relationships between leaders (managers) and followers (subordinates), the commissioner agrees to the plan.

Over a two-week study period, a survey is made available electronically to all staff members, including leaders. The study uses a full network design methodology in which staff members are included without a control group. At the start of the study period, all staff receive an e-mail explaining the general purpose of the study and assuring them of anonymity and confidentiality.

By the conclusion of the study period, 49.8 percent of the 582 staff members have responded to the survey. In addition to the CTI items, the survey included a series of demographic questions to record the gender of the employee and supervisor, the race/ethnicity of the respondent, the respondent's job classification, the respondent's status as full- or part-time, the respondent's age, and the number of years the respondent has worked for MCMHD. The study found that the gender breakdown of the respondents was 85 percent female and 15 percent male, whereas the gender of the respondents' supervisors was 61 percent female and 39 percent male. The respondents were 57 percent white, 38 percent black, 3 percent Asian, and 1 percent Hispanic, whereas the supervisors were 64 percent white, 29 percent black, and 2 percent Asian.

John has assessed the CTI responses in relation to the gender and race/ethnicity data and finds the results to be instructive. Black employees rated supervisors lower than white employees did on the trust dimensions of supervisor availability, supervisor consistency, supervisor integrity, and supervisor loyalty, but higher on the dimension of supervisor fairness. In an analysis of employee–supervisor race concordance, nonconcordant pairs consistently scored lower in trust dimensions than did concordant pairs, with statistically significant and meaningful differences for the dimensions of supervisor availability, supervisor consistency, supervisor integrity, and supervisor loyalty. The findings confirm that MCMHD faces a number of trust differences related to employee race, supervisor race, and employee–supervisor race concordance.

As John reviews the data, he wonders how differences in trust might affect staff performance and turnover in his division, and across all of MCMHD. Furthermore, he worries that issues with employee trust, satisfaction, retention, and turnover might adversely influence the outcome of MCMHD's impending PHAB accreditation. He is particularly concerned about the lack of trust in white supervisors by black employees. Sitting in his office, John thinks: How can I use these results to improve the organizational culture of my followers and those of the rest of the department?

1. Analyze how John can use the results of his study to improve the level of trust MCMHD employees have for their leaders.
2. How would you deal with the trust issues raised by this study?
3. Why is trust such an important part of leadership?
4. Could the use of LMX theory have prevented the issues uncovered by John's study? If so, how?
5. Assess the applicability of the individualized leadership approach to the different levels of workers in John's division.

Chapter 7 Application: Tears in the Office

The staff of the division of epidemiology work diligently and strive to be innovative in carrying out their epidemiologic surveillance mission. As a result, the section chiefs in the division often feel a certain pressure to demonstrate their technical expertise.

Recently, several section chiefs have noted that Dr. Jacob Chadwick, the Bracken City section chief, has been talking repeatedly about the new approaches, protocols, and procedures in his section and claiming the innovations as his own. He has a tendency to say "*I* developed this model" or "*I* thought of this new procedure," rather than sharing credit with others in his section. Jacob's statements have become a common topic of discussion in the organization's informal channels, and John is considering how he might engage Jacob to change his leadership style. John is certain that, if the chatter surrounding Jacob is remotely true, the Bracken City section has significant personnel problems.

In Jacob's time with the epidemiology division, he has not gained a reputation for creativity. Discussion in the organization's informal channels tends to credit Bracken City's assistant section chiefs, rather than Jacob, with maintaining the section's reputation. Unfortunately, the assistant section chief position for Bracken City has had a high attrition rate in recent years, with several people coming and going. Chatter within the informal organization attributes the rapid turnover in this position to several causes, notably Jacob's obsessive micromanagement and Jacob's taking personal credit for the work of others. Jacob not only fails to give or share credit for successes; he also readily assigns blame to others for any failures. In addition, he has been said to use various forms of manipulation to retain dissatisfied staff members.

Exit interviews with departing staff members have further revealed aspects of Jacob's coercive and micromanaging leadership style. This time, Juliet Morgan, Bracken City's current assistant section chief, is leaving after only six months in the position. John is hopeful that he can gather credible information during her exit interview to help him engage Jacob in a discussion about his leadership style. Juliet walks slowly into John's office. John explains the exit interview process and is about to ask the first question when Juliet bursts into tears: "I wish I didn't have to leave!"

1. Assess the type of leadership style used by John.
2. Describe Jacob's approach to leading the Bracken City section.
3. Analyze how John should approach a discussion of leadership with Jacob.
4. Describe what Jacob should do to become an authentic transformational leader. How would his staff members view such a leadership style?
5. Analyze how John's application of transformational leadership theory reflects his self-confidence in leadership.

Chapter 8 Application: A Breach of Trust

The MCMHD epidemiology laboratory serves as the central laboratory for the cities of Jefferson, Wilmore, Bracken, Nicholasville, Norfolk, and Anderson. Before John was appointed as director of the epidemiology division, his predecessor had applied for a Centers for Disease Control and Prevention (CDC) prevention and wellness grant for the purchase of a Siemens Intelligent Laboratory System.

The MCMHD has now received the CDC grant for $225,000 to purchase the new equipment, and John, having weathered some tough decisions since his appointment, is determined to get the assignment right. Following department protocol, he assigns a committee to review bids and to recommend specifically which equipment to purchase. The committee is required to make a public call for sealed bids, with a minimum of two bids. It then must evaluate the bids, both technically and financially, and make a recommendation to the division director, who participates in the purchase and negotiation process with the final two competitors. The director's final recommendation is forwarded to MCMHD's finance and purchasing department, and the purchase contract is signed, closing the process.

The committee has recommended two companies, ArcTech and Precision, to make their sales presentations. Both quotes are competitively priced for the same piece of equipment. John is meeting with the vice president of ArcTech, Mark Wilson, and his sales team. During the presentation, John realizes that ArcTech knows the amount bid by Precision. He is taken by complete surprise when Mark proposes that, if John refers ArcTech to the finance and purchasing department, he will receive an honorarium.

1. How should John respond?
2. Apply the moral reasoning process to identify the justice component of the situation.
3. Analyze the situation, and describe your recommendations.
4. Analyze the moral outcomes of the situation.
5. Should John report the breach of trust? If so, to whom?

Chapter 9 Application: John Marshall's Three Rubrics

John is aware that his predecessor as epidemiology director left under adverse circumstances. Several months before John joined MCMHD, a disagreement between the director and the senior section chief, the epidemiologist for Wilmore, erupted into a major clash at a division staff meeting, leaving a bitter aftertaste among the meeting's attendees. John's next staff meeting is coming up.

John is thinking about how to develop a strong culture that he can sustain at the division of epidemiology. John knows that integration and cohesion are included in the division's core values, but he feels that such values are currently not clearly enunciated. John's personal core values, which are a part of his own approach to work and which he intends to integrate into the division's culture, consist of three rubrics: (1) Do the right thing, the right way, the first time; (2) quality work is always the least expensive; and (3) everything accomplished should be legal, moral, and ethical.

As John contemplates his upcoming staff meeting, he concludes that his best approach would be to address the issues he inherited head-on but in a tangential manner. By doing so, he expects to establish that the epidemiology division has only one team—his. John understands that not all the people reporting to him directly will be comfortable with his leadership, but he intends to give them all the opportunity to demonstrate their professional capabilities.

John intends to offer staff members a six-month period to demonstrate their knowledge, skills, and ability to accomplish assigned tasks. In the meantime, he will personally interact with the section chiefs and discuss progress toward the sections' goals in an effort to facilitate teamwork.

1. What steps should John take to integrate his three rubrics into the division's culture?
2. Assess John's three rubrics, and determine whether they are sufficient to create an effective organizational culture.
3. Is John's staff meeting an appropriate place to begin developing his desired organizational culture?
4. How would you go about the task of developing an organizational culture based on John's rubrics?
5. Choose the appropriate leadership style to be used by John in leading this group.

Chapter 10 Application: The Performance Rating

John is in his office working on the annual performance evaluations of the six section chiefs. Since this round of evaluations represents John's first time rating his direct reports, he wants to make every effort to honestly and fairly assess each individual.

John is currently reviewing the technical, interpersonal, and conceptual skills criterion for Dr. Rebecca Anderson, the Nicholasville section chief. Rebecca scores very well on knowledge about methods, processes, procedures, and techniques for specialized activities, and has strong conceptual skills, such as general analytical ability, logical thinking, proficiency in concept formation, and ability to recognize opportunities and potential problems—core traits of a good leader.

However, John recalls a presentation from his last TPHLI session that emphasized that "good leaders are good followers." John reflects on his vertical dyadic relationship with Rebecca and carefully thinks through their professional interactions and the feedback he has received from the deputy section chief of her section. Ultimately, he concludes that she does not always meet this requirement. John feels that Rebecca has been detached and uninvolved in her interactions with him for more than a few months. He has worked diligently to match his leadership style to her developmental level, but to no avail. She comes across as uninformed during their weekly meetings, and she seems disinterested in the division's long-range planning meetings. John wonders if she feels powerless in the core team and therefore remains silent.

John feels that Rebecca has good leadership characteristics but poor followership attributes. John is fully aware he himself has been a difficult follower at times in his career, but he senses a certain difference in Rebecca's pattern. In their dyadic relationship as leader and follower, she engages in a minimal fashion and appears uninterested in the tasks he assigns her. He thinks highly of Rebecca's ability to get the section's work accomplished, but her lack of engagement with him is of significant concern.

Filling out the performance evaluation, he thinks: What rating should I give her?

1. Based on Kellerman's followership model, what type of followership does Rebecca exhibit?
2. Assess the actions that John can take to change her approach.
3. How would you approach a similar situation?
4. Describe the integration of the followership model with the concept of shared influence.
5. How would you rate yourself on Kellerman's model of followership?

Chapter 11 Application: The Big Blow-Up

Over time, John has developed a sense of camaraderie with his team of six section chiefs. At an early staff meeting, he established a "one-team" policy for the group, making clear that he expected each section chief to be a fully functioning member of his team. Through his experience at the TPHLI program, John understands that leaders and team members may or may not find working together to be satisfactory and that either leaders or team members may desire to terminate a relationship. Fortunately, John and his section chiefs have found working together to be mutually beneficial and enjoyable. John has continued to develop his team as a cohesive group.

At one of the team's regularly scheduled meetings, discussion over shared financial resources turns ugly, much to John's surprise. The section chiefs begin to angrily yell at each other, hurling accusations and unpleasant comments. John, horrified by the behavior, seems to have momentarily lost control of the team. His staff assistant is perplexed and anxiously awaits a reaction from John.

As minutes pass and the anger continues, John rises from his chair and lets out an uproarious laugh—a trademark of his. His laughter gets everyone's attention, and a sudden silence takes over. One could hear a pin drop as John walks over to his bookshelf and takes out Ken Blanchard's *The One Minute Manager Builds High Performing Teams*.[1] He opens the book, turns to the situational leadership team development diagram, and points out that the team is exhibiting an R2 performance readiness level. At this level, regarded as the "storming" stage, competence as a group is slowly but surely increasing, but members often become divided and compete for recognition. Commitment to the group and its processes, which began on a high note, steadily wanes because of intrateam dissonance.

John tells his section chiefs that he will buy each of them a copy of the book and that he expects them to read it and discuss it in a week's time. He feels the exercise will help the group find ways to work with one another to fulfill the department's mission.

1. Will John's approach of providing information on team development be effective in resolving the challenges of the R2 level?
2. Considering that resolution of the R2 level requires high levels of direction and support, assess the effectiveness of John's approach.
3. Analyze the leadership style required to move a group through the "storming" phase.
4. How would you apply Hill's team leadership model to the situation?
5. Explain the steps that should be taken to resolve the group's dysfunction.

Chapter 12 Application: Gone by Midnight

A potential outbreak of equine encephalitis has John worried. He is not certain that the commissioner of health's response to the situation is adequate, and he is trying to find an appropriate venue in which to bring up the subject with the commissioner. At the same time, John is informed that a city council member will be visiting the epidemiology division. The council member is a former public health practitioner who wants to know more about the work of the division, especially against the backdrop of recent equipment purchases.

John leads the council member through the division and briefs him on the nature of the work and the recent incidences in the community. The council member appreciates John's work and asks what he can do to be helpful. In his response, John mentions his recent frustration with trying to engage at a higher level on the potential outbreak issue. John does so without making any disparaging remarks about the commissioner, and he explicitly states that the problem is not currently significant for the Missouri City population and that his concern is based only on the need to be fully prepared in case an outbreak occurs. The council member takes an interest in the situation, requests additional details, and, later, discusses the situation with the mayor of Missouri City. The mayor is concerned that the city might not be fully prepared and angry that the MCMHD commissioner did not inform him of the issue.

The commissioner discusses the situation with Jack Jones, his principal staff assistant, who in turn calls John and berates him for not following the proper chain of command in reporting the situation. John had worked closely with Jack and is stunned by the outburst, especially as Jack remarks, "John, if this was anyone but you, I would have him out of town by midnight!"

John sits at his desk in a quandary over how to deal with the situation.

1. Under what type of authority does Jack function, and who possesses it?
2. Using the French-Raven taxonomy of power, analyze the type of power Jack is exercising, and assess its effectiveness in relation to John.
3. Describe the ethical implications of the type of power used by Jack.
4. Describe the options available to John following the telephone conversation, and discuss how you would deal with the situation.
5. Categorize the proactive influence tactics you would employ in a similar situation.

Chapter 13 Application: Is It All Over?

Prior to working at MCMHD, John had served as an assistant professor and research associate at the state university's school of public health. The demanding workload during this time created a difficult work–life balancing act for John, but he received valuable guidance from Dr. Paul Reynolds, his department chair and personal mentor. Over time, Dr. Reynolds and John developed a close mentor–mentee relationship, with Dr. Reynolds supporting John during tough times and celebrating his successes. John reveres Dr. Reynolds and feels fortunate to have had such a strong mentor.

Sitting at his desk at the end of a hectic week, John recollects with fondness the good times he had with his mentor. He picks up the phone to call Dr. Reynolds but then hesitates; he is not sure that the timing for the call is right. The timing of his interactions with Dr. Reynolds had never been a concern in the past, but John now realizes that their relationship has changed somewhat since John moved to Missouri City. Their interactions have become less frequent; the tone of recent conversations has at times been sharp, even curt; and Dr. Reynolds has been difficult to engage over key issues, whether personal or professional.

John recalls that Dr. Reynolds had strongly recommended that he apply for the division director position at MCMHD and shared in his excitement about the Blankenship Institute and TPHLI training programs. However, John soon became heavily engaged in his work and training programs, and he no longer had a significant need for Dr. Reynolds's assistance or suggestions. Their more recent conversations have been more relational than professional, perhaps making Dr. Reynolds feel he is no longer needed as a mentor. John wonders if Dr. Reynolds is unwilling to adjust to the change in their relationship or unable to accept John's development as an independent epidemiologist and a key leader in a large metropolitan health department.

John asks himself: Should I call Dr. Reynolds? Is it all over?

1. Describe the benefits that John has received through his mentoring experience with Dr. Reynolds.
2. Assess John's current stage in the mentoring process.
3. Describe how the situational leadership mentoring model can be applied to the situation between John and Dr. Reynolds.
4. Identify what key aspect of the mentoring process has not occurred in the relationship between John and Dr. Reynolds.
5. What can John do at this point in the mentoring process to improve the situation?

Reference

1. Blanchard, K. H., D. Carew, and E. Parisi-Carew. 1990. *The One Minute Manager Builds High Performing Teams.* Escondido, CA: Blanchard Training and Development.

THE BASIS FOR EFFECTIVE PUBLIC HEALTH PRACTICE

1

THE NATURE OF EFFECTIVE PUBLIC HEALTH LEADERSHIP

James W. Holsinger Jr.

Learning Objectives

Upon completion of this chapter, you should be able to

- summarize the various definitions of *leadership*,
- describe the three core functions of public health and their relationship to public health leadership,
- identify the ten essential public health services,
- discuss the public health leadership competencies,
- differentiate between traditional and systems thinking,
- describe networking and its key components,
- discuss the importance of power in the practice of leadership and distinguish between personal and position power,
- understand the difference between leadership and management, and
- identify the key leader ethical shadows.

Focus on Leadership Competencies

This chapter emphasizes the following Association of Schools and Programs of Public Health (ASPPH) leadership competencies:

- Describe the attributes of leadership in public health.
- Describe alternative strategies for collaboration and partnership among organizations, focused on public health goals.
- Communicate an organization's mission, shared vision, and values to stakeholders.

(continued)

It also addresses the following Council on Linkages public health leadership competencies:

- Describes public health as part of a larger inter-related system of organizations that influence the health of populations at local, national, and global levels.
- Explains the ways public health care and other organizations can work together or individually to impact the health of a community.
- Modifies organizational practices in consideration of changes.

Note: See the appendix at the end of the book for complete lists of competencies.

Introduction

As the twenty-first century unfolds, a clear understanding of the key concepts of effective leadership is essential for all current and prospective public health practitioners. Following significant lapses of leadership in the for-profit world, leaders in governmental and not-for-profit agencies must learn from others' failures. The practice of public health entered the modern era with the publication of the 1988 Institute of Medicine (IOM) report *The Future of Public Health*, which stated that public health in the United States was at such a low ebb that the nation's health was in jeopardy.[1] Over the past 20 years, a number of American universities have developed new schools or colleges of public health or started new departmental public health programs.[2] In addition, national and regional institutes of public health leadership have equipped today's practitioners with skills that their predecessors often lacked. As the health of the public continues to evolve and the field of public health develops to meet these changes, familiarity with the principles and attributes of leadership is of foremost importance.

The 1988 IOM report[4] provided a clear description of the state of public health leadership at the end of the twentieth century. The authors commented on the lack of specificity in the training of public health practitioners for their leadership roles, and they stated that the need for well-trained public health leaders was simply too

Check It Out

The 1988 Institute of Medicine report is available at www.nationalacademies.org/hmd/Reports/1988/The-Future-of-Public-Health.aspx.

Consider This

"But men who followed must have the right leadership. . . . These men needed leadership. . . . No, they should have it as a right."

—Alexander Kent[3(p262)]

Do you think a person has the right to effective leadership? If so, why?

important to leave to chance. They argued that greater emphasis must be placed on academic preparation across a variety of leadership skills. The report's future vision for public health centered on the development of leaders with substantial technical competence in dealing with public health issues, the ability to manage complex organizations, strong communication skills, and an understanding of the political dimensions of the public decision-making process. In addition, leaders would need the ability to bring together a variety of constituencies for concerted action.

A key portion of the report identified three **core functions of public health** for agencies at all levels of government. The first function, **assessment**, involves systematically collecting, assembling, analyzing, and making available information about the health of the community. **Policy development**, the second core function, involves acting in the public interest to develop comprehensive public health policies through decisions that are based on scientific knowledge. The third core function is to provide **assurance** to constituents that they will be provided with the necessary services—either from the agency itself or through another public or private entity—to meet agreed-upon health goals; it involves guaranteeing high-priority personal and community health services to every member of the community. The IOM report provided the groundwork for the ten essential public health services, as identified by the Core Public Health Functions Steering Committee[5]:

1. Monitor health status to identify and solve community health problems.

2. Diagnose and investigate health problems and health hazards in the community.

3. Inform, educate, and empower people about health issues.

4. Mobilize community partnerships and action to identify and solve health problems.

5. Develop policies and plans that support individual and community health efforts.

6. Enforce laws and regulations that protect health and ensure safety.

7. Link people to needed personal health services and assure the provision of health care when otherwise unavailable.

8. Assure competent public and personal health care workforce.

9. Evaluate effectiveness, accessibility, and quality of personal and population-based health services.

10. Research for new insights and innovative solutions to health problems.

The eighth essential service, in particular, highlights the need for effective public health leadership training.

The 1988 IOM report observed that schools of public health had become isolated from the practice of public health and that, as a result, they were no

---

core functions of public health
Three central tasks—assessment, policy development, and assurance—to be carried out by all public health agencies at every level of government.

assessment
Systematically collecting, assembling, analyzing, and making available information about the health of the community.

policy development
Acting in the public interest to establish comprehensive public health policies based on scientific knowledge.

assurance
Ensuring that necessary personal and community health services are provided to every member of the community.

longer training public health practitioners effectively. In 2002, the IOM followed up its earlier findings with a new report titled *The Future of the Public's Health in the 21st Century*. Among other recommendations, that report stated that "leadership training, support, and development should be a high priority for governmental public health agencies and other organizations in the public health system and for schools of public health that supply the public health infrastructure with its professionals and leaders."[6] The two IOM reports together set the stage for significant changes in the education and training of public health practitioners. Core competencies have since been developed for public health practitioners, as well as lists of competencies for specific academic degrees. (The IOM was later renamed the National Academy of Medicine.)

In 2001, the Council on Linkages Between Academia and Public Health Practice promulgated core competencies for leaders functioning at various levels in public health organizations. The council developed the leadership and systems thinking domain to establish the core competencies for frontline, senior-level, and supervisory and managerial staff. By 2010, the council had revised the original core competencies and added several additional ones at each staff level.[7] In 2004, the Association of Schools of Public Health (ASPH)—later renamed the Association of Schools and Programs of Public Health (ASPPH)—set out to develop the competencies that individuals completing various public health degrees should possess.[8] Subsequently, the ASPPH developed specific master of public health (MPH),[9] doctor of public health (DrPH),[10] and bachelor's degree[11] competencies (see appendix).

✓ Check It Out

Visit www.aspph.org for more information about the Association of Schools and Programs of Public Health and the various professional public health degree programs.

In 1991, the Centers for Disease Control and Prevention (CDC) initiated support for the National Public Health Leadership Institute, creating the foundation for a system of state, regional, and national public health leadership institutes. The system's one- to two-year leadership programs have offered public health practitioners the opportunity to enhance their leadership skills while providing essential public health services.[7] Regional and national institutes make up the National Public Health Leadership Development Network (NLN), which has developed a Conceptual Model for Leadership Development[12] and a Public Health Leadership Competency Framework.[13] The framework consists of four overarching leadership areas: core transformational leadership competencies, legal and political competencies, transorganizational competencies, and team leadership

✓ Check It Out

Visit www.ncbi.nlm.nih.gov/pmc/articles/PMC 1446322/pdf/10936996.pdf for more information on the NLN's Public Health Leadership Competency Framework.

and dynamics competencies.[7] Within these four areas are 79 competencies that incorporate key elements of leadership, such as developing team-building skills and leading across organizational and system boundaries.

Since the 1988 IOM report, numerous other reports have recognized the need for a competent public health workforce and better education and training for public health leaders. Core competencies have been identified for the practice of public health, for effective public health leadership, and for specific academic degrees, and the CDC has begun supporting national and regional public health leadership institutes. As a consequence, the practice of public leadership is now a critical requirement in the education of public health practitioners.

> ### Consider This
>
>
> "Leadership [is] the art of getting someone else to do something that you want done because he wants to do it."
>
> —Dwight David Eisenhower[14]
>
> Why should you want to do what your leader wants you to do?

The Definition of *Leadership*

Defining *leadership* may be like defining *beauty*: It "lies in the eyes of the beholder."[15] As Yukl[16(p2)] has stated, "The term *leadership* is a word taken from the common vocabulary and incorporated into the technical vocabulary of a scientific discipline without being precisely redefined." As early as 1960, Janda[17] found that the term *leadership* was ambiguous because of the various extraneous concepts associated with it. At the same time, Bennis[18(p260)] succinctly stated: "Always, it seems, the concept of leadership eludes us or turns up in another form to taunt us again with its slipperiness and complexity. So we have invented an endless proliferation of terms to deal with it: leadership, power, status, authority, rank, prestige, influence, control, manipulation, domination, and so forth, and still the concept is not sufficiently defined." By 1974, Stogdill[19(p259)] was able to state, "There are almost as many definitions of leadership as there are persons who have attempted to define the concept."

Regardless of the diversity of interpretations, the term is central to our discussion and therefore must be defined here. For our purposes, **leadership** is a process that occurs whenever an individual intentionally acts to influence another individual or group, regardless of the reason, in an effort to achieve a common goal, which may or may not contribute to the success of the organization.

A key word in our definition of *leadership* is *process*. Leadership is a transaction between leaders and the people who follow them, not a trait or characteristic of the leader.[20] Leadership is an interactive process, not a one-way process, as leaders and followers affect one another. It is not confined to

leadership
A process in which an individual intentionally acts to influence another individual or group, regardless of the reason, in an effort to achieve a common goal, which may or may not contribute to the success of the organization.

the person who is formally designated as the leader of a group; in practice, anyone can be a leader.

Leadership is an *intentional* process in that the person leading does so deliberately. Leaders want to lead. To state that an individual *attempts* to lead simply recognizes the fact that leaders are not always successful in this process of influencing others. *Influencing* another individual or group is based on the manner in which a leader engages with the other person; leadership does not exist if influence does not occur. Leaders engage *another individual or group*, normally with a common purpose.

Groups being led can be of various sizes, depending on the situation or context. The influence process can occur within a group of any size as well as between individuals. An individual attempting to influence others may do so for a wide variety of reasons that may or may not be considered appropriate; history is replete with examples both good and bad. A *common goal* is a prerequisite for leadership, because leading involves one or more individuals having a mutual purpose and achieving something together. Unfortunately, the common goal does not necessarily contribute to the *success* of the organization. Surely, people intend for their work to be successful, but the lack of success does not necessarily interfere with the process of leadership.

Effective Public Health Leaders . . .

". . . learn that a leader without followers is simply a [person] taking a walk."

—John Boehner[21]

Describing Leadership

Leadership in public health requires that skillful individuals meet the health challenges of communities and the population as a whole. But before we examine leadership in that field, we must further describe the concept of leadership as a whole.

Traits or Process

All too often, leadership is described in terms of personal traits. People might emphasize that a particular leader is tall (e.g., President Abraham Lincoln), extroverted (e.g., Surgeon General M. Jocelyn Elders), intelligent (e.g., Surgeon General C. Everett Koop), or skilled at speaking (e.g., President Ronald Reagan). Individuals are often described as natural or born leaders. This approach considers certain attributes or properties to be **leadership traits** and suggests that leadership is restricted to those individuals believed to possess such special talents.[22] People often take for granted that individuals have certain innate or inborn qualities that fit them for leadership positions.

leadership traits
Personal attributes or characteristics that are commonly associated with the ability to lead.

As noted, our definition considers leadership to be a process, not a collection of traits. Approaching leadership in this manner focuses on the interactions between leaders and followers and highlights practices that can be learned from leaders' behavior. Thus, leadership can be available to everyone, not just people with desired characteristics.

> ### Leadership Application Case: Getting Started
>
>
>
> The Leadership Application Case at the beginning of this book provides realistic scenarios for the application of key leadership concepts covered in the text. See the section marked "Chapter 1 Application" for the scenario and discussion questions that correspond with this chapter.

Assigned and Emergent Leadership

The structures of formal organizations result in certain individuals becoming leaders due to their assigned positions. This type of **assigned leadership** is certainly common in public health, most obviously among the directors of state, territorial, county, or city public health organizations. However, in practice, an individual assigned to a leadership position is not always the actual leader in every situation or context. Based on our definition of leadership, we would expect the most influential member of the organization to function in a leadership role.

assigned leadership
Leadership based on a person's assigned position in an organization.

Emergent leadership occurs when people exercise leadership even though they have not been assigned to formal leadership roles. Such a leader may emerge from a work group over time as other individuals in the group come to recognize and support the individual's leadership. Fisher writes that certain communication behaviors play a major role in the development of emergent leaders: verbal involvement, initiation of new ideas, firmness without rigidity, being informed, and seeking the opinions of others.[23] Personality has also been found to play a key role. Smith and Foti[24] used a multivariable pattern approach to study three traits that were associated with individuals who emerged as leaders: dominance, intelligence, and general self-efficacy. They found that leaders who were rated high in all three areas (HHH) emerged as leaders more often than individuals who were low in all three (LLL). Furthermore, Hogg[25] postulated, using social identity theory, that emergent leaders arise from groups based on the degree to which they match the identity of the group as a whole. A prototype of a group member develops, and emergent leaders become attractive to the group if they have a strong resemblance to the group prototype. As a result, the group allows those individuals to exhibit influence.

emergent leadership
Leadership exercised by an individual who is not assigned to a leadership role.

As we examine the various aspects of leadership in this text, we maintain that leaders may be both assigned and emergent.

Power and Leadership

Power is a key ingredient in the influence process at the center of our definition of *leadership*. When leaders are able to influence their followers' beliefs,

power
A leader's ability to influence followers' beliefs, attitudes, and courses of action.

attitudes, and courses of action, they are said to have power.[20] Leaders use that power to produce change in their followers.

French and Raven[26] examined the roots of power as it exists between two individuals in the influence relationship (i.e., the person influencing and the person being influenced). In 1959, they identified five bases of power[27]:

1. **Referent power**, based on followers' identification with and liking for the leader. A teacher who is adored by students has referent power.

2. **Expert power**, based on followers' perceptions of the leader's competence. A tour guide who is knowledgeable about a foreign country has expert power.

3. **Legitimate power**, associated with status or formal job authority. A judge who administers sentences in the courtroom exhibits legitimate power.

4. **Reward power**, derived from one's capacity to provide rewards to others. A supervisor who gives rewards to employees who work hard is using reward power.

5. **Coercive power**, derived from one's capacity to penalize or punish others. A coach who sits players on the bench for being late to practice is using coercive power.

French and Raven's five bases of power are commonly used to increase the influence of leaders on the behaviors, attitudes, and values of followers.

French and Raven's bases of power are closely related to two key aspects of power in organizations: personal power and position power. When followers perceive a leader to be knowledgeable and likable, they confer **personal power** on the leader. Personal power is based on the perception of the followers and includes both referent and expert power as delineated by French and Raven. **Position power**, on the other hand, refers to the power conferred on an individual based on a particular rank or office within a formal organization. As such, it corresponds with French and Raven's legitimate, reward, and coercive bases of power.

Leadership Versus Management

Controversy has reigned for many years over the relationship between leadership and management. To address this issue, we must first define *management*. **Management** in its simplest form is the act of working with and through people in order to complete the work at hand in an effective and efficient manner.[28] Comparing that definition with our definition of *leadership*, we can clearly see that the two terms are not synonyms: A manager does not have to be a leader,

referent power
Power based on followers' identification with and liking for a leader.

expert power
Power based on followers' perceptions of a leader's competence.

legitimate power
Power associated with status or formal job authority.

reward power
Power derived from one's capacity to provide rewards to others.

coercive power
Power derived from one's capacity to penalize or punish others.

personal power
Power based on a leader's effective use of skills and attributes, as perceived by the followers.

position power
Power based on a leader's assigned role in the organization.

management
Working with and through people in order to complete the work at hand in an effective and efficient manner.

nor does a leader have to be a manager. However, disagreement continues as to the degree of overlap between the two terms.

Describing the difference between management and leadership, Pascale[29(p65),30] states, "Managers do things right, while leaders do the right things." Zaleznik[31] maintains that management and leadership are mutually exclusive, and some other authors do not believe that leadership and management coexist in the same person. Most people, however, do not take such extreme positions; thus, our approach will assume that, although the roles of leaders and managers are distinct, leaders and managers are not different types of people.

Some scholars, such as Mintzberg,[32] consider leadership simply to be one of the key managerial roles. Kotter[33] states that managers seek to develop order and predictability, whereas leaders, on the other hand, create organizational change. Kotter argues that both roles are essential but that balance between the two must be maintained. If the emphasis on managing is paramount, risk taking will be inhibited, and the bureaucracy created will lack a clear purpose. If the emphasis on leadership is paramount, the order of the organization can be upset and unrealistic change produced.[16] Rost[34] writes that management is based on an authority relationship between managers and subordinates, whereas leadership is based on an influence relationship between leaders and followers. Management may lead to coercion, whereas leadership is based on mutual influence within the leader–follower relationship.

Because management is based on attaining an organization's goals through five classic functions (i.e., planning, organizing, staffing, directing, and controlling), we must consider how management and leadership interact to reach these goals. Some managers are outstanding leaders, and some leaders are outstanding managers. In public health organizations, practitioners must develop not only managerial skills but also the qualities necessary for effective leadership. Management cannot be replaced by leadership; thus, leadership should always be in addition to management.[35]

High-performing organizations require both management and leadership. Leadership maintains a long-term view and provides direction to the organization, establishing a vision, strategy, and organizational values. Leaders align followers and work to reduce boundaries to the organization's shared culture. Management, on the other hand, is deeply involved in the day-to-day functions of planning and budgeting, always keeping the bottom line in mind. It engages in the functions of organizing, staffing, directing, and controlling, without which organizations cannot succeed. Managers create boundaries in order to provide better control. With regard to relationships, leaders focus on people and strive to inspire and motivate their followers. Leadership is based on personal power, and leaders serve as coaches, facilitate interaction within the group, and provide support to followers. Management, meanwhile, focuses on position power, considering that managers are often bosses. Instead of focusing on people, managers focus more on objects, or the products of the organization.

Personal qualities associated with leadership include heart (emotional connections), mindfulness (open mindedness), communication (listening), courage (nonconformity), and character (insight into self). The personal qualities of managers differ from those of leaders in that managers maintain emotional distance and value conformity. Managers seek to develop an expert mind and maintain insight into the organization. Both managers and leaders focus on the outcomes of their actions: Managers strive to maintain stability while creating a culture of efficiency; leaders aim to create change and develop a culture of integrity.[33]

Leadership Competencies

As we approach leadership, we must remember that it is an art as well as a science. The art of leadership for public health practitioners encompasses a number of key concepts. Much of the art revolves around interpersonal relationships, because of the constant networking and broad array of stakeholder relationships required of public health leaders. When leadership is approached as an art, its practice is embedded in people, and decisions are based primarily on the leader's perceptions of people. The image the leader maintains in interactions with public health stakeholders is highly important. The art of leadership also requires a keen understanding of timing. As musician Tommy Shaw[36] once said, "Timing is everything," and the tempo of a public health organization is an art in and of itself. Finally, intuition plays a major role in the art of leadership in public health organizations, especially as it applies to the skillful use of power.

The science of leadership, on the other hand, also encompasses a variety of elements. In public health organizations, it includes such technical skills as budgeting, forecasting, and controlling costs; the ability to apply analytic skills in decision making; and the development of expert systems and systems thinking (discussed later in this chapter). The key to effectively leading public health organizations lies in maintaining a strong working relationship and balance between the art and the science of leadership.[37] Establishing this balance, however, can be challenging for new leaders.

Ledlow and Stephens[38] outlined six key characteristics that lay the foundation for an individual to be a successful leader: (1) communication, (2) consistency, (3) comprehension of the relationship between trust and understanding, (4) the ability to be adaptive, (5) emotional intelligence, and (6) integrity. The ability of leaders to communicate must surpass basic-level communication knowledge and skills; it must also include an understanding of how, what, and when to communicate with critical stakeholders, as well as how to project oneself in an authentic and genuine manner. Leaders need to appropriately understand, interpret, and use nonverbal as well as symbolic and verbal communication skills. Furthermore, a leader should strive for consistency in both actions and character. Consistency is a highly valued leadership characteristic that helps to establish and increase trust between leaders and their subordinates and superiors, which in turn builds increased understanding and trust for the future. At the same time, leaders must be able to adapt their leadership styles to specific situations, which will allow for success in the rapidly changing environment of public health practice. Many of the traits already described contribute to emotional intelligence, which consists of a leader's self-awareness, self-regulation, motivation, empathy, and social skills. Studies have shown that high emotional intelligence is at least as important to successful leadership as technical skills and cognitive ability.[39] Integrity, the final characteristic needed to establish a foundation for successful leadership, encompasses and expands upon the previous five. Leaders should strive to communicate and act with integrity in all facets of life. In addition, leaders show integrity by balancing the interests of the organization with the rights and feelings of the individuals involved, as well as by putting the needs of others above their own.

When integrity is combined with competence and other key personal and technical skills, an effective public health practitioner establishes the foundation to become a successful public health leader. In public health, practitioner leaders can be gifted in a variety of ways, with different skills and personalities. Because we do not assume that leaders possess inherent leadership skills, we maintain that all public health leaders can grow and develop in both the art and science of leadership. In doing so, public health leaders can increase their effectiveness as they grow in competence.

Check It Out

Visit www.mindtools.com/pages/main/newMN_LDR.htm for additional information about leadership skills and the requirements for being an effective leader.

Principles of Public Health Leadership

Public health leadership is best approached as a lifelong learning process. It should be viewed within the context in which it occurs, since the context determines the skills and tools necessary to lead.[7] Certain skills must be mastered as the leader advances professionally over time. The public health leader is first required to obtain discipline-specific knowledge and core public health skills, which serve as the foundation for the leadership competencies that follow. The development of management skills is essential for an efficient and effective organization, and the development of core individual leadership skills enables the leader to put team leadership into practice.

Public health practitioners often have difficulty shifting from management to leadership, largely because the concepts have contrasting orientations: Management is based on the internal requirement that the organization function efficiently and effectively, whereas leadership is outwardly focused and engaged with community public health activities. As practitioners master each step of the learning process, leadership performance improves, strengthening the public health infrastructure by building capacity. As practitioners develop leadership competencies as individuals, the practice of such leadership engages their teams. The sum of these competencies prepares public health practitioners to provide effective crisis leadership, followed by the development of public health best practices. An understanding of this model is essential for meeting the requirement of having a well-trained public health workforce.[40] Unfortunately, too many practitioners at the local, state, and national levels have no formal public health education or training.

 Spotlight

Leadership as an influence process requires the development of skills that can be used by public health practitioners across a variety of contexts. Efforts to perfect such skills will result in effective engagement with the three core public health functions and the development of the ten essential public health services, considering that leadership is required for both.

Systems Thinking

systems thinking
A leadership practice that emphasizes the system components required to meet an organization's short- and long-term needs.

Systems thinking, a key practice in effective public health leadership in the twenty-first century, focuses on the system components required to meet the organization's short- and long-term needs.[41] A central element of systems thinking is recognizing the importance of becoming a public health learning organization.[42] Public health organizations have long been traditional in nature; thus, the transformation into a learning organization requires redirection and rethinking.

To develop systems thinking, public health practitioners must orient themselves around five learning disciplines: (1) personal mastery, (2) mental models, (3) shared vision, (4) team learning, and (5) systems thinking. Personal mastery requires leaders to enhance their own learning as well as encourage the learning of their followers. Effective public health leaders are aware of the deeply ingrained mental models that influence how people see the world, and they understand the cultural context of their organizations, recognizing the importance of cultural norms and values in decision making, organizational actions, and problem solving.[7] A shared vision encourages buy-in from constituents and stakeholders, as well as followers. Team learning—in which a team rather than an individual is the fundamental learning unit—produces a synergistic process that will enable the public health organization to produce extraordinary results. Finally, systems thinking requires public health leaders to understand that the framework for future change is the entire community being served. They use this mind-set to locate leverage points, where small efforts can result in significant changes.

Traditional thinking is usually linear in nature, following a causal chain from point A to point B. As patterns develop, leaders move toward systems thinking. As combinations of patterns emerge and connections become established, systems thinking occurs. Because every system has a purpose (mission) and every system is tied or related to other systems, all parts of a system must be present and properly arranged for the system to work. However, parts can be replaced or adapted to a new level of functioning. Change occurs because information is constantly received, guiding the system's operation (feedback). Systems can remain stable only if they make adjustments based on feedback.[7,43]

Systems thinking analysis occurs in a stepwise manner, as shown in exhibit 1.1. As a leader or team works through the process, leverage and learning occur. The analysis begins with the events—and the telling of the story of events—that are involved in the issue being analyzed. The second step involves graphing trends and identifying key variables, thereby revealing patterns. Simultaneously with the identification of variables, the focusing question is clarified. By the third step, the leader is beginning to understand key system structures through the identification of core loops or archetypes. Loops may be reinforcing, in which the leader would expect an intervention to have resulted in some impact, or balancing. When combined, two or more loops may produce an archetype, which is a pattern seen over and over in a specific environment. As archetypes occur, they fall into eight key types: (1) drifting goals, (2) escalation, (3) fixes that fail, (4) growth and underinvestment, (5) limits to success, (6) shifting the burden, (7) success to be successful, and (8) tragedy of the commons.

Systems thinking provides a useful toolbox for public health leaders as they consider the methods and means by which they will lead and move their

EXHIBIT 1.1
The Steps in Systems Thinking Analysis

Events	Patterns		Structure			
			Systems Thinking Analysis			
Tell the story	Identify key variables and graph the trends	Clarify the focusing question	Identify a core loop or archetype	Develop additional loops (ensure complete diagram explains graph)	Apply the Going Deeper™ questions	Identify potential leverage points (explain how they would work throughout the system)

← An iterative process →

← Learning and leverage →

Source: Data from Goodman, M., and R. Karash. 1995. "Six Steps to Thinking Systemically." *Systems Thinker* 6 (2): 16–18.

Check It Out

Visit www.phf.org/resourcestools/Documents/ Core_Competencies_for_Public_Health_ Professionals_2010May.pdf for more information about essential leadership and systems thinking skills as defined by the Council on Linkages Between Academia and Public Health Practice.

organizations ahead.[44] The development of public health leadership institutes across the United States has significantly increased the opportunities for practitioners to enhance leadership and systems thinking skills.

Action Plans

Public health leadership intersects with the three core functions of public health, as illustrated in exhibit 1.2.[7,41] The work of public health can be viewed in terms of both planning and action. The systems components of public health provide the basis for meeting the identified needs of communities and populations. Thinking systemically, as well as strategically, is an important aspect of public health leadership. Use of a systems approach to public health leadership and application of the three core functions of public health require innovative approaches.

Assessment, the first core function, continues throughout the systems process, as represented by the arrow extending across the top of exhibit 1.2. In applying the assessment function, the effective public health leader establishes goals and objectives for the organization being led. The second core function, policy development, incorporates team building, a key aspect of public health leadership. Assurance, the third core function, involves action plans based on the goals and objectives.

EXHIBIT 1.2
A Systems Approach to Public Health Leadership and Applications of the Core Functions

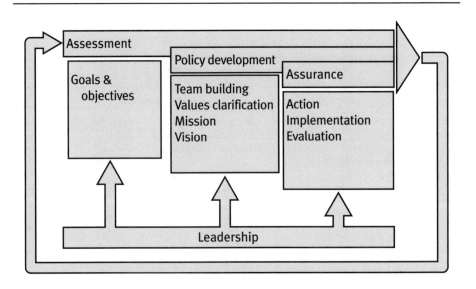

Source: Data from Institute of Medicine, Committee for the Study of the Future of Public Health. 1988. *The Future of Public Health*. Washington, DC: National Academies Press.

When difficult situations arise, an appropriate response is to develop a committee, team, or coalition to study the problem; develop a plan for dealing with the situation; implement the plan; and, finally, evaluate the result of the action(s) taken. Policy development begins with the establishment of the team and continues as the team clarifies its values and the issues facing it. The purpose of the team must be clearly identified through the development of a mission and a vision of the future it seeks; the mission and vision provide a vector (direction and force) for the team process. Policy development addresses long-term goals and short- to mid-term objectives, and the assessment function is engaged as the goals and objectives are developed. As action plans are developed from the goals and objectives, a key aspect is the determination of the real costs associated with the solution to the issue. The assurance function begins as the action plans are implemented, and it continues through the team's evaluation of the entire process. As the process unfolds, the three core functions of public health—assessment, policy development, and assurance—are fully engaged.[7]

Public health has no true status quo, because change is the norm and constant adaptation is necessary.[41] In developing an action plan that leads to change, effective public health leaders must be creative; the action plan will most certainly require innovative approaches to meeting the goals and objectives. Structural tension occurs between the vision and the current situation, and public health leaders develop a means to resolve this tension in order to move their organization forward.[45] Fritz has divided this creative process into three stages: (1) germination, during which the leader's personal excitement in addressing the situation aids in the development of the action plan; (2) adaptation, during which the organization and its employees adapt to the leader's agenda; and (3) process completion, in which the creative process comes to completion—though often at this point the leader begins the process again in an iterative manner.[46]

For some situations, the action plan process may be too narrow an approach, and strategic thinking may need to be added to ensure effectiveness. Strategic thinking should not be separated from the attainment of the goal. Public health leaders need to recognize that bringing a plan to fruition may be difficult if the plan is too complex. However, developing an action plan that addresses a few important areas may work best while keeping in mind the need to think strategically. Strategies alone will not provide the required result for a specific situation. However, strategies are important in guiding the public health organization toward its desired future state.

Perhaps now more than ever, effective public health leaders must be flexible and resilient. Wheatley[47] has proposed that chaos must occur in order for change to happen. Public health leaders certainly sense that they live in a chaotic world, even though a bounded system may appear ordered and even predictable. But chaos today results in future order, because it is based on culture, values and belief systems, ethics, and even vision.[7]

Due to the constant change in the public health system, leaders must look to other perspectives for dealing with system change. One such perspective is based on syndemics. A **syndemic**—a word derived by merging the prefix *syn-* (together) and *epidemic*—is an aggregation of two or more diseases in a population in which some biological interaction exacerbates the negative effects of the diseases.[48] Applying this perspective to public health systems would suggest that many public health issues or problems are interrelated and may exacerbate one another. For example, substance abuse, violence, and AIDS—collectively referred to as the SAVA syndemic—disproportionately affect individuals living in poverty in US cities. To control a syndemic, public health practitioners must prevent or limit each disorder as well as the impetus that links the disorders together.[49]

Such an effort is difficult because many public health issues are multidimensional, and making a change in one area can result in a number of unintended consequences. The public health community includes a variety of complex partner interactions, and engaging one community partner without considering the impact on others can result in a less than satisfactory result. Thus, a broad-based approach to problem solving may produce better results than a single-dimensional approach.

Collaboration

Clearly, effective public health leadership requires skills related to team building and collaboration. Winer and Ray[50] define **collaboration** as a mutually beneficial and well-defined relationship between two or more individuals or organizations that is created to achieve results that would not have occurred if these parties had not worked together. As public health leaders collaborate, they discover that people participate in group relationships in a series of stages that increase in intensity. As the intensity increases, people's commitment and involvement also increase, and more resources are dedicated to the collaboration.

Networking is the first stage of collaboration. Effective public health leaders possess extensive networks of colleagues, and they engage their networks on a day-to-day basis. The discussion of public health actions and the sharing of information benefit all parties in the relationship. As the relationship between parties grows closer and becomes more formal, the coordination phase begins. Information exchange continues to occur in this phase of the group relationship, but now activities are being changed because of the interactions that occur. Modification of the activities in the relationship begins as the parties initiate cooperation, thus intensifying the engagement. The sharing of resources also begins at this point in the relationship, and it becomes more intense as the parties enter the collaboration phase. By the collaboration phase, all the

syndemic
An aggregation of two or more diseases in a population in which some biological interaction exacerbates the negative effects of the diseases.

collaboration
A mutually beneficial, well-defined relationship between two or more organizations or individuals that achieves results through working together.

activities that were engaged in previous phases continue to intensify, and the capacity of others is significantly enhanced.

As a result of collaboration, effective public health leaders will discover that they share responsibilities, resources, risks, and rewards with their colleagues, partners, or constituents.[51] Lamberth and Rowitz[7(p435)] have found that "most discussions of collaboration involve a concern for the structure of the interactions. Just because people work together does not mean that collaboration is occurring. Coalitions tend to operate primarily at the networking level, although attempts at coordination may occur. Alliances and partnerships tend to be more intense and work at the coordination and collaboration levels, although networking and coordination may occur at the earlier stages of work before trust develops." Further, Senge and colleagues point out that reinventing relationships is a key to developing collaborative efforts.[52]

The work of public health encompasses a wide array of disciplines in addition to the core areas of epidemiology, biostatistics, health services management, health behavior, and environmental health. Engagement and collaboration by public health leaders across a wide variety of disciplines contributes to a deeper and broader understanding of the environment in which they lead and manage.

Rowitz[41] has proposed a list of 16 public health leadership principles, shown in exhibit 1.3. Internalizing these principles should be a priority for all public health practitioners, but especially for public health leaders, as the principles will help to instill an ethical culture in the organizations they lead. A key element in the principles is recognition that the members of populations and communities are interdependent and that such interdependence is crucial to the growth and development of communities.

Ethical Leadership

Moral reasoning and ethical decision making lie at the heart of effective public health leadership.[53] Public health leaders often serve as role models; thus, when they take seriously their ethical responsibilities, positive outcomes can develop and spread in the groups and organizations they lead. Such outcomes may include reduction in stress, lower staff turnover, improved attendance rates, higher employee satisfaction and commitment, and a desire by followers to put in extra effort on the job. **Ethical leadership** can also lead to increased trust and collaboration, higher performance and productivity, and, ultimately, a positive public image.[54]

In recent years, various ethical failures—and the misery those failures have caused—have highlighted the importance of ethical leadership. Effective public health leaders take responsibility in their own inner consciousness, their own inner self, to do more good than harm.[55] When leadership is toxic, however, leaders act out of the "shadow" side of their ethical position. Kellerman[56] describes seven types of bad leaders—incompetent, rigid, intemperate, callous, corrupt, insular, and evil—and notes that their leadership can be either

ethical leadership
Leadership based on moral reasoning and ethical decision making.

EXHIBIT 1.3

Leadership
Principles
to Guide the
Public Health
Practitioner

1. Strengthen the infrastructure of public health by utilizing the core functions and essential public health services framework.
2. Improve the health of each person in the community.
3. Build coalitions for public health.
4. Work with leaders from culturally diverse backgrounds.
5. Collaborate with boards for rational planning.
6. Learn leadership through mentoring and coaching.
7. Commit to lifelong learning.
8. Promote health protection for all.
9. Think globally and act locally.
10. Manage as well as lead.
11. Walk the talk.
12. Understand the importance of community.
13. Be proactive and not reactive.
14. See leadership everywhere.
15. Know that leaders are born and made.
16. Live our values.

Source: Rowitz, L. 2014. *Public Health Leadership: Putting Principles into Practice*, 3rd ed. Sudbury, MA: Jones & Bartlett.

ineffective, unethical, or both ineffective and unethical. The ethical dilemmas faced by public health leaders often involve issues of power, privilege, information, consistency, loyalty, or responsibility. Johnson[54] lists the following shadows: (1) power, (2) privilege, (3) mismanaged information, (4) inconsistency, (5) misplaced or broken loyalties, and (6) irresponsibility. The way leaders handle their difficult challenges will determine whether they cause more harm than good—whether they cast light or shadow on the issues at hand.

Effective public health leadership cannot exist without power; thus, the shadow side of leadership is determined by how the leader utilizes it. Leaders are often reluctant to admit that they even possess power, let alone use it. However, failing to acknowledge this reality makes leaders more prone to leading from the shadow side, causing more harm than good. Leaders almost always possess greater privileges than followers do, and rewards for leaders (e.g., pay, fringe benefits) are often based on their amount of power. Abuse of privilege can have the same negative results that abuse of power does.[54] Leaders also possess significant amounts of information; without information, they simply cannot function. But information is power, and the way it is used will determine whether leaders cast light or shadow. Leaders must understand issues of confidentiality, which play a major role in determining how information should be used or not used.

The need for consistency can be an additional ethical burden for public health leaders, especially as it relates to the diversity of the workforce. Does the leader treat all followers the same, even when they have a variety of backgrounds and skill sets? When considering consistency, the perceptions of followers may be closer to reality than leaders care to admit. A lack of consistency can cast a long shadow across the organization.

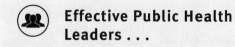

Effective Public Health Leaders . . .

. . . suppress the urge "to blow off steam—shout at people—all the time."

—Robert M. Gates[57(p266)]

Ethical shadows may also be cast by misplaced or broken loyalties. Misplaced loyalties by corporate leaders have come to be considered commonplace in recent years, but broken loyalties can result in even greater dilemmas. The issue is always with the leader. Who or what comes first? Does duty really come before self? To whom do I owe loyalty and for how long? How do I honor the trust of others? Leaders have a greater breadth of responsibility than followers do, which raises the risk of a shadow of irresponsibility. Unlike followers, who are responsible chiefly for their own actions, leaders bear the responsibility of others—the team, the group, the division, or even the entire organization. Public health leaders can fail in their ethical responsibilities in a variety of ways, such as by failing to prevent followers' misdeeds, ignoring ethical problems, not holding themselves accountable for ethical lapses, and failing to accept responsibility for their actions.[58]

The practice of public health leadership is built on a number of small decisions, which can be made ethically or unethically. The nature of these decisions will determine whether leadership is used for the good of the organization or for its harm.[59]

Case Study: US Surgeon General C. Everett Koop's Response to HIV/AIDS

Dr. C. Everett Koop served as US Surgeon General from January 1982 through October 1989. Though he possessed little statutory authority, Dr. Koop's vigorous efforts to address smoking, intimate partner violence, disability rights, and HIV/AIDS, as well as his reinvigoration of the Commissioned Corps of the US Public Health Service (PHS), provided his lasting legacy and demonstrated the immense potential of effective public health leadership.

Just months before Dr. Koop was officially sworn in, the Centers for Disease Control (CDC) issued two reports identifying clusters of extremely rare diseases occurring among homosexual men. Not until 1983 did French and American scientists identify the human immunodeficiency virus (HIV) as the root cause. Scientists soon identified the ways that AIDS was spread: via sexual intercourse; through the sharing of contaminated needles among intravenous drug users; by transfusion of infected blood; and through transmission from

(continued)

pregnant mother to child in utero, during birth, or during nursing. Still, for more than two years, Dr. Koop was excluded from President Ronald Reagan's Executive Task Force on AIDS. Not until 1986, fully five years after the epidemic began, was he authorized to prepare a surgeon general's report on the issue.

Dr. Koop's approach to this epidemic provided a powerful example of public health leadership. With neither vaccine nor cure in his toolbox, he knew that public health education was the sole means available to him to stem the epidemic. He immediately began engaging critical stakeholder groups and experts. Importantly, he met personally with AIDS patients. Throughout this process, he tactfully treated AIDS as a public health issue, rather than a moral one, and fought to protect his independence from any stakeholders, including his superiors and even the president. Dr. Koop released the report at a press conference in October 1986. More than 20 million copies of the 36-page report were eventually distributed through various media, public policy, public health, and other stakeholder avenues.

Over the next two years, Dr. Koop delivered numerous speeches and provided interviews about AIDS. He met with the World Health Organization and other international bodies that were concerned about the epidemic. In 1988, by congressional mandate, he mailed an informational brochure about AIDS to every American household—nearly 110 million of them. He argued vociferously against mandatory testing and quarantine, and he denounced discrimination by any means or in any circumstance against people with AIDS. In his opinion, quarantine was both unconstitutional and epidemiologically unnecessary, and confidential, voluntary testing was most likely to encourage the highest-risk people to seek care. More than any other public official, Dr. Koop's efforts shifted the debate about AIDS away from moral politics and toward the ethics of care and compassion.

Discussion and Application Questions

1. How did Dr. Koop demonstrate effective public health leadership?
2. What political barriers did Dr. Koop experience as surgeon general, especially relating to the AIDS epidemic? How did he overcome those barriers?
3. How might Dr. Koop's response have been different had this case occurred today?

Summary

Leadership behavior is a much-discussed—and, at the same time, much-maligned—topic in twenty-first century America. The literature surrounding this topic grows constantly as people try to better understand how leaders develop and how they function in their organizations. We define *leadership* as a process that occurs whenever an individual intentionally acts to influence another individual or group, regardless of the reason, in an effort to achieve a common goal that may or may not contribute to the success of the organization.

Leadership is certainly a major challenge for public health practitioners, who find themselves working in an ever-changing environment. Since 1988, numerous reports have detailed the need for trained and effective public health leaders, and various leadership competencies have been developed in response. Certain core competencies are required to complete academic degrees in public health, which are rapidly becoming entry-level educational requirements for working in the field.

Certain key elements are central to the understanding of effective public health leadership. An important distinction is the difference between assigned leadership, which is based on a person's assigned position, and emergent leadership, which is practiced by people outside of formal leadership roles. Public health practitioners typically understand the structure of their organizations and the titles that designate position, so assigned leadership is generally well understood. Practitioners, however, may have greater difficulty grasping the importance of emergent leadership, which develops through support from followers and is based on what a person does instead of what position the person holds.

Another important aspect of leadership is power—particularly, the way power is used by the public health leader. Inappropriate use of power is a key contributor to the "shadow" side of leadership practice. Power can be divided into two forms—position power and personal power—which are connected with the assigned and emergent forms of leadership. French and Raven[27] identify five bases of power: (1) referent power, (2) expert power, (3) legitimate power, (4) reward power, and (5) coercive power. The legitimate, reward, and coercive bases represent position power, whereas the referent and expert bases represent personal power. Position power is attained through the title of one's assigned position, whereas followers grant personal power to leaders because they recognize that the leaders provide something of value to them. Some leaders consider coercion a valid form of leadership, but coercion fails to treat followers as partners in reaching goals.

Effective public health leadership is both an art and a science. Communication skills—including the skills for nonverbal and symbolic communication—are extremely important for engaging followers, constituents, and collaborators. Outstanding public health leaders understand the importance of emotional intelligence, and they use it to monitor themselves and govern their own behavior. In addition, trust and understanding are powerful elements of effective leadership. The importance of integrity in public health leadership cannot be overstated.

Leadership and management overlap in many ways, but the two concepts are different: Leadership emphasizes influence, whereas management focuses on the traditional aspects of organizing and running an organization. Both leaders and managers work to influence others to achieve common goals. Some managers are outstanding leaders, and some leaders are outstanding managers. High-performing organizations rely on the skills of both leadership and management, and those skills may be found in the same individual or in multiple people.

Systems thinking has become a core leadership skill for the twenty-first century. The practice of public health occurs within a variety of overlapping systems, and leaders must be able to adapt to constant change and remain resilient in a chaotic environment. Leaders must know the requirements of group relationships and the stages of networking, coordination, cooperation, and collaboration. Successful public health leaders engage their networks daily to maintain valuable relationships.

Finally, public health leaders must practice ethical leadership. Leaders must be regarded by their followers as authentic and genuine, and they must demonstrate consistency in their behaviors, particularly in their interactions with the diverse individuals who make up the public health workforce. Because of the fragile nature of trust, leaders must remain vigilant as they carry out their daily tasks and responsibilities.

Discussion Questions

1. Discuss the need for public health practitioners to be educated and trained leaders.
2. What are the leadership competencies for educating and training public health practitioners?
3. Describe leadership as it is defined in this text.
4. What is the difference between leadership traits and processes?
5. Outline the differences between management and leadership as concepts. How do they interrelate?
6. Distinguish between networking, coordinating, cooperating, and collaborating. What is the importance of networking to the public health practitioner?
7. Describe the relationship between networking, coordinating, cooperating, and collaborating. Explain the importance of group relationships.
8. What are the differences between leadership and systems thinking skills?
9. Explain the shadows of leadership. How do they affect the ethical practice of public health leadership?

10. For deeper thought: You are the state commissioner of public health, and you have discovered a systematic effort by the Division of Vital Statistics to underreport the number of cases of childhood disease in an effort to mask the low rate of immunizations. As an effective public health leader, how would you deal with this ethical dilemma?

Web Resources

Council on Linkages Between Academia and Public Health Practice. 2014. "Core Competencies for Public Health Professionals." Published June. www.aspph.org/app/uploads/2015/01/Core_Competencies_for_Public_Health_Professionals_2014June.pdf.

Institute of Medicine. 1988. *The Future of Public Health.* Published January. www.nationalacademies.org/hmd/Reports/1988/The-Future-of-Public-Health.aspx.

Mind Tools. 2017. "Leadership Skills." Accessed April 17. www.mindtools.com/pages/main/newMN_LDR.htm.

Wright, K., L. Rowitz, A. Merkle, W. M. Reid, G. Robinson, B. Herzog, D. Weber, D. Carmichael, T. R. Balderson, and E. Baker. 2000. "Competency Development in Public Health Leadership." *American Journal of Public Health.* Published August. www.ncbi.nlm.nih.gov/pmc/articles/PMC1446322/pdf/10936996.pdf.

References

1. Holsinger, J. W., Jr., and F. D. Scutchfield. 2012. "Introduction: History and Context of Public Health Care." In *Contemporary Topics in Public Health*, edited by J. W. Holsinger Jr., 1–24. Lexington, KY: University Press of Kentucky.

2. Keck, C. W., F. D. Scutchfield, and J. W. Holsinger Jr. 2012. "Conclusion: Future of Public Health." In *Contemporary Topics in Public Health*, edited by J. W. Holsinger Jr., 251–76. Lexington, KY: University Press of Kentucky.

3. Kent, A. 1970. *Enemy in Sight!* New York: Putnam.

4. Institute of Medicine Committee for the Study of the Future of Public Health. 1988. *The Future of Public Health.* Published January. www.nationalacademies.org/hmd/Reports/1988/The-Future-of-Public-Health.aspx.

5. Centers for Disease Control and Prevention. 2017. "The Public Health System and the 10 Essential Public Health Services." Accessed April 14. www.cdc.gov/nphpsp/essentialservices.html.

6. Institute of Medicine Committee on Assuring the Health of the Public in the 21st Century. 2002. *The Future of the Public's Health in the 21st Century.* National Academies Press. Published November 11. http://nationalacademies.org/hmd/Reports/2002/The-Future-of-the-Publics-Health-in-the-21st-Century.aspx.

7. Lamberth, C. D., and L. Rowitz. 2009. "Leadership in Public Health Practice." In *Principles of Public Health Practice*, 3rd ed., edited by F. D. Scutchfield and C. W. Keck, 418–44. Clifton Park, NJ: Delmar Cengage.

8. Keck, C. W., and F. D. Scutchfield. 2009. "Emergence of a New Public Health." In *Principles of Public Health Practice*, 3rd ed., edited by F. D. Scutchfield and C. W. Keck, 36–56. Clifton Park, NJ: Delmar Cengage.

9. Association of Schools of Public Health Education Committee. 2006. *Master's Degree in Public Health Core Competency Model, Version 2.3.* Published August. www.aspph.org/app/uploads/2014/04/Version2.31_FINAL.pdf.

10. Association of Schools of Public Health Education Committee. 2009. *Doctor of Public Health (DrPH) Core Competency Model, Version 1.3.* Published November. www.aspph.org/app/uploads/2014/04/DrPHVersion1-3.pdf.

11. Association of Schools and Programs of Public Health. 2017. "Undergraduate Learning Outcomes Model." Accessed January 27. www.aspph.org/educate/models/undergraduate-learning-outcomes/.

12. Wright, K., L. Rowitz, and M. Adelaide. 2001. "A Conceptual Model for Leadership Development." *Journal of Public Health Management & Practice* 7 (4): 60–66.

13. Wright, K., L. Rowitz, A. Merkle, W. M. Reid, G. Robinson, B. Herzog, D. Weber, D. Carmichael, T. R. Balderson, and E. Baker. 2000. "Competency Development in Public Health Leadership." *American Journal of Public Health* 90 (8): 1202–7.

14. Eisenhower, D. D. 1954. Remarks at the Annual Conference of the Society for Personnel Administration, May 12. www.eisenhower.archives.gov/all_about_ike/quotes.html.

15. Plato. n.d. "Quotes." Goodreads. Accessed April 4, 2014. www.goodreads.com/quotes/346491-beauty-lies-in-the-eyes-of-the-beholder.

16. Yukl, G. A. 2013. *Leadership in Organizations*, 8th ed. Upper Saddle River, NJ: Prentice Hall.

17. Janda, K. F. 1960. "Towards the Explication of the Concept of Leadership in Terms of the Concept of Power." *Human Relations* 13 (4): 345–63.

18. Bennis, W. G. 1959. "Leadership Theory and Administrative Behavior: The Problem of Authority." *Administrative Science Quarterly* 4 (3): 259–301.

19. Stogdill, R. M. 1974. *Handbook of Leadership: A Survey of Theory and Research*. New York: Free Press.

20. Northouse, P. G. 2016. *Leadership: Theory and Practice*, 7th ed. Los Angeles: Sage.

21. Rauch, J. 2016. "What's Ailing American Politics?" *The Atlantic* 318 (1): 51–63.

22. Jago, A. G. 1982. "Leadership: Perspectives in Theory and Research." *Management Science* 28 (3): 315–36.

23. Fisher, B. A. 1974. *Small Group Decision Making: Communication and the Group*. New York: McGraw-Hill.

24. Smith, J. A., and R. J. Foti. 1998. "A Pattern Approach to the Study of Leader Emergence." *Leadership Quarterly* 9 (2): 147–60.

25. Hogg, M. A. "A Social Identity Theory of Leadership." *Personality and Social Psychology Review* 5 (3): 184–200.

26. French, J. R., Jr., and B. Raven. 1959. "The Bases of Social Power." In *Studies in Social Power*, edited by D. Cartwright, 150–67. Ann Arbor, MI: Institute for Social Research.

27. French, J. R., Jr., and B. Raven. 1962. "The Bases of Social Power." In *Group Dynamics: Research and Theory*, edited by D. Cartwright, 259–69. New York: Harper & Row.

28. Faculty of Information Studies, University of Toronto. 1995. "Development of Management Thought." Accessed February 5, 2017. http://choo.fis.utoronto.ca/fis/courses/lis1230/lis1230sharma/history4.htm.

29. Pascale, R. 1990. *Managing on the Edge*. London, UK: Penguin.

30. Bennis, W. G., and B. Nanus. 1985. *Leaders: The Strategies for Taking Charge*. New York: Harper & Row.

31. Zaleznik, A. 1977. "Managers and Leaders: Are They Different?" *Harvard Business Review* 55 (5): 67–78.

32. Mintzberg, H. 1973. *The Nature of Managerial Work*. New York: Harper & Row.

33. Kotter, J. P. 1990. *A Force for Change: How Leadership Differs from Management*. New York: Free Press.

34. Rost, J. C. 1993. *Leadership for the Twenty-First Century*. Westport, CT: Praeger.

35. Daft, R. L. 2015. *The Leadership Experience*, 6th ed. Mason, OH: South-Western.

36. Shaw, T. n.d. "Tommy Shaw Quotes." Brainy Quote. Accessed February 6, 2017. www.brainyquote.com/quotes/quotes/t/tommyshaw294384.html.

37. Lynn, L. E., Jr. 1994. "Public Management Research: The Triumph of Art over Science." *Journal of Policy Analysis and Management* 13 (2): 231–87.

38. Ledlow, G. R., and J. H. Stephens. 2018. *Leadership for Health Professionals: Theory, Skills, and Applications*, 3rd ed. Sudbury, MA: Jones & Bartlett Learning.

39. Goleman, D. 1998. "What Makes a Leader?" *Harvard Business Review* 76 (6): 93–102.

40. Rowitz, L. 2006. *Public Health for the 21st Century: The Prepared Leader*. Sudbury, MA: Jones & Bartlett.

41. Rowitz, L. 2014. *Public Health Leadership: Putting Principles into Practice*, 3rd ed. Sudbury, MA: Jones & Bartlett.

42. Senge, P. M. 2006. *The Fifth Discipline*, revised ed. New York: Doubleday.

43. Systems Thinker. 2002. *What Is Systems Thinking?* Waltham, MA: Pegasus Communications.

44. Goodman, M., and R. Karash. 1995. "Six Steps to Thinking Systemically." *Systems Thinker* 6 (2): 16–18.

45. Fritz, R. 1999. *The Path of Least Resistance for Managers*. San Francisco: Berrett-Kohler.

46. Fritz, R. 1989. *The Path of Least Resistance*. New York: Fawcett.

47. Wheatley, M. J. 2006. *Leadership and the New Science: Discovering Order in a Chaotic World*. San Francisco: Berrett-Koehler.

48. Merrill, S. 2009. *Introducing Syndemics: A Critical Systems Approach to Public and Community Health*. Hoboken, NJ: Wiley.

49. Sullivan, K. A., L. C. Messer, and E. B. Quinlivan. 2015. "Substance Abuse, Violence, and HIV/AIDS (SAVA) Syndemic Effects on Viral Suppression Among HIV Positive Women of Color." *AIDS Patient Care and STDs* 29 (Suppl. 1): S42–S48.

50. Winer, M., and K. Ray. 1997. *Collaboration Handbook*. St. Paul, MN: Amherst H. Wilder Foundation.

51. Himmelman, A. T. 1996. *Collaboration for a Change: Definitions, Models, Roles and a Guide to the Collaboration Process*. Minneapolis, MN: Himmelman Consulting Group.

52. Senge, P. M., A. Kleiner, C. Roberts, R. B. Ross, and B. J. Smith. 1994. *The Fifth Discipline Fieldbook: Strategies and Tools for Building a Learning Organization*. New York: Doubleday.

53. Ciulla, J. (ed.). 2004. *Ethics: The Health of Leadership*. Westport, CT: Praeger.

54. Johnson, C. E. 2015. *Meeting the Ethical Challenges of Leadership: Casting Light or Shadow*, 5th ed. Los Angeles: Sage.

55. Palmer, P. 1996. "Leading from Within." In *Insights on Leadership: Service, Stewardship, Spirit, and Servant-Leadership*, edited by L. C. Spears, 197–208. New York: Wiley.

56. Kellerman, B. 2004. *Bad Leadership: What It Is, How It Happens, Why It Matters*. Boston: Harvard Business School Press.

57. Gates, R. M. 2016. *A Passion for Leadership*. New York: Alfred A. Knopf.

58. Goleman, D., R. Boyatzis, and A. McKee. 2002. *Primal Leadership: Realizing the Power of Emotional Intelligence*. Boston: Harvard Business School Press.

59. Daft, R. L. 2016. *Management*, 12th ed. Mason, OH: South-Western.

PROFESSIONALISM FOR THE EFFECTIVE PUBLIC HEALTH LEADER

Donna J. Schmutzler and James W. Holsinger Jr.

Learning Objectives

Upon completion of this chapter, you should be able to

- describe the characteristics of a profession,
- apply the professional attributes to public health practice,
- describe medical professionalism as outlined in the *Physician Charter*,
- apply the values of medical professionalism to the practice of public health,
- analyze Priester's framework of healthcare values,
- apply Priester's framework to the practice of public health, and
- apply the public health professionalism framework to the practice of public health leadership.

Focus on Leadership Competencies

This chapter emphasizes the following Association of Schools and Programs of Public Health (ASPPH) leadership competencies:

- Describe the attributes of public health leadership.
- Articulate an achievable mission, set of core values, and vision.
- Demonstrate a commitment to personal and professional values.
- Influence others to achieve high standards of performance and accountability.

It also addresses the following Council on Linkages public health leadership competencies:

(continued)

> - Modifies organizational practices in consideration of changes.
> - Advocates for the role of public health in providing population health services.
>
> *Note: See the appendix at the end of the book for complete lists of competencies.*

Introduction

Although, historically, public health in the United States was strongly influenced by the medical model, it developed almost entirely outside of the practice of medicine. Years ago, the medical community distanced itself from public health in an attempt to keep public health agencies from providing individual healthcare services, which would increase competition. Public health played only a limited role in the planning and organizational development of the modern healthcare system, and the practice of public health, for many years, was not recognized as a distinct profession with the same status afforded to physicians.[1] As a result, public health practice had difficulty becoming established as a profession, and a chasm developed between the two fields. However, both professions—medicine and public health—have a powerful impact on the health of the American people, and a focus on conflict resolution and collaboration is vital for improving the health of individuals and society at large.[2]

The health-related professions have evolved over time as a result of technological advancements and changes in professional responsibilities.[3] Today, the relationship between the public health practitioner and professionalism, on its surface, appears straightforward. However, as we begin our discussion, certain key terms—including *public health*, *public health system*, *practitioner*, *profession*, and *professionalism*—require definition.

public health
A science and art of protecting and improving the health of populations and communities.

Public health is the science and art of protecting and improving the health of populations and communities through education, research, and an emphasis on healthy personal lifestyles and injury prevention. It aims to improve people's health and well-being from the local level to the global level by focusing on primary prevention of health problems.[4] Modeste and Tamayose[5(p104)] define *public health* as "Preventing disease, prolonging life, and promoting health and efficiency through organized community efforts for the sanitation of the environment, control of communicable infections, education in personal hygiene, organization of medical and nursing services, and development of the social machinery to ensure everyone a standard of living adequate for the maintenance of health." Public health focuses on the health of populations and communities rather than the care of individuals. It may serve as a safety net within the healthcare system, providing such essential healthcare services as childhood immunizations and prenatal care to disadvantaged populations (e.g., people with low incomes or no insurance). A nation's socioeconomic status and public health practices, such as education in environmental sanitation and personal hygiene, benefit the health of a population more than all biomedical interventions combined.[6]

The **public health system** in the United States consists of a variety of governmental and nongovernmental agencies. Governmental public health agencies form the core of the public health system and are present at the federal, state, and local levels.[7] The public health agencies of the federal government form the umbrella under which state and local health departments receive guidance, regulations, and funding. At the federal level, the US Department of Health and Human Services is the primary agency overseeing the health of Americans and providing essential public health services.[8] Other public health organizations at the national level include the Centers for Disease Control and Prevention (CDC), the Food and Drug Administration (FDA), and the National Institutes of Health (NIH). State departments of public health, as well as regional and local public health departments, operate throughout the United States. Nongovernmental public health agencies include hospitals, universities, grassroots consumer organizations, national professional organizations, and other private-sector organizations.[9] The American Public Health Association (APHA), for instance, was established in 1872 partly in response to urban development but also to reduce the health and safety risks faced by factory workers during the Industrial Revolution.[10]

The word *practitioner* refers to an individual who practices a profession; thus, to understand the work of practitioners across the various segments of the public health system, we must first examine what constitutes a profession. According to Gruen and colleagues,[11] the basic criteria that characterize **professions** are (1) altruistic service to others at the individual and societal levels, (2) **autonomy** and **self-regulation**, (3) monopoly on the usage of specialized knowledge, and (4) preservation and expansion of professional skills and knowledge. Cruess and Cruess[12] list the key characteristics of a profession (see exhibit 2.1), and they categorize those characteristics into three areas: knowledge, organizations and legalities, and ethics. The expertise of a profession stems from the formal education process required of practitioners, as well as from the constant renewal of knowledge and skills through research.[13] Trustworthy individuals are attracted to the life of public service offered by the various professions.[14] Practitioners demonstrate **altruism** when they use their unique knowledge and skills to deliver services to others.

Public health has all the essential characteristics of a profession.[15,16] Practitioners possess a monopoly over a distinctive body of skills and knowledge, they self-regulate as authorities in the affairs of their profession, and they have personal autonomy.[11,12] Members of the public health workforce represent various professional disciplines, such as medicine, nursing, and public health, and they provide health-related services at the community, state, and national levels.

Gebbie and colleagues[17] describe a career ladder in public health with the following levels: (1) frontline workers educated at community colleges; (2) entry-level program staffers with baccalaureate degrees in public health; and (3) master's- and doctoral-prepared practitioners with extensive knowledge

public health system
The various governmental and nongovernmental agencies, including advocacy groups, focused on the health of populations and communities.

practitioner
An individual who practices a profession.

profession
A field characterized by specialized knowledge and skills, altruism, self-regulation, and the preservation and expansion of knowledge.

autonomy
Practitioners' freedom to establish criteria for entry into a profession, to control a body of knowledge and skills, and to oversee professional standards and certification.

self-regulation
Practitioners' control over the practice of a profession under the guidance of a professional organization independent of direct governmental supervision.

altruism
An unselfish concern for the welfare of others.

EXHIBIT 2.1
Characteristics
of a Profession

Knowledge

Extended time period for education and training

Provision of services within the area of expertise to the public

Organizations and Legalities

Exclusive control over a unique body of knowledge and skills

Organization and control of work independent of state and capital

Formal documents, including laws governing regulations and licensure

Status as the ultimate authorities within their domains of personal, social, cultural, economic, and political affairs

Efforts to influence public policy and educate the public about area of expertise

Control number of persons admitted into profession, as well as qualifications and educational requirements

Control over terms, conditions, and goals of the profession

Disciplinary action for professionals exhibiting unprofessional conduct

Development of ethical standards and evaluation criteria for professionals

Ethics

Right to personal autonomy as established by professional organizations and legal regulations

Higher value placed on performance than on one's own reward

Professionals held to higher standards of conduct than nonprofessionals

Source: Data from Cruess, S. R., and R. L. Cruess. 1997. "Professionalism Must Be Taught." *BMJ* 315 (7123): 1674–77.

and experience in health fields. Tilson and Gebbie[16] have questioned, however, whether classification as a public health professional is dependent on the worksite or on the credentials possessed by the individual. According to the Committee on Educating Public Health Professionals for the 21st Century,[18(p1)] "a public health professional is a person educated in public health or a related discipline who is employed to improve health through a population focus." According to the Institute of Medicine (IOM),[7] a public health professional is a person who possesses a degree in public health or a related discipline (e.g., medicine, nursing, law) and whose employment position focuses on the improvement of the health and well-being of individuals at the community, state, or national level. Since definitions of *public health professional* vary, we will use the term *public health practitioner* for our discussion in this book.

The concept of **professionalism** is highly applicable to the public health practitioner. McNair[19] writes that professionalism occurs when an individual practices a profession with competence, skill, and a commitment to serving the interests of other people either individually or collectively as a society. The Association of Schools of Public Health Education Committee[20(p11)] listed professionalism as a "cross-cutting" competency of public health and defined it as the "ability to demonstrate ethical choices, values and professional practices implicit in the public health decision-making process; [to] consider the effect of choices on community stewardship, equity, social justice and accountability; and to commit to personal and institutional development." Establishing professionalism as a core principle for public health practitioners at both the individual and organizational levels is essential.[3]

Professionalism is reflected in a code of ethics that originated with the Hippocratic Oath. Hippocrates (c. 460 BC–c. 375 BC) has long been regarded as the "father of medicine," largely because of his acknowledgment of the clinical signs of illness and his use of rational reasoning. The application of moral values to the practice of medicine can also be traced to Hippocrates, and these values are similarly applicable to the practice of public health.[21] Values are thus a key component of professionalism, and they refer to ideas about what is desirable or what should be—not what is or what might be.[22]

Professionalism focuses on relationships and collaboration.[23] The relationship between the public health practitioner and society is the foundation on which other relationships are built. Other relationships include those between practitioners and clients, resulting in high-quality service; between practitioners and the public health system, resulting in efficient use of finite resources; between practitioners and colleagues, resulting in collaboration; and between practitioners and themselves, resulting in personal development. Thus, public health practitioners practice professionalism at societal, collegial, and personal levels.[23]

Professionalism in public health is based on a collaborative model in which practitioners work as team members while offering leadership to colleagues in the public health system. Each practitioner brings unique knowledge and strengths to the multidisciplinary team, and all members are committed to providing high-quality service. Whereas the traditional physician–client relationship typically denotes one physician and one individual, the public health practitioner–client relationship is more complex. In public health, the client could be an individual using services provided by the local health department (e.g., water testing), or it could be a target group, such as a group of schoolchildren taking part in an influenza

professionalism
The manner of practicing a profession with competence, skill, and a commitment to serving the interests of other people either individually or collectively as a society.

Effective Public Health Leaders . . .

. . . understand that quality work is always the least expensive.

vaccination program. Practitioners in the field of public health must exhibit professionalism on a daily basis in both their personal and professional lives.[23]

Public Health as a Profession

The development of the public health workforce gained widespread attention with the publication of a 1988 IOM report titled *The Future of Public Health*. That report stated that the mission of public health is "fulfilling society's interest in assuring conditions in which people can be healthy."[9(p7)] A 2002 IOM report titled *The Future of the Public's Health in the 21st Century* highlighted a need for both governmental and nongovernmental public health agencies, as well as university programs in public health, to provide the training, leadership, support, and development required by public health organizations and the field's leaders and practitioners.[7]

 Consider This

"Too many people overvalue what they are not and undervalue what they are."
— Malcolm S. Forbes[24]

Why is it important that public health practitioners not undervalue what they achieve in providing support for communities and populations?

Public health has long been misunderstood, and it has lagged behind other healthcare professions in gaining respect and recognition from members of the community. Since public health agencies often act as a safety net for individual healthcare services, members of the public often view the public health system as a part of the larger US healthcare system but not as a distinct professional practice. Even healthcare leaders have been found to lack a basic working comprehension of public health.[25] However, as public health evolves, it is increasingly becoming established as a professional community. To be classified as a "community of profession," as described by Goode,[26] public health should seek to produce the next generation of leaders through the community's selection and training processes; determine a set of clear social limits; develop shared values among community members; understand that, typically, once a member joins the community, that person is always a member; establish a "sense of identity" binding members together; exert control over the members of the community; develop a unique language; and establish defined roles for both members and nonmembers.

Public Health Practice

In 1927, Frances W. Peabody, addressing graduating students at Harvard Medical School, stated his position that the practice of medicine required a "hands-on" approach. When individuals seek healthcare services, they expect their providers to take a hands-on approach to care while also using advanced technology. Peabody's ideas similarly apply to health-related services provided at the population level. Public health practitioners use technology daily, but they also apply a hands-on approach in interactions with colleagues and the community. Through their professionalism and the set of values incorporated in that professionalism, they demonstrate respect for colleagues and community members.

The distinction between medicine and public health can be clarified by emphasizing the phrases "cure of disease," which pertains to the practice of medicine, and "maintenance of health," which represents the public health mission of ensuring the health of communities and the population at large.[9,27] In its pursuit of that mission, the practice of public health impacts the lives of all Americans. The ten most common services and activities provided by local health departments are the following: adult immunizations, child immunizations, communicable/infectious disease surveillance, environmental health surveillance, food safety education, food-service establishment inspection, school and day care center inspection, tobacco use prevention, tuberculosis prevention, and tuberculosis screening.[28]

Local public health activities, such as communicable/infectious disease surveillance and food-service establishment inspections, provide valuable information about cases of **notifiable disease**. Notifiable diseases are those for which frequent and timely information about individual cases is deemed necessary for public health.[29] Information about such cases is reported annually to the CDC's National Notifiable Diseases Surveillance System, which is operated in partnership with the Council of State and Territorial Epidemiologists (CSTE).[29,30,31] Required notifiable conditions can vary from state to state, but a list of national notifiable conditions—the *CSTE List of Nationally Notifiable Conditions*—is determined through collaboration between state public health officials, the CSTE, and the CDC.[29,31]

notifiable disease
A disease for which frequent and timely information about individual cases is deemed necessary for public health.

Public Health Practitioners

Studies have shown that as many as four out of five public health workers have no formal training in public health.[32,33] Frequently, practitioners are hired for public health teams with minimal, if any, knowledge of or experience in the field.[34]

Given the breadth of public health activities at the local, state, and federal levels, developing a clear statistical estimate of the public health workforce is challenging, though recent efforts to quantify public health professions have provided a useful taxonomy.[35] A 2014 study[36] that aggregated public health workforce data from six sources—including the 2013 National Association of County and City Health Officials and the 2012 Association of State and Territorial Health Officials profile surveys—estimated the total governmental public health workforce at 290,988 (range: 231,464–341,053). Although the Bureau of Health Professions lists more than 30 professional disciplines in the public health workforce, current enumeration methods identify only 14, plus a fifteenth category for "other" or uncategorized public health professions. Administrative or clerical personnel (55,644) formed the largest discipline, followed by public health nurses (47,720), environmental health workers (23,838), and public health managers (18,394). Other/uncategorized public health professionals (86,431) made up nearly 30 percent of the enumerated workforce.

Notably, data indicate that the size of the public health workforce is shrinking.[37] An earlier workforce enumeration, *The Public Health Work Force Enumeration 2000*,[38] estimated that the public health workforce consisted of 448,254 salaried individuals. The newer enumeration statistics therefore reflect a reduction of 24 to 48 percent. Such a significant shift in the size and composition of the public health workforce has important implications for the public health leaders who must staff the various functions and services within their purview. Leaders may also need to determine whether the traditional workforce disciplines can meet the evolving demands of public health systems and services.

The measurement of population health outcomes through research projects and data collection can help ensure accountability for public health practitioners. It can also provide resources with which health outcomes can be analyzed and evaluated. The US Department of Health and Human Services (HHS) operates a decennial initiative called Healthy People, which aims to improve the health of the American people by establishing 10-year goals and objectives related to health promotion and disease prevention; the current version, Healthy People 2020, was launched in December 2010.[39] Public health practitioners are held accountable for the various steps in gathering, analyzing, interpreting, and reporting health outcomes as they strive to implement the HHS initiative.

 Consider This

"My idea of professionalism is probably a lot of people's idea of obsessive."
—David Fincher[40]

Why do you think individuals who practice a profession might be obsessive in their work?

Frameworks of Professionalism

A variety of professional organizations have emphasized the importance of professionalism in public health and worked to identify the key components of public health's development as a profession. Such organizations include the American Public Health Association, the Association for Prevention Teaching and Research, the Association of Schools and Programs of Public Health, the Association of State and Territorial Health Officials, the Council on Education for Public Health, the Council on Linkages Between Academia and Public Health Practice (often referred to simply as the Council on Linkages) within the Public Health Foundation, the National Association of County and City Health Officials, and the National Board of Public Health Examiners. These organizations have established professional standards and requirements for credentialing public health practitioners and accrediting public health organizations and educational programs.

Certification in Public Health

In 2005, five national public health organizations started NBPHE as an independent organization with the aim of establishing public health as a recognized profession with certified practitioners.[10] NBPHE developed the Certified in Public Health (CPH) examination, which was first administered in August 2008, both within the United States and internationally.[41] To be eligible to take the CPH exam, an individual must meet at least one of the following criteria: (1) enrollment in or completion of the five core content courses for a public health graduate degree at a CEPH-accredited school or program, (2) completion of the requirements for a master's or doctoral degree at a CEPH-accredited school or program, (3) possession of a bachelor's degree and completion of at least five years of public health work experience.[10] Public health practitioners who have passed the credentialing exam are automatically placed in a recertification program that requires 50 CPH recertification education credits every two years.[42] The aims of recertification are to encourage the continued development of the practitioner through lifelong learning and to promote the profession of public health. NBPHE has also developed a code of ethics for the CPH practitioner, shown in exhibit 2.2.

Council on Linkages

The Council on Linkages Between Academia and Public Health Practice, established in 1992, is a coalition of organizations that promotes collaboration between academic settings and practice sites, thereby increasing the relevance of

---

Key Professional Organizations in Public Health, with Abbreviations and Websites

American Public Health Association (APHA)
www.apha.org

Association for Prevention Teaching and Research (APTR)
www.aptrweb.org

Association of Schools and Programs of Public Health (ASPPH)
www.aspph.org

Association of State and Territorial Health Officials (ASTHO)
www.astho.org

Council on Education for Public Health (CEPH)
www.ceph.org

Council on Linkages Between Academia and Public Health Practice within the Public Health Foundation (PHF)
www.phf.org/programs/council/Pages/default.aspx

National Association of County and City Health Officials (NACCHO)
www.naccho.org

National Board of Public Health Examiners (NBPHE)
www.nbphe.org

EXHIBIT 2.2
Certified in
Public Health
Code of Ethics

- Place the safety and health of the public above all other interests.
- Demonstrate integrity, honesty, and fairness in all activities and strive for excellence in all matters of ethical conduct.
- Undertake work utilizing skills that ensure competent performance.
- Act truthfully and speak in good faith in an objective manner based on knowledge of facts and competence of subject matter.
- Protect confidential information that may bring harm to an individual or a community.
- Act in a timely manner in disseminating information that protects the health of the public.
- Act in a manner free of bias with regard to religion, ethnicity, gender, age, national origin, or disability, and respect the rights of individuals in the community.
- Accurately represent academic and professional qualifications.
- Maintain competency requirements through recertification.
- Acknowledge that the credential is the property of NBPHE.
- Uphold and abide by the policies and procedures required by NBPHE to remain in good standing.
- Use the NBPHE logo and credential as authorized by NBPHE.

Source: National Board of Public Health Examiners (NBPHE). 2017. "Code of Ethics." Accessed April 25. www.nbphe.org/codeofethics.cfm.

public health education to public health practice. The council's aim is to ensure a well-trained and competent public health workforce and a solid, evidence-based public health infrastructure.[43] In 2001, the Council on Linkages adopted its first set of competencies for public health practitioners.[44] Since then, additional competencies for other areas of the public health workforce—including public health informatics, public health nursing, epidemiology in government agencies, and bioterrorism/emergency readiness—have been developed.

Cultural Competence

Although medicine and public health operate separately, they are connected in that practitioners in both fields develop policies and deliver services that affect the health and well-being of individuals and populations. Thus, practitioners preparing to enter either field have a similar need for cultural competence training, to ensure that they can effectively engage with diverse communities and demonstrate inclusion and cultural awareness in their interactions. In 2012, the Association of American Medical Colleges and the Association of Schools of Public Health (now the Association of Schools and Programs of Public Health)[45] convened an

 Check It Out

Visit www.aspph.org/app/uploads/2014/04/11-278-CulturCompet-Interactive-final.pdf to read the full list of joint medical and public health cultural competencies.

expert panel to develop a set of cultural competencies that are expected of both graduating medical students and graduate students in public health programs.

The Medical Model

The practice of medicine has a well-established model of professionalism. Physicians are assumed to have a clear understanding of professionalism, and they apply this understanding to their personal and professional lives.[1,12] Professional medical organizations such as the American College of Physicians (ACP), the Accreditation Council for Graduate Medical Education (AGME), the American Board of Internal Medicine (ABIM), and the European Federation of Internal Medicine (EFIM) have worked to promote professionalism in the practice of medicine, and many of the materials developed by these organizations are applicable to the practice of public health.

Medical Professionalism in the New Millennium: A Physician Charter[46]—commonly known simply as the **Physician Charter**—was published in 2002 through a collaboration between the ABIM Foundation, the ACP Foundation, and EFIM. The charter outlines the fundamental professional principles and responsibilities for physicians and, by extrapolation, other healthcare practitioners. The preamble of the *Physician Charter* states that "professionalism is the basis of medicine's contract with society." The charter was developed to promote dedication to the practice of medicine and to reaffirm physicians' active commitment to the values of professionalism, thereby strengthening society's loyalty to physicians. Practitioners are encouraged to progress beyond the charter to embrace its ideals and deep commitment to members of society.[3,46]

Physician Charter
A document that outlines fundamental professional principles and responsibilities for physicians and other healthcare practitioners.

The Educational Basis of Public Health Professionalism

Public health educational programs have the distinct role of preparing individuals to be public health practitioners.[47] The majority of public health educational institutions, including both schools of public health and programs of public health at the departmental level, are of more recent vintage than programs in the other healthcare professions.[17] Although courses in public health were offered within other educational programs during the 1800s, schools of public health were not established in the United States until the early twentieth century. The first professional training program specifically for public health opened in 1913 as a joint venture between the Massachusetts Institute of Technology (MIT) and Harvard University, with students in the Harvard-MIT School of Health Officers taking courses at both universities.[48] The Johns Hopkins School of Hygiene and Public Health—the first school of public health in the United States—was established in Baltimore, Maryland, in 1916, and it emphasized practical training in public health and excellence in research.[17] Early schools of public health had departments of biostatistics, environmental health, health administration, and public health practice.

The Council on Education in Public Health Accreditation

The Association of Schools of Public Health and the American Public Health Association established the Council on Education for Public Health in 1974.[49] CEPH is recognized by the US Department of Education as an independent accrediting agency for public health educational programs. It has both accredited and associate members: Accredited members are programs or schools of public health that have passed a rigorous peer-review accreditation process, whereas associate members are programs or schools undergoing the peer-review process.[50]

Programs and schools of public health must demonstrate a number of characteristics to be considered for an accreditation review by CEPH.[51] They must use an ecological perspective that supports interdisciplinary communication; promote development of public health professional values; endorse a broad intellectual framework for problem solving; and address the health of populations through instruction, research, and service. In addition, the programs must possess adequate human, learning, physical, and financial resources to deliver an in-depth educational experience in the areas applicable to public health. By applying this framework across various programs and schools, CEPH provides an educational basis for the practice of public health professionalism.

Attendance at a CEPH-accredited public health institution provides a number of benefits to students—notably, a well-rounded, high-quality education and excellent preparation for practice in the field.[50] Some public health positions require graduation from an accredited school or program. Many, if not most, institutions now offer bachelor's degrees in public or population health. Master's degree programs are offered in five core areas of public health: social and behavioral science, biostatistics, environmental health sciences, epidemiology, and health policy and administration. Doctoral programs are offered in at least three of these areas. Students in satisfactory academic standing are assisted when transferring between accredited schools of public health. Also, graduates of accredited programs may sit for the certification examination administered by NBPHE and are eligible for federally funded public health internships and fellowships.

Association of Schools and Programs of Public Health

Originally established in 1953 as the Association of Schools of Public Health, the Association of Schools and Programs of Public Health represents and serves as a national resource for schools and programs accredited by CEPH. It promotes public health as a career and improves the public's health through the advancement of higher education, service, and research. It supports partnerships with both governmental and nongovernmental organizations within the healthcare system to assist accredited schools and programs, and it facilitates cooperative initiatives among accredited schools and programs, such as the committee to develop competencies for students obtaining a master of public health (MPH) degree. ASPPH also encourages and promotes practice-based training opportunities for students.[50]

When schools and programs of public health develop curricula pertaining to the principle of professionalism for bachelor's, master's, and doctoral degrees, they draw information from a variety of resources, including textbooks, professional organizations and boards, professional journals, and fellowships.[3] The importance of professionalism is reflected by its inclusion in the core competency models developed for all public health degree graduates.[20,52]

Core Competencies

In 2004, ASPPH initiated the development of a **core competency model** for MPH graduates. A number of factors influenced the model's development, including new twenty-first century challenges in the practice of public health, the expansion of recommended competency-based training and the inclusion of competencies into program accreditation criteria, increased attention on accountability in higher education, and the development of a credentialing exam for graduates of CEPH-accredited programs. In 2006, ASPPH published the Master's Degree in Public Health Core Competency Model, Version 2.3.[20]

The MPH core competency model includes the five core areas of social and behavioral sciences, biostatistics, epidemiology, environmental health sciences, and health policy and management; the seven cross-cutting areas of diversity and culture, communication and informatics, leadership, professionalism, program planning, systems thinking, and public health biology; and a number of additional competencies reflecting the baseline of knowledge and skills expected of an emerging public health practitioner with an MPH degree.[20] For the MPH model, the ASPPH Education Committee determined that the cross-cutting competencies of professionalism and leadership were key elements in developing effective public health practitioners.[20]

The doctor of public health (DrPH) degree is available for students who wish to receive advanced education in evidence-based leadership in public health, as well as practice-based research.[7] During the mid-1980s, Roemer proposed that the DrPH curriculum should concentrate on healthcare systems management, protecting the health of populations and preventing disease, and developing social analytic tools.[17,53] The ASPPH's Doctor of Public Health (DrPH) Core Competency Model, Version 1.3,[52] was published in 2009. According to the model, graduates with a DrPH degree should be competent in the domains of advocacy, communication, community/cultural orientation, critical analysis, leadership, management, and professionalism and ethics.

core competency model
A framework developed by the Association of Schools and Programs of Public Health that establishes a baseline of knowledge required of candidates for various public health degrees.

✓ Check It Out

ASPPH's MPH Competency Model can be found at www.aspph.org/educate/models/mph-competency-model/.

ASPPH's DrPH Competency Model can be found at www.aspph.org/educate/models/drph-model/.

ASPPH's Undergraduate Learning Outcomes Model can be found at www.aspph.org/educate/models/undergraduate-learning-outcomes/.

Further efforts from ASPPH's Framing the Future initiative can be found at www.aspph.org/educate/framing-the-future/.

Leadership Application Case: The Other Side of the Story

The Leadership Application Case at the beginning of this book provides realistic scenarios for the application of key leadership concepts covered in the text. See the section marked "Chapter 2 Application" for the scenario and discussion questions that correspond with this chapter.

The model signifies that practitioners with a DrPH degree should be leaders thoroughly educated in the development and implementation of evidence-based public health practice, public health research techniques, and the principle of professionalism.

In 2012, ASPPH assembled an expert panel as part of an initiative titled Framing the Future: The Second 100 Years of Education for Public Health, and the panel identified the critical component elements (CCEs) of an undergraduate degree in public health.[54] The panel determined that undergraduate students should be proficient in the humanities, mathematics, and a variety of sciences and also possess skills related to communication and information literacy. It further concluded that undergraduate students should be introduced to nine public health domains and also engage in a capstone experience. Cross-cutting areas identified by the model included professionalism as a core concept. The panel's initial effort has since been transformed into ASPPH's Undergraduate Learning Outcomes Model, mirroring its MPH and DrPH cousins.

The Practice of Professionalism

For both practitioners and educators, professionalism and its values will be critical to public health leadership in the twenty-first century. Professionalism must be instilled both in practice and in academic settings.[55] Relevant information about professionalism can be drawn not only from the practice of medicine, but also from such disciplines as economics, philosophy, political science, and sociology.[12] A thorough understanding of professionalism can thus renew the practice of public health in rewarding and exciting ways.[3]

The Institute of Medicine Committee on Assuring the Health of the Public in the 21st Century[7] has pointed out that challenges will arise as professionalism is subjected to the forces of uncertainty and rapid change, which are common among public health agencies, the healthcare system, academia, and other areas of public health. The practice of public health as an independent profession continues to evolve and expand, with a workforce that includes such diverse professional groups as physicians, environmental health specialists, epidemiologists, nurses, case managers, social workers, health education specialists, dentists, and laboratory technicians.[9,33] In fact, the American Public Health Association today boasts more than 30 membership sections for various disciplines and special interests. The constant change across the various segments of the public health workforce may at times seem debilitating; however, the ability to acknowledge, accept, and actively participate in change is a basic requirement for any public health practitioner.[56] During periods of intense change, the professionalism of public health practitioners is a key to maintaining continuity and stability across the system. Just as the principle of professionalism has been integral to the practice of medicine, it is indispensable to the effective practice of public health leadership.[3]

The rapid development of public health as a profession and its growing recognition as an important part of American life have created the need to teach the principle of professionalism to public health students. Some schools have introduced professionalism education courses.[57] However, the importance of professionalism is best reinforced for students when professionalism as a value is not only taught in a didactic setting but also reflected in the daily lives of faculty members and practitioners. Professional organizations, such as APHA and ASPPH, are working together to promote professionalism as a core discipline in public health.

 Effective Public Health Leaders . . .

. . . understand that "silence and restraint are essential, if undervalued, tools of leadership."
—Robert M. Gates[58(p167)]

A Values Framework

Public health practitioners must remember that to be esteemed as a professional is a privilege, not a right.[12] Ethical behavior results from a distinctive blend of values and standards.[15] When professionalism is emphasized as a principle and embraced by all public health practitioners, higher standards and increased performance levels result.[12]

As public health continues its development as a professional discipline, it must have a **values framework** that includes the principle of professionalism. The formal code of ethics used in the medical profession—set forth by the American Medical Association (AMA)[59]—provides a useful starting point for our consideration of professionalism in public health. Since the origination of the AMA code, medical organizations have further developed and updated the profession's values system. We discuss medical professionalism alongside public health professionalism for several reasons. First, the values systems for medicine and public health have similarities because both disciplines provide health-related services either to the individual, the community, or the population

values framework
A basic structure of principles and standards of behavior.

at large. Second, familiarity with professionalism in the medical profession can assist in the development of professionalism as a priority in public health. Third, an understanding of professionalism for all health professions can be based on its application for many years in the practice of medicine.[60]

The principle of professionalism incorporates a variety of values, including accountability, altruism, commitment to personal and professional development, community stewardship, equity, self-regulation, and social justice. These values, which have defined professionalism for many years,[61] provide a moral foundation for public health practitioners; from this foundation, practitioners can develop an understanding of themselves, their professional responsibilities, and their ways of providing services to the population or community.[3] Physicians have traditionally practiced the values of professionalism while applying a specialized body of knowledge and maintaining internally developed standards.[56]

Public health practitioners practice altruism by providing services unselfishly to others in a population or community, especially during times of natural or human-made disaster. Altruism is demonstrated when an environmental health specialist trudges through a forest, risking exposure to ticks and poisonous snakes, to evaluate a possible location for a water well or when field epidemiologists investigate an outbreak of contagious disease, such as Ebola, even at the risk of being exposed to the disease themselves.

Professionalism and Society

Often, healthcare enterprises face pressures related to material concerns—such as competition, consumerism, financial responsibility to stockholders, market-driven services, and efforts to provide society with the medical services "it thinks it wants"—that can clash with the traditional values of professionalism.[56] At the same time, society has its own expectations, including community awareness, social justice, and solidarity across all healthcare practitioners, including those practicing public health.[3] When "provider autonomy" results in the neglect of community-oriented values, the dignity and well-being of all individuals—and of society at large—suffer.[22]

The relationship between medical practitioners and members of society can be considered a social contract, and the basis for that contract is professionalism.[13,46] According to the *Physician Charter*,[46] professionalism is practiced by establishing and maintaining standards of competency and integrity, placing the client's interest above the physician's interest, and providing society with expert advice on health-related matters. In a similar fashion, the relationship between public health practitioners and society can also be considered a social contract, with professionalism as part of its moral foundation.[8]

One sociological approach to professionalism suggests that it is not a principle to be taught or assessed but rather something that develops socially through personal interactions.[60] Public health practitioners must be sensitive to cultural diversity (see chapter 9), and they must take time to listen to the public health needs of varied populations. The practice of professionalism opens the door for collaboration between public health practitioners and colleagues in the healthcare system, as practitioners in both fields aim to provide appropriate services to culturally diverse populations.[3] Krieger and Birn [61(p1603)] write that "social justice is the foundation of public health," such that those drawn to work in public health have a "desire to make the world a better place, free of misery, inequity, and preventable suffering, a world in which we all can live, love, work, play, ail, and die with our dignity intact and our humanity cherished." Thus, the principle of professionalism is at the center of effective public health practice, defining public health practitioners and the work they perform.[43]

Autonomy and Self-Regulation

The concepts of autonomy and self-regulation support the idea that a profession has the power to determine what is in the best interest of its members and to practice independently from outside influences.[15] Practitioners in a number of fields enjoy the ability to self-regulate within their professions; however, that ability is especially beneficial for the large multiprofessional group of practitioners that makes up the public health workforce.

Governmental public health agencies are the largest purchaser of services provided by public health practitioners. This arrangement presents a potential barrier to self-regulation, because such agencies may require strict compliance with bureaucratic regulations.[1] Nevertheless, self-regulation remains a viable option. Active-duty armed forces physicians, for instance, are regulated through state and national medical regulatory bodies—representing self-regulation—even while working for a government entity. Before an occupation can practice self-regulation, it must have recognized status as a profession. A public health work site may include some employees whose positions are not professional in nature; therefore, self-regulation may not be possible in all instances. But self-regulation is possible if the professional classification requires the individual to possess a degree in the discipline of public health or a related field. Public health practitioners must be able to communicate effectively with legislators and policy makers if they wish to effectively lobby for policies and legislation that affect the public's health.[18]

Priester's Framework of Healthcare Values

In 1992, Reinhard Priester[22] reviewed the fundamental values of the American healthcare system and presented them in a new framework with a strong emphasis on professionalism. **Priester's values framework** (shown in exhibit 2.3) examines six **influential values**, or "former values," that were already embraced in US healthcare and adds a set of **proposed values** that look to the

Priester's values framework
A model developed by Reinhard Priester in 1992 to show the values that underlie the health system and should be used to guide reform.

influential values
A category in Priester's values framework that includes six values that were emphasized in US healthcare during the twentieth century.

proposed values
A category in Priester's values framework that includes essential values and instrumental values for meeting society's healthcare needs in the future.

future. The framework provides a useful tool for the development of a model of professionalism for public health practitioners.

Influential Values

The six influential values identified by Priester[22] are the ones that shaped US healthcare through much of the twentieth century. They are (1) professional autonomy, including both self-regulation and clinical autonomy; (2) patient autonomy, particularly patients' ability to make informed decisions about their health status and options for care, aided by the sharing of pertinent information by healthcare providers; (3) consumer sovereignty, which allows individuals to freely choose not only their healthcare plan but also their healthcare provider; (4) patient advocacy, which represents such values as beneficence, benevolence, caring, fidelity, and service; (5) high-quality care, as demonstrated in both practice settings and client outcomes, with a focus on achieving "best practice" care through research and continuing education; and (6) access to care, which has at times been an area of confusion, because the phrase may be considered in terms of universality (the people receiving care) or comprehensiveness (the services being offered). Unfortunately, Priester points out, these six values have functioned as ideals more than as realities in US healthcare. Professional autonomy is the only one that has been fully implemented. Access to care has lagged behind the other five.

Priester retains these six former values in his proposed framework, though he reorders and redefines several of them.

Spotlight

1992, the year in which Priester presented his values framework, was a presidential election year in which healthcare reform was a major campaign issue. Priester described the values that underlay the healthcare system at that time and also presented a collection of new values that should be used to guide reform of that system. In our current era of healthcare reform, Priester's framework remains useful and maintains its freshness.

Proposed Values

essential values
Fundamental values, proposed in Priester's values framework, that are required for a healthcare system.

instrumental values
Values, proposed in Priester's values framework, that are necessary to support the essential values.

The new values that Priester[22] proposed for his framework represented societal needs that had previously been neglected by the US healthcare system. The proposed values were divided into two categories: essential values and instrumental values. The **essential values** are basic values that Priester considered fundamental for any healthcare system; the **instrumental values** are used to achieve those values. Without the instrumental values, the essential values are unobtainable.

Essential Values

The essential values, as proposed by Priester[22], consist of the following: (1) fair access to an adequate level of healthcare for all people, with the acknowledgment that society cannot afford every required individual healthcare service; (2) quality of care, which involves maximizing the chances of desired outcomes

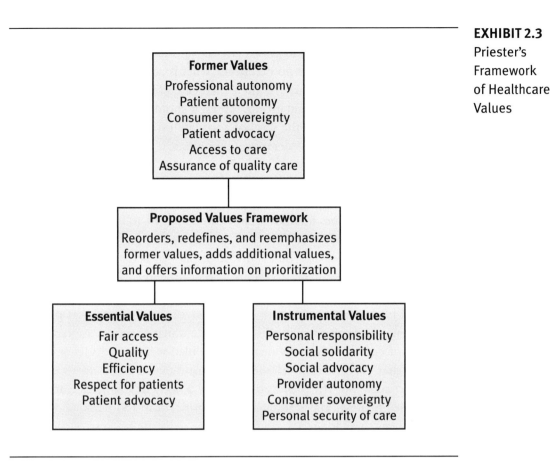

EXHIBIT 2.3
Priester's
Framework
of Healthcare
Values

Source: Data from Priester, R. 1992. "A Values Framework for Health System Reform." *Health Affairs* 11: 84–107.

at both the individual and population level, using practices that reflect current professional knowledge, and providing services in a respectful and humane manner; (3) efficiency, which occurs when the greatest benefit related to health outcomes occurs at the least expensive cost; (4) respect for clients, which covers such areas as a patient's right to informed consent, a healthcare provider's disclosure of conflicts of interest, a patient's right to refuse recommended treatment when properly informed of options and risks, a patient's right to access personal medical records in a manner that protects health and healthcare information, and the right of patients to be treated with dignity; and (5) client advocacy, meaning that providers advocate in the client's best interest by taking into consideration the fair and judicious use of finite resources, as well as providing treatment to the extent that would be provided to all other individuals under the same circumstances.

A number of critical issues must be considered when determining the "adequate" level to which each individual should have access to healthcare. Priester[22] makes clear that the adequate level of access should not be based on the financial budget. The definition of *adequate* should be determined first, with budgeting considerations later. Priester also states that, to ensure accountability, the people who determine what is adequate should be bound by that definition as it relates to their own care. The adequate level should not be defined by one special group; rather, it should be determined by what is adequate for all. Finally, the level of adequate care should be continuously evaluated to take into consideration technological advances and changes in societal needs and preferences.

Instrumental Values

The instrumental values identified by Priester[22] are the following: (1) personal responsibility, meaning both that individuals are responsible for sharing the cost of their own care and that individuals play an active role in their own health, with assistance from providers, the healthcare system, and society at large; (2) social solidarity, or a sense of community that results from every individual having access to care; (3) social advocacy, meaning that providers acknowledge the health needs of individuals and make services available to all, including disenfranchised individuals and populations; (4) provider autonomy, meaning that every health-related profession has the freedom to establish entrance criteria into the profession, control a body of knowledge and skills, and oversee professional standards and certification; (5) personal security, which ensures that individuals do not become destitute because of the cost of required healthcare needs; and (6) consumer sovereignty, meaning that the healthcare system is receptive to client preferences regarding such elements as the time and setting of service.

The framework includes both individual-oriented and community-oriented values. Whereas the former values listed professional autonomy first, Priester instead places access to care—the first essential value—at the pinnacle of his framework. Professional autonomy continues as a value in the framework, though patient autonomy has been removed.[3] Consumer sovereignty is closely related to patient autonomy, in that it ensures that ultimate authority in making final healthcare decisions falls to the client or patient; however, it fails to ensure that the decision-making process will occur without external influence, which had previously been a feature of patient autonomy.

Professionalism in a New Century

Economic and political circumstances in the twenty-first century have brought far-reaching reform to the US healthcare system, and that reform includes matters of public health. Reform efforts may result in expansion in the provision of public health services, in part because of the demands of human-made and natural crises. Such crises have traditionally resulted in conflict between public health and other organizations and professions, some of which have sought to limit the jurisdiction of public health practitioners.[1] However, as the public health portion of healthcare expenditures increases, the practice of medicine and public health may be expected to draw closer together. Advances in medical science and technology that began in the twentieth century have carried over into the twenty-first, and they have been embraced by the public health system. Technical knowledge in the field of public health has increased rapidly through research and its associated data analysis, and, despite limited financial resources, new health-related technologies will continue to be incorporated into public health services over time. The principle of professionalism will need to be applied as public health practitioners adapt to these changes and address new challenges.[18]

By applying the principle of professionalism, public health practitioners strengthen relationships with stakeholders—including individual clients, community special interest group members, and legislators, as well as colleagues. By doing so, they can ensure that they will not fall prey to pursuing priorities advocated within the profession at the expense of the values expected by individual clients and society at large.[62] Swick[56] has expressed concerns about the future of medicine and the potential clash between business and medical values, and similar concerns can be can be applied to the future of public health. If and when future occurrences—such as acts of bioterrorism or environmental crises[1]—present challenges to public health or disagreements over responsibility, practitioners will benefit from avoiding a defensive posture and implementing the value of professional collaboration. As the structure of the healthcare system continues to change, the time-honored principle of professionalism may need to be redefined to meet the needs of the twenty-first century.

A New Professionalism Framework for Public Health Practitioners

Although several values frameworks have been developed for public health, none of them, either singly or collectively, has become the framework of choice for the discipline.[5] In this section, we present a professionalism framework that can support public health leaders and practitioners in their relationships with other healthcare practitioners and the general population. The framework is illustrated in exhibit 2.4.

The public health professionalism framework involves four interactive entities—(1) the public health system; (2) the public health leader; (3) the client, whether an individual or a population; and (4) society—and practitioners must appreciate the significance of collaborative relationships between these entities.

EXHIBIT 2.4
Public Health
Professionalism
Framework

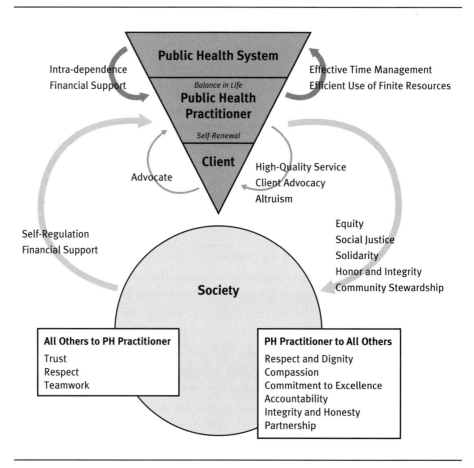

Source: Schmutzler, D. J., and J. W. Holsinger Jr. 2011. "New Professionalism." In *Professionalism in Mental Healthcare: Experts, Expertise and Expectations*, edited by D. Bhugra and A. Malik, 115–26. Cambridge, UK: Cambridge University Press. Used by permission.

The framework also identifies key values that practitioners must understand and commit to incorporating into their personal lives and professional careers.

To succeed in their roles and to actively reflect the principle of professionalism, public health practitioners must maintain a balance between their personal and professional lives while continuing to expand self-awareness and knowledge.[3] Covey[63] states that self-renewal of the mind (emotional), body (physical), relationships (social), and spirit (spiritual) are essential for balance in an individual's life. The public health practitioner must be a lifelong learner who uses research to develop knowledge of current evidence-based practices and who participates in various forms of continuing education, such as conferences, webinars, and activities with professional organizations. Research and continual learning enable public health practitioners to provide high-quality services that result in improved health outcomes for their communities and the populations they serve.

The arrows in exhibit 2.4 represent the various influences directed by the public health practitioner to the other three entities, as well as the feedback influences directed from these entities back to the practitioner. The public health practitioner influences the public health system through effective time management and the efficient use of the finite resources provided by the community. The practitioner influences society at large through the application of the principles of equity, social justice, solidarity, and honor and integrity, as well as by understanding community stewardship. The practitioner influences the client, either individually or as a collective community or population, by providing high-quality service, client advocacy, and the practice of personal altruism. In return, the client advocates for the public health practitioner, and society allows for self-regulation of the profession. Society also provides personal financial support to the practitioner. The public health system likewise provides financial support to the practitioner, with intradependence between the two producing a symbiotic relationship.

Also included in the framework are several values significant to the principle of professionalism. These values are implemented by the public health practitioner in interactions with clients, the public health system, and society as a whole; in return, the other entities provide benefits to the practitioner. By practicing in a professional manner, the practitioner provides the values of respect and dignity, compassion, commitment to excellence, accountability, integrity and honesty, and partnership to all others. In return, the public health practitioner is accorded trust and respect by those served. The field of public health focuses on ensuring conditions necessary for the promotion of health for all persons, and success depends on a strong foundational relationship between the practitioner and society. Teamwork must occur between all four entities in the framework, and the practitioner must promote collaboration with various public health stakeholders. Team members are found among colleagues, individual clients, policy makers, professional organizations, and grassroots organizations. Since governments provide a significant portion of public health's funding, practitioners must skillfully and efficiently utilize finite fiscal resources while at the same time advocating for equal access for all Americans to the services provided by public health agencies.

The moral foundation of public health practice must be grounded in the principle of professionalism. As exhibit 2.4 shows, more values are required of public health leaders and practitioners than are provided to them by the other three entities. The practitioner benefits from the self-regulation, financial support, and advocacy provided by members of society, but these elements are secondary to what the practitioner provides to the individuals, communities, and populations receiving public health services. With professionalism, practitioners can maintain a healthy perspective with regard to the benefits and values represented in the framework; in turn, public health will be perceived as a profession that is respected and trusted by colleagues and the general public.

Case Study: Dr. D. A. Henderson and the Death of a Disease[64]

In 1967, Dr. D. A. Henderson was appointed the director of the global effort to eradicate smallpox, a 3,000-year-old human scourge that historically had killed as many as two million people each year.

The effort to end smallpox had begun at the World Health Assembly in 1953, when Dr. Brock Chisholm, the first director-general of the World Health Organization (WHO), proposed that WHO develop a global effort to eradicate smallpox. Although a modest five-year budget was proposed, the plan failed to find fertile ground. No country expressed an interest in the project until the World Health Assembly of 1958, when the Soviet Union's deputy minister of health, Dr. Viktor Zhdanov, presented a report detailing the global value of eradicating smallpox and proposing a four- to five-year vaccination campaign. The Soviet Union offered to provide large quantities of heat-stable, freeze-dried vaccine in an effort to move forward with the campaign. Although WHO's director-general at that time, Marcelino Candau, reported favorably on the proposal, WHO's efforts were miniscule initially. Several years later, in response to the faltering WHO effort, Director-General Candau forced the 1966 World Health Assembly to decide whether it was serious about the eradication effort.

In 1965, Dr. Henderson was serving as the chief of the surveillance section at the Communicable Disease Center (now the Centers for Disease Control and Prevention), and WHO sought his assistance in creating a plan for smallpox eradication. Soon thereafter, Dr. Henderson received a call from US Surgeon General James Watt. Dr. Henderson had been directing the effort to eradicate smallpox in West Africa, but he was now ordered to assume responsibility for the program globally.

The smallpox global eradication program required more than just mass vaccination efforts. Dr. Henderson and his international staff encountered such challenges as floods, impassable roads, civil wars, and refugees, and they struggled against entrenched bureaucracies, cultural barriers, inadequate budgets, and shortages of field personnel. In a remarkable display of leadership and professionalism, Dr. Henderson was able to work closely with the health leadership of the Soviet Union, during one of the most difficult periods of the Cold War, while leading a staff of practitioners from more than 70 nations.

The world's last case of smallpox was reported on October 26, 1977. Thus, in just ten short years, Dr. Henderson had taken charge of the global eradication effort and brought it to a successful conclusion—still the most remarkable global health achievement to date.

Discussion and Application Questions
1. How did Dr. D. A. Henderson demonstrate effective public health leadership?
2. How did Dr. Henderson engage the public health system, his clients, and society globally?
3. Which of the issues facing Dr. Henderson during his period of leading the global effort to eradicate smallpox do you think posed the most difficulty? Why?
4. In what ways did Dr. Henderson exhibit the professional values of public health?

Summary

Recognition of public health as a profession has increased dramatically during the late twentieth and early twenty-first centuries, thanks in large part to efforts by organizations to develop competency sets for practitioners and other specialists, core competency models for public health graduates, certification for public health practitioners, and accreditation for programs and schools of public health. As a profession, public health must embrace the principle of professionalism and its values framework, which ensure continuity, stability, and commitment to standards of excellence as practitioners serve the interests of the public's health from the local level to the global arena.

Public health practitioners are educated in public health or a related discipline (e.g., medicine, nursing, law), and their work focuses on improving the health of communities and populations. In practicing the principle of professionalism, practitioners must be committed to client-focused values such as quality service and altruism, and they must advocate for their clients' best interests. A public health practitioner who provides services in this manner will, in turn, benefit from their clients, who will become their strongest public supporters.

Public health practitioners must be prepared to engage culturally diverse populations while functioning as good stewards of the community's health. Their attention to society-focused values, such as social justice and equitable access to health-related services, will improve the health status of their communities and populations. Individual clients and society at large will support public health's professional-focused values, such as self-regulation, when the services provided by practitioners concentrate on the community's or population's health needs.

Each of the professional disciplines in the public health workforce plays a unique and active role in preventing disease and promoting the health of individuals at the community, state, or national level. Within the public health system, practitioners specializing in various areas and skills maintain relationships characterized by interdependence and collaboration.

A new framework of professionalism for public health identifies key values that public health practitioners extend to the public health system, to clients, and to society. Practitioners demonstrate respect, honesty, and compassion toward others, and they show commitment to excellence by delivering high-quality service, pursuing continual professional development, and encouraging active participation by stakeholders. Public health leaders and practitioners who demonstrate professionalism will be accorded trust and respect from those with whom they interact.

Discussion Questions

1. What are the characteristics of a profession?
2. What are the key professional attributes of a public health practitioner?
3. Apply the fundamental elements of the *Physician Charter* to the practice of public health.
4. Why should medical professionalism and public health professionalism be discussed together?
5. List and discuss the values that make up the principle of professionalism.
6. Compare and contrast the values of professionalism with the practices that result in the destruction of professionalism.
7. Review Priester's framework of healthcare values, and compare the former healthcare values with the ones Priester added.
8. How does Priester's framework of healthcare values apply to the practice of public health?
9. Apply the public health professionalism framework to the practice of public health leadership.
10. For deeper thought: You have recently been employed by your hometown department of public health. Discuss how the public health professionalism framework applies to your practice of public health leadership.

Web Resources

Association of Schools and Programs of Public Health. 2017. "DrPH Model." Accessed April 27. www.aspph.org/educate/models/drph-model/.

———. 2017. "Framing the Future." Accessed April 27. www.aspph.org/educate/framing-the-future/.

———. 2017. "MPH Core Competency Model." Accessed April 27. www.aspph.org/educate/models/mph-competency-model/.

———. 2017. "Undergraduate Learning Outcomes Model." Accessed April 27. www.aspph.org/educate/models/undergraduate-learning-outcomes/.

References

1. Holsinger, J. W., Jr., and F. D. Scutchfield. 2012. "Introduction: History and Context of Public Health Care." In *Contemporary Topics in Public Health*, edited by J. W. Holsinger Jr., 1–24. Lexington, KY: University Press of Kentucky.

2. Swick, H. M., C. S. Bryan, and L. D. Longo. 2006. "Beyond the Physician Charter: Reflections on Medical Professionalism." *Perspectives in Biology and Medicine* 49 (2): 263–75.

3. Schmutzler, D. J., and J. W. Holsinger Jr. 2011. "New Professionalism." In *Professionalism in Mental Healthcare: Experts, Expertise and Expectations*, edited by D. Bhugra and A. Malik, 115–26. Cambridge, UK: Cambridge University Press.

4. Association of Schools and Programs of Public Health. 2017. "Discover: What Is Public Health?" Accessed February 6. www.aspph.org/discover/.

5. Modeste, N., and T. Tamayose. 2004. *Dictionary of Public Health Promotion and Education: Terms and Concepts*, 2nd ed. San Francisco: Jossey-Bass.

6. Lee, L. M. 2012. "Public Health Ethics Theory: Review and Path to Convergence." *Journal of Law, Medicine & Ethics* 40 (1): 85–98.

7. Institute of Medicine Committee on Assuring the Health of the Public in the 21st Century. 2002. *The Future of the Public's Health in the 21st Century.* National Academies Press. Published November 11. http://nationalacademies.org/hmd/Reports/2002/The-Future-of-the-Publics-Health-in-the-21st-Century.aspx.

8. US Department of Health and Human Services. 2017. "About HHS." Accessed April 19. www.hhs.gov/about/index.html.

9. Institute of Medicine Committee for the Study of the Future of Public Health. 1988. *The Future of Public Health.* Published January. www.nationalacademies.org/hmd/Reports/1988/The-Future-of-Public-Health.aspx.

10. National Board of Public Health Examiners (NBPHE). 2017. "Certified in Public Health: Eligibility Requirements." Accessed January 20. www.nbphe.org/eligibility.cfm.

11. Gruen, R. L., J. Arya, E. M. Cosgrove, R. L. Cruess, S. R. Cruess, A. B. Eastman, P. J. Fabri, P. Friedman, T. D. Kirksey, I. J. Kodner, F. R. Lewis, K. R. Liscum, C. H. Organ, J. C. Rosenfeld, T. R. Russell, A. K. Sachdeva, E. G. Zook, and A. H. Harken. 2003. "Professionalism in Surgery." *Journal of the American College of Surgeons* 197 (4): 605–8.

12. Cruess, S. R., and R. L. Cruess. 1997. "Professionalism Must Be Taught." *BMJ* 315 (7123): 1674–77.

13. Irvine, D. 1997. "The Performance of Doctors. I: Professionalism and Self Regulation in a Changing World." *BMJ* 314 (7093): 1540–42.

14. Kultgen, J. H. 1988. *Ethics and Professionalism.* Philadelphia, PA: University of Pennsylvania Press.

15. Cruess, R. L., and S. R. Cruess. 2008. "Expectations and Obligations: Professionalism and Medicine's Social Contract with Society." *Perspectives in Biology and Medicine* 51 (4): 579–98.

16. Tilson, H., and K. M. Gebbie. 2004. "The Public Health Workforce." *Annual Review of Public Health* 25: 341–56.

17. Gebbie, K. M., M. A. Potter, B. Quill, and H. Tilson. 2008. "Education for the Public Health Profession: A New Look at the Roemer Proposal." *Public Health Reports* 123 (Suppl. 2): 18–26.

18. Gebbie, K. M., L. Rosenstock, and L. M. Hernandez (eds.). 2003. *Who Will Keep the Public Healthy? Educating Public Health Professionals for the 21st Century.* Washington, DC: National Academies Press.

19. McNair, R. P. 2005. "The Case for Educating Health Care Students in Professionalism as the Core Content of Interprofessional Education." *Medical Education* 39 (5): 456–64.

20. Association of Schools of Public Health Education Committee. 2006. *Master's Degree in Public Health Core Competency Model, Version 2.3.* Published August. www.aspph.org/app/uploads/2014/04/Version2.31_FINAL.pdf.

21. Yapijakis, C. 2009. "Hippocrates of Kos, the Father of Clinical Medicine, and Asclepiades of Bithynia, the Father of Molecular Medicine. Review." *In Vivo* 23 (4): 507–14.

22. Priester, R. 1992. "A Values Framework for Health System Reform." *Health Affairs* 11 (1): 84–107.

23. Bhugra, D., and A. Malik. 2010. "Professionalism and Psychiatry: The Way Forward." In *Professionalism in Mental Healthcare: Experts, Expertise and Expectations*, edited by D. Bhugra and A. Malik, 188–93. Cambridge, UK: Cambridge University Press.

24. Forbes, M. S. n.d. "Malcolm S. Forbes Quotes." Thinkexist.com. Accessed February 6, 2017. http://thinkexist.com./quotes/Malcolm_S._Forbes/.

25. Carlton, E. 2014. "Answering the Call for Integrating Population Health: Insights from Health System Executives." *Advances in Health Care Management* 16: 115–38.

26. Goode, W. J. 1957. "Community Within a Community: The Professions." *American Sociological Review* 22 (2): 194–200.

27. Fee, E. 1992. "The Welch-Rose Report: Blueprint for Public Health Education in America." In *The Welch-Rose Report: A Public Health Classic*, prepared by the Delta Omega Honorary Public Health Society. Accessed April 19, 2017. www.deltaomega.org/documents/WelchRose.pdf.

28. National Association of County and City Health Officials (NACCHO). 2009. *2008 National Profile of Local Health Departments.* Published July. http://naccho.org/topics/infrastructure/profile/resources/2008report/upload/NACCHO_2008_ProfileReport_post-to-website-2.pdf.

29. Adams, D. A., K. M. Gallagher, R. A. Jajosky, J. Ward, P. Sharp, W. J. Anderson, J. P. Abellera, A. E. Aranas, M. Mayes, M. S. Wodajo, D. H. Onweh, and M. Park. 2012. "Summary of Notifiable Diseases—United States, 2010." *Morbidity and Mortality Weekly Report* 59 (53): 1–116.

30. Centers for Disease Control and Prevention (CDC). 2016. "Foodborne Germs and Illnesses." Updated September 1. www.cdc.gov/foodsafety/foodborne-germs.html.

31. Council of State and Territorial Epidemiologists (CSTE). 2012. "CSTE List of Nationally Notifiable Conditions." Published August. www.cste.org/resource/resmgr/PDFs/CSTENotifiableConditionListA.pdf.

32. Perlino, C. M. 2006. *The Public Health Workforce Shortage: Left Unchecked, Will We Be Protected?* American Public Health Association issue brief. Washington, DC: American Public Health Association.

33. Association of State and Territorial Health Officials (ASTHO). 2014. *Information to Action: The Workforce Data of Public Health WINS.* Accessed February 2, 2016. www.astho.org/phwins/National-Summary-Report-of-Workforce-Data/.

34. Gebbie, K. M., and B. J. Turnock. 2006. "The Public Health Workforce, 2006: New Challenges." *Health Affairs* 25 (4): 923–33.

35. Boulton, M. L., A. J. Beck, F. Coronado, J. A. Merrill, C. P. Friedman, G. D. Stamas, N. Tyus, K. Sellers, J. Moore, H. H. Tilson, and C. J. Leep. 2014. "Public Health Workforce Taxonomy." *American Journal of Preventive Medicine* 47 (5 Suppl. 3): S314–23.

36. Beck, A. J., M. L. Boulton, and F. Coronado. 2014. "Enumeration of the Governmental Public Health Workforce, 2014." *American Journal of Preventive Medicine* 47 (5 Suppl. 3): S306–13.

37. Leider, J. P., G. H. Shah, B. C. Castrucci, C. J. Leep, K. Sellers, amd J. B. Sprague. 2014. "Changes in Public Health Workforce Composition." *American Journal of Preventive Medicine* 47 (5 Suppl. 3): S331–36.

38. Gebbie, K. M. 2000. *The Public Health Workforce Enumeration 2000.* Washington, DC: Health Resources and Services Administration.

39. US Department of Health and Human Services (HHS). 2010. "HHS Announces the Nation's New Health Promotion and Disease Prevention Agenda." Published December 2. www.healthypeople.gov/sites/default/files/DefaultPressRelease_1.pdf.

40. Fincher, D. n.d. "David Fincher Quotes." BrainyQuote. Accessed February 6, 2017. www.brainyquote.com/quotes/authors/d/david_fincher.html.

41. National Board of Public Health Examiners (NBPHE). 2017. "Eligibility Requirements." Accessed April 26. www.nbphe.org/eligibility.cfm.

42. National Board of Public Health Examiners (NBPHE). 2017. "Why Get Certified?" Accessed April 26. www.nbphe.org/getcertified.cfm.

43. Council on Linkages Between Academia and Public Health Practice. 2017. "Membership." Accessed February 6. www.phf.org/programs/council/Pages/Council_on_Linkages_Members.aspx.

44. Council on Linkages Between Academia and Public Health Practice. 2014. "Core Competencies for Public Health Professionals." Accessed February 7, 2016. www.phf.org/resourcestools/Pages/Core_Public_Health_Competencies.aspx.

45. Joint Expert Panel Convened by the Association of American Medical Colleges and the Association of Schools of Public Health. 2012. *Cultural Competence Education for Students in Medicine and Public Health.* Published July. https://members.aamc.org/eweb/upload/Cultural%20Competence%20Education_revisedl.pdf.

46. ABIM Foundation. 2002. "The Physician Charter." Accessed February 6, 2017. www.abimfoundation.org/Professionalism/Physician-Charter.aspx.

47. Fineberg, H. V., G. M. Green, J. H. Ware, and B. L. Anderson. 1994. "Changing Public Health Training Needs: Professional Education and the Paradigm of Public Health." *Annual Review of Public Health* 15 (1): 237–57.

48. Harvard School of Public Health. 2017. "History of the School." Accessed February 6. www.hsph.harvard.edu/history-of-the-school/.

49. Council on Education for Public Health (CEPH). 2017. "CEPH." Accessed February 6. www.ceph.org.

50. Association of Schools and Programs of Public Health. 2017. "Preparing Tomorrow's Public Health Leaders by Advancing Education, Research, Practice, and Advocacy." Accessed January 28. www.aspph.org.

51. Council on Education for Public Health (CEPH). 2017. "Accreditation Criteria and Procedures." Accessed February 6. http://ceph.org/criteria-procedures/.

52. Association of Schools of Public Health Education Committee. 2009. *Doctor of Public Health (DrPH) Core Competency Model, Version 1.3.* Published November. www.aspph.org/app/uploads/2014/04/DrPHVersion1-3.pdf.

53. Roemer, M. I. 1986. "The Need for Professional Doctors of Public Health." *Public Health Reports* 101 (1): 21–29.

54. Wykoff, R., D. Petersen, and E. M. Weist. 2013. "The Recommended Critical Component Elements of an Undergraduate Major in Public Health." *Public Health Reports* 128 (5): 421–24.

55. Swick, H. M. 2007. "Viewpoint: Professionalism and Humanism Beyond the Academic Health Center." *Academic Medicine* 82 (11): 1022.

56. Swick, H. M. 1998. "Academic Medicine Must Deal with the Clash of Business and Professional Values." *Academic Medicine* 73 (7): 751–55.

57. Levy, M., D. Gentry, and L. M. Klesges. 2015. "Innovations in Public Health Education: Promoting Professional Development and a Culture of Health." *American Journal of Public Health* 15 (Suppl. 1): S44–S45.

58. Gates, R. M. 2016. *A Passion for Leadership.* New York: Alfred A. Knopf.

59. American Medical Association (AMA). 2017. "AMA Code of Medical Ethics." Accessed February 6. www.ama-assn.org/about-us/code-medical-ethics.

60. Martimianakis, M. A., J. M. Maniate, and B. D. Hodges. 2009. "Sociological Interpretations of Professionalism." *Medical Education* 43 (9): 829–37.

61. Krieger, N., and A. E. Birn. 1998. "A Vision of Social Justice as the Foundation of Public Health: Commemorating 150 Years of the Spirit of 1848." *American Journal of Public Health* 88 (11): 1603–6.

62. Holsinger, J. W., Jr., and B. Beaton. 2006. "Physician Professionalism for a New Century." *Clinical Anatomy* 19 (5): 473–79.

63. Covey, S. R. 2004. *The 7 Habits of Highly Effective People: Powerful Lessons in Personal Change*, revised ed. New York: Free Press.

64. Henderson, D. A. 2009. *Smallpox: The Death of a Disease*. Amherst, NY: Prometheus Books.

LEADERSHIP THEORIES
AND CONCEPTS

TRAITS, SKILLS, AND STYLES OF LEADERSHIP

James W. Holsinger Jr.

Learning Objectives

Upon completion of this chapter, you should be able to

- appraise the key role played by an individual's personal traits;
- describe the traits model of leadership and explain the importance of traits in the practice of public health leadership;
- explain the importance of leadership traits for the effective practice of public health leadership;
- discuss leadership skills and the skills model of leadership;
- identify key personality factors that affect the practice of leadership;
- define and contrast the different cognitive styles;
- explain the importance of social appraisal skills and emotional intelligence in the practice of leadership;
- describe the behavioral model of leadership and understand its importance in the twenty-first century;
- explain the importance of leadership styles in the practice of public health leadership; and
- compare leadership traits, skills, and styles and understand the difference between them.

Focus on Leadership Competencies

This chapter emphasizes the following Association of Schools and Programs of Public Health (ASPPH) leadership competencies:

- Describe the attributes of leadership in public health.

(continued)

- Develop strategies to motivate others for collaborative problem solving, decision-making, and evaluation.
- Create a shared vision.

It also addresses the following Council on Linkages public health leadership competency:

- Analyzes internal and external facilitators and barriers that may affect the delivery of the 10 Essential Public Health Services.

Note: See the appendix at the end of the book for complete lists of competencies.

Introduction

trait
A distinguishing characteristic or quality possessed by a person.

intelligence
The capacity for understanding, reasoning, and perception, including the aptitude for grasping facts and the relationships between them.

Dating back to early civilizations, personal **traits** have been regarded as a key factor determining a person's ability to lead.[1] The Chinese philosopher Lao-Tzu wrote about the traits of effective leaders as far back as the sixth century BC.[2] Traits commonly associated with leadership have included ambition, conscientiousness, integrity, persistence, and honesty, among others. In the early period of leadership research, such traits were thought to define successful leaders, and investigators worked to identify the characteristics that contributed to leaders' effectiveness and advancement within organizations.

The first empirical leadership research was conducted in 1904, when scientists observed schoolchildren and sought to identify the qualities that differentiated leaders from nonleaders. The attributes found to characterize young leaders included congeniality, verbal fluency, **intelligence**, goodness, low emotionality, liveliness, and daring.[3] These early studies advanced the idea that certain personal qualities are inherent in leaders and distinguish them from nonleaders; they also supported the belief that these traits can be identified and assessed. However, this line of thinking soon fell out of favor. As early as 1948, Stogdill[4] found that possession of a certain combination of traits did not necessarily result in a person becoming a leader. Based on Stogdill's studies, researchers soon came to understand that models based solely on traits failed to explain the emergence of leadership or leader effectiveness.

Nonetheless, leadership trait research continued, and it has experienced a resurgence in an evolved form (with renewed interest stemming from research into various models of leadership, which will be discussed in later chapters). People bring certain strengths, qualities, and characteristics to their leadership roles,[5] and these traits are apparent in the patterns of behavior that leaders exhibit.

Consideration of these traits helps us better understand individual leadership styles and the ways that various behaviors relate to effective leadership. A cursory glance at successful leaders suggests that, even though certain characteristics may overlap, key traits, skills, and styles are in many ways unique to each individual. All public health leaders should understand their own leadership style and recognize their personal strengths as determined by their traits and skills.

Definition of Key Terms

The term *trait* has been variously defined by different investigators. Yukl[6(p135)] says the term refers "to a variety of individual attributes, including aspects of personality, temperament, needs, motives, and values." Daft[5(p36)] describes traits as "the distinguishing personal characteristics of a leader, such as intelligence, honesty, self-confidence, and appearance." Antonakis and colleagues[3(p104)] define the term as "relatively stable and coherent integrations of personal characteristics that foster a consistent pattern of leadership performance across a variety of group or organizational situations." For our purposes, traits are various attributes possessed by individuals—including personality, temperament, abilities, needs, motives, disposition, and values—that produce consistent leadership performance regardless of the organizational situation. Qualities such as physical appearance and demographic attributes also play a role in effective leadership; however, for this discussion, we will focus on less tangible personal traits.

A thorough discussion of leadership traits requires that we clarify the definitions of key personal attributes. An individual's **personality** is a combination of qualities and characteristics that form a distinctive character and tend to influence behavior in a particular manner. Examples of personality attributes include adaptability, emotional balance, enthusiasm, objectivity, resourcefulness, and **self-confidence**. **Temperament** deals with the individual's level of emotionalism, irritability, or excitability, especially when displayed openly. **Abilities** represent the knowledge and skills that an individual possesses or acquires over time; for our purposes, we are focusing on intellectual abilities. **Needs** represent requirements or desires that are usually physiological in nature, such as hunger or thirst. **Motives** are similar to needs but social in nature; they are a response to certain social experiences or stimuli. Motives may include power, independence, esteem of others and self, personal achievement, or social affiliation. **Disposition** refers to the individual's inclinations or tendencies toward a certain temperament. **Values** are the attitudes an individual holds concerning what is right and wrong, ethical and unethical, and moral and immoral. They influence the individual's perceptions, preferences, and behavior choices.[6] These attributes are distinguishing features of a leader's personal nature, and they are reflected in the leader's performance regardless of the organizational situation.

personality
The combination of qualities and characteristics that form an individual's distinctive character.

self-confidence
Realistic certainty in one's own judgment, ideas, ability, power, decision making, and skills.

temperament
A person's nature, particularly with regard to emotionalism or excitability.

ability
Possession of the manner or skill to do something.

need
Something essential or strongly desired, usually physiological in nature.

motive
A reason for doing something in response to social experiences or stimuli.

disposition
A person's inclinations or tendencies toward a certain temperament.

value
An attitude or belief dealing with ethics, morals, or what is right and wrong.

skill
The ability to perform activities in an effective manner.

technical skills
Skills relating to the use of things, such as tools and equipment.

interpersonal skills
Social skills and skills involving people.

conceptual skills
Skills that are cognitive in nature and based on concepts and ideas.

great man theory
An approach to leadership study, popular prior to 1950, that focused on the traits of individuals who were thought to be great men.

Skills—the ability to perform activities in an effective manner—are determined through a combination learning and heredity.[7] Yukl[6(p191)] has described skills "at different levels of abstraction, ranging from general, broadly defined abilities (e.g., intelligence, interpersonal skill) to narrower, more specific abilities (verbal reasoning, persuasive ability)." Building on the work of Katz[8] and Mann,[9] Yukl[6] developed a taxonomy of skills that uses three main categories: technical skills, interpersonal skills, and conceptual skills. **Technical skills** are concerned with the use of things, such as tools and equipment. **Interpersonal skills** are social skills, and they involve people. **Conceptual skills** are based on concepts and ideas and are cognitive in nature. Other skill sets—such as administrative and strategic management skills—have also been proposed, though these areas tend to be directed more toward management than leadership.

The Trait Approach to Leadership

Prior to 1950, the trait approach to leadership was known as the **great man theory**, because it focused on the traits of individuals who were thought to be great men. The individuals who developed this model sought to identify the traits associated with leaders in comparison with the traits of individuals not deemed to be leaders. Over time, however, research demonstrated poor correlation between personal traits and successful leadership, and studies of effective leaders suggested that leadership ability was not genetically based.[3] By midcentury, researchers were using aptitude and psychological tests to study personality traits, as well as social and work-related characteristics.

In a seminal literature review, Stogdill[4] examined 124 trait studies that had been conducted between 1904 and 1948. He demonstrated a pattern in which the concept of a leader was based on people acquiring status in an organization by exhibiting the ability to work with a group in attaining mutual goals. Stogdill found that relevant leadership traits included intelligence, self-confidence, alertness to others' needs, understanding of tasks, initiative and persistence in addressing problems, and desire to take responsibility and hold positions of dominance and control.[6] The key result of Stogdill's work was the discovery that each trait was dependent on the specific situation and that none of the traits were themselves required to produce success in every situation. Thus, Stogdill hastened the demise of the great man theory of leadership.

 Consider This

"A person does not become a leader by virtue of the possession of some combination of traits, but the pattern of personal characteristics of the leader must bear some relevant relationship to the characteristics, activities, and goals of the followers."
—Ralph Stogdill[4(p64)]

If a combination of traits does not make a person a leader, why do you think that the traits found in leaders are important?

In 1974, Stogdill[10] conducted a second literature review of 163 trait studies that had been conducted between 1949 and 1970. This review covered a wider variety of studies than the first one and included more skills and traits presumed to be related to leadership, as well as extensive measurement techniques. The review produced strong results, identifying many of the same traits as the first review and also finding additional traits and skills to be relevant. However, the review provided no evidence for universal leadership traits. Stogdill noted that some personal traits did appear to contribute to effective leadership, but he stressed that the organizational situation was key. Following Stogdill's work, some investigators moved away from attempting to identify universal leadership traits. Others turned their attention to the behavior of leaders and the consideration of leadership situations.

After Stogdill's first review, Mann[11] examined more than 1,400 findings dealing with personality and small-group leadership. His research avoided Stogdill's emphasis on contextual factors, and it suggested that the traits of intelligence, dominance, and masculinity were significantly related to perceived leadership, regardless of the situation. (The inclusion of masculinity reflects the fact that male leadership was dominant in the United States at this time.) Following Stogdill's 1974 review, Lord, DeVader, and Alliger[12] used meta-analysis to reassess—and largely support—Mann's findings. In 1991, Kirkpatrick and Locke[13] found that, without doubt, leaders are not like other people. They proposed that traits differentiating leaders from nonleaders included drive, motivation, integrity, confidence, cognitive ability, and task knowledge. They also stated that these traits can be either inborn or learned.

During the 1990s, the study of leadership traits focused on understanding an individual's own behaviors, thoughts, and feelings, as well as those of others, and the appropriate actions pertaining to them. Studies during this period looked at a variety of social intelligence attributes, including social awareness, social acumen, and self-monitoring. By 2004, Zaccaro, Kemp, and Bader[14] had included social intelligence attributes in their study of leadership traits. In 2013, Northouse[15] conducted a review of past studies and examined lengthy lists of traits that had accumulated over a 60-year period. He ultimately proposed a set of five major leadership traits that individuals should possess or seek to develop: intelligence, self-confidence, determination, integrity, and sociability.

Leadership Traits
Intelligence

Intelligence, or intellectual or cognitive ability, includes mental capacity for understanding, reasoning, and perception, as well as the aptitude for grasping facts and the relationships between them. Zaccaro, Kemp, and Bader[14] support the notion that leaders have higher intelligence than nonleaders, and the attributes of intelligence do generally appear to make individuals better leaders. However, research suggests that leadership may become impeded if a leader's intellectual ability is significantly different from that of the followers. Effective leaders must be able to explain complex concepts in a manner that meets the needs of the followers.

Self-Confidence and Determination

Leaders who possess self-confidence have realistic certainties in their own judgment, ideas, ability, power, decision making, and skills. Such leaders know and trust themselves without pride or arrogance. They have a positive attitude about themselves and are able to press ahead with the belief that, if and when they make a wrong decision, any setback can be overcome. Effective leaders have self-assurance and self-esteem. They understand that their leadership can and will make a difference to their organizations and that the influence they have on others is right and appropriate.[15]

determination
The motivation a leader needs to come to a decision, to persevere in the face of obstacles, and to see a job through to completion.

Determination is the motivation a leader needs to come to a decision, and it includes such characteristics as energy, initiative, persistence, and tenacity. Leaders with determination have the persistence needed to see a job through to completion and to persevere in the face of obstacles.

Personal Integrity

personal integrity
Adherence to personal values in day-to-day behavior; the quality of being ethical, trustworthy, and honest.

Personal integrity—simply, the adherence to personal values in day-to-day behavior—is a predominant aspect of interpersonal trust.[6] Effective leaders show their character by being ethical, trustworthy, and honest. With regard to integrity, leaders truly must "walk the talk." Integrity is foundational in relationships between public health leaders and followers: Leaders who demonstrate integrity receive admiration, respect, and loyalty from followers. But if leaders are not deemed trustworthy, they receive no loyalty from followers, and relationships with peers and superiors will be impossible to maintain. Being of service to followers and recognizing that loyalty is a two-way street are both signs of leadership integrity. Effective leaders live by the same rules that they establish for followers; to do otherwise violates the followers' trust.

Clearly, deception or lying to followers results in a loss of leadership credibility. Exploitation, manipulation, and failure to keep promises likewise compromise the leader's effectiveness. Leaders who act in their own self-interest lose the trust of their followers. If leaders fail to maintain the confidence of followers, effective communication and the flow of useful information become hampered. Leaders who refuse to take responsibility for their own actions and decisions are perceived as undependable or worse, especially if they try to cast blame on others for their own failures. When a breach of personal integrity becomes obvious, effective leadership ceases.

When 1,500 managers were asked to name the most desired traits in leaders, integrity was at the top of the list.[16] Kouzes and Posner[16(p8)] write: "Honesty is absolutely essential to leadership. If people are going to follow someone willingly, whether into battle or into the boardroom, they first want to assure themselves that the person is worthy of their trust. They want to know that the would-be leader is truthful, ethical, and principled." To be an effective public health leader, one must demonstrate ethical convictions in the daily routine of leading.

Leadership Skills

Leadership skills are the competencies and knowledge that a leader possesses and uses to successfully reach goals and objectives.[15] Katz[8] determined that effective leadership is based on three types of personal skills: technical skills, interpersonal or human skills, and conceptual skills. These skills are significantly different from leaders' personal traits: Whereas traits define who the leaders are, skills determine what the leaders are able to accomplish.

Technical Skills

Technical skills include knowledge about an organization's work, structure, and rules; proficiency in specialized activities; and an understanding of the methods, processes, and equipment used by organizational units. Technical skills may be acquired through a variety of means, including formal education and on-the-job training and experience. Katz[8] notes that technical skills are important for leaders in supervisory and middle management positions but somewhat less important for senior leaders and those in top management positions.

Effective Public Health Leaders . . .

. . . know that "the leader of an organization needs to be a role model."

—Robert M. Gates[17(p170)]

Interpersonal or Human Skills

Whereas technical skills involve working with things, interpersonal or human skills are all about working with people. Leaders should have a knowledge of human behavior and group processes, and they should be able to understand the feelings, attitudes, and motives of their followers. Interpersonal skills enable public health leaders to work cooperatively with subordinates, peers, and superiors, as well as with constituents and collaborators. One crucial component of the interpersonal skill set is **empathy**—the capacity to understand the values, motives, and emotions of other people. Empathy also involves the social insight to determine what behaviors are acceptable in particular situations.[6] The ability

empathy
The capacity to understand the values, motives, and emotions of another person.

to select an appropriate influence strategy as a leader depends on knowing what followers want and how followers perceive a situation. Leaders who continually monitor themselves better understand their own behavior and the way it affects their followers.[18] Such leaders can adjust their behavior to match specific situations. Other interpersonal skills useful in the leadership influence process include oral communication ability and persuasiveness.

Effective leadership is fundamentally based on interpersonal competence.[1] Leaders with strong interpersonal skills enhance group cooperation, support the pursuit of common goals, and have success with influence and impression management tactics.[19] Katz[8(p34)] states: "Real skill in working with others must become a natural, continuous activity, since it involves sensitivity not only at times of decision making but also in the day-to-day behavior of the individual. . . . Because everything a leader says and does (or leaves unsaid or undone) has an effect on his associates, his true self will, in time, show through. Thus, to be effective, this skill must be naturally developed and unconsciously, as well as consistently, demonstrated in the individual's every action."

For public health leaders, interpersonal or human skills can be summarized simply as the ability to get along with followers as they go about their own work. Such skills are important at all levels, from supervisors and middle management to the organization's top management positions.

Consider This

"Interpersonal competence is fundamental to successful and effective leadership."
—Bernard M. Bass[1(p122)]

Why might one say that interpersonal competence—rather than technical or conceptual competence—is fundamental to effective public health leadership?

Conceptual Skills

Just as technical skills involve working with things and interpersonal skills involve working with people, conceptual skills involve working with ideas and concepts. Conceptual skills incorporate a variety of attributes, including judgment, intuition, creativity, and foresight. Some conceptual skills, such as inductive or deductive reasoning, logical thinking, analytical ability, and concept formation—can be measured using aptitude tests.[6]

Public health leaders must have significant conceptual skills to understand how their organizations operate and where the organizations should be going. Effective strategic planning—a key responsibility for shaping an organization's future, particularly in economically difficult times—requires that leaders have the ability to predict the future based on current trends. Public health leaders must be able to deal with a variety of constituencies and complex relationships. They must understand how various organizational parts work together and how a change in one area might affect elements in a number of different areas. Intuition also plays an important role, and it develops in the leader's repertoire through experience with certain types of problems.[21] Effective leaders often blend conscious reasoning with intuition, depending on the situation.

Conceptual skills are the most important skill set for senior public health leaders and upper-level managers. Without strong conceptual skills, senior leaders can place the entire organization at risk. Conceptual skills are of less importance for supervisory-level leaders (see exhibit 3.1).

> **Effective Public Health Leaders . . .**
>
> . . . remember that "half-finished work generally proves to be labor lost."
>
> —Abraham Lincoln[20]

Personality

A leader's personality is a set of processes and characteristics that reflects a relatively stable behavior approach that responds to people, objects, or ideas in the environment.[3] Leadership effectiveness is influenced both by the leader's own personality and by the leader's ability to understand the personalities of followers. A number of investigators have examined the various aspects of personality, and over time they have identified the "big five" personality dimensions: (1) extraversion (or surgency), (2) agreeableness, (3) conscientiousness (or dependability), (4) emotional stability (or neuroticism), and (5) openness (or intellectance). This taxonomy was developed in the early 1990s, and particular versions are known by slightly different titles (e.g., the five-factor model).[22,23] The big five dimensions correspond with specific personality traits as shown in exhibit 3.2. The dimensions can be viewed as continuums, and individual leaders may demonstrate a high, moderate, or low degree of each.

	Supervisory Management	Middle Management	Senior Management
Technical skills Knowledge or proficiency in specialized tasks and activities	High	High	Low
Interpersonal skills Understanding of people being led and of group processes	High	High	High
Conceptual skills Ability to work with ideas and concepts, including long-range vision	Low	High	High

EXHIBIT 3.1 Importance of Leadership Skill Sets at Different Levels

Source: Data from Katz, R. L. 1955. "Skills of an Effective Administrator." *Harvard Business Review* 33 (1): 33–42.

EXHIBIT 3.2
The Big Five Dimensions and Specific Personality Traits

Big Five Personality Dimensions	Specific Traits	
	Positive	Negative
Extraversion (surgency)	Energy level Assertion Expressiveness	Aloofness Shyness Passivity
Agreeableness	Cooperation Empathy Flexibility	Belligerence Rudeness Callousness
Conscientiousness (dependability)	Organization Precision Persistence	Disorganization Inconsistency Aimlessness
Adjustment (neuroticism)	Emotional stability Self-control Independence	Insecurity Instability Gullibility
Openness (intellectance)	Curiosity Insight Creativity	Unimaginativeness Imperceptiveness Shallowness

Source: Data from Goldberg, L. R. 1990. "An Alternative 'Description of Personality': The Big-Five Factor Structure." *Journal of Personality and Social Psychology* 59 (6): 1216–29.

Extraversion

extraversion
One's degree of concern and engagement with what is outside the self.

Extraversion (also spelled *extroversion*) is one's degree of concern and engagement with what is outside the self. The traits and characteristics that make up this dimension strongly influence a leader's behavior in group settings. The degree to which individuals are comfortable talking with and meeting people is based on their sociability and the outgoing nature of their personality. Individuals who like to be in control and influence others often have a high degree of dominance and assertiveness. They have the self-confidence to seek positions of authority and are prepared to become competitive in doing so. Meanwhile, introverts may become physically or emotionally drained by social encounters and require time alone to reflect and regain energy.

Dominance, assertiveness, and other traits associated with extraversion are valuable to many leaders, but not every public health leader will possess a high degree of extraversion. In fact, one investigator found that four in ten top executives classify as introverts.[24] Thus, extraversion may not be as significant a leadership trait as is often thought. Furthermore, dominance can be a negative attribute if it is not offset by other dimensions such as agreeableness and emotional stability.

Agreeableness

agreeableness
The ability to get along with other people; a key characteristic for resolving conflict and gaining followers.

Agreeableness is the ability to get along with other people, and it is generally understood to include such characteristics as compassion, trust, cooperativeness, and having a good nature. Leaders who rate high in this dimension tend to come across as cheerful, approachable, optimistic, nurturing, and sympathetic. In short, they are seen as having warm personalities. Agreeableness is an especially important characteristic for public health leaders because of the collaborative nature of public health practice. A leader who is friendly and cooperative will typically be well liked and well equipped to resolve conflicts within the organization. Also, because public health leaders are often in the public eye, agreeableness can help them generate support and gain adherents to their cause. Individuals with high agreeableness often find a need for affiliation, both with other individuals and with organizations.

Conscientiousness

Conscientiousness, or dependability, is the degree to which a person is responsible, possesses personal integrity, and has a high need for achievement. Conscientious individuals can maintain focus on specific goals and pursue them in a purposeful manner; by contrast, people with low conscientiousness are often impulsive and easily distracted from the task at hand. With the dimension of conscientiousness, work is the object, not people. Public health leaders are drawn toward conscientiousness because of the nature of their practice. Intense focus is often necessary to resolve various community and population health issues that arise.

conscientiousness
The ability to remain focused on goals and to pursue them in a purposeful manner.

Emotional Stability

The personality dimension of **emotional stability** has been labeled as *neuroticism* in some versions of the taxonomy. Regardless of the phrasing, the dimension reflects how calm, secure, and well-adjusted a person is. Key components of this dimension include self-esteem, self-control, and self-confidence. Emotionally stable leaders are able to handle stress, deal with criticism, and take failures and mistakes in stride; leaders with low emotional stability, on the other hand, are often tense, irritable, anxious, depressed, or lacking in self-confidence. Emotional stability helps public health leaders develop good interpersonal relationships.

emotional stability
The degree to which a person is calm, secure, and well adjusted.

Openness

Openness—sometimes called *intellectance*—is the degree to which an individual is intellectually curious, inquisitive, open-minded, and learning oriented. Individuals with high degrees of openness tend to be imaginative, creative, and willing to consider fresh approaches and new ideas. Individuals with low openness, meanwhile, tend to have narrower interests and often prefer to do things the way they have always been done. Openness is an important quality in public health, particularly because the field so heavily emphasizes change over stability.

openness
The quality of being intellectually curious and inquisitive, open-minded and learning oriented, and experience based.

Research on the Big Five Dimensions and Leadership

The big five personality dimensions have been the subject of much research. In one meta-analysis of 78 leadership and personality studies, Judge and colleagues[25] found a strong relationship between the personality factors and leadership, and they determined that the dimensions varied in the strength of their association with effective leadership. Extraversion showed the strongest relationship to leadership, followed by conscientiousness, emotional stability, openness, and agreeableness.[3] Similarly, Hogan, Curphy, and Hogan[26] summarized 70 years of leadership and personality research and determined that four of the five dimensions were consistently related to effective leadership. Leaders scoring high in extraversion, conscientiousness, agreeableness, and emotional stability were found to be most effective and successful. Openness was linked to higher performance in some leaders but not in others.

Additional research will help us more fully understand the degree to which the big five dimensions—as well as other factors—are predictive of leadership effectiveness. In the meantime, public health leaders can use their understanding of the big five dimensions to assess their own personalities, emphasize the positive aspects, and deemphasize the negative.[3]

Cognitive Style

cognitive style
The way one perceives, processes, interprets, and uses information.

Cognitive style is the manner in which individuals perceive, process, interpret, and use information. It plays an important role in leadership behavior as well as in leaders' efforts to relate to followers, peers, superiors, collaborators, and constituents. People differ in the ways they perceive and assimilate data, make decisions and solve problems, and relate to others; their preferred habits in these areas are based on their cognitive styles.

Many discussions of cognitive style have distinguished between "left-brain" and "right-brain" thinking patterns. A linear approach to thinking, emphasizing analytical and logical tendencies, is said to be based in the left side of the brain, whereas creative and intuitive thinking is said to be based in the right side. This construct oversimplifies complex physiological processes and is not entirely accurate, but it provides a useful model for two contrasting approaches to thinking. Left-brain individuals tend to possess strong language skills, whereas right-brain individuals are more likely to use visual images in thinking. In reality, all leaders use both left- and right-brain processes, but most have a dominant style.

Individuals' cognitive styles can also be assessed using two other approaches that we will discuss at length: Herrmann's Whole Brain Thinking model and the Myers-Briggs Type Indicator.

Herrmann's Whole Brain Thinking Model

The Whole Brain Thinking model, developed by Ned Herrmann[27] in the 1970s, uses a four-quadrant approach to represent four styles of thinking, as shown in exhibit 3.3. Quadrants A, B, C, and D have distinct characteristics, and an individual's preferences for each quadrant influence patterns of leadership, behavior, and communication. An assessment called the Herrmann Brain Dominance Instrument (HBDI) is used to determine an individual's preference for each style. Research has shown that some individuals favor a single quadrant whereas others use any or all of the styles found in the model.

Quadrant A focuses on logical and analytical thinking, analysis of facts, and quantitative processing. People who favor Quadrant A think critically and rationally and engage strongly in technical matters, including work with numbers. They enjoy knowing how things work and are willing to follow procedures. Public health leaders utilizing this thinking style are often authoritative and directive in nature; they focus on the task at hand using specific information, often placing less importance on the opinions and feelings of others.

Quadrant B thinkers take a highly organized approach, developing detailed plans and working through problems in a sequential, linear manner. They use deadlines to ensure that tasks are completed on time. Such individuals are reliable and highly traditional, and therefore usually conservative, in their approach. Public health leaders favoring this quadrant are risk averse, seek a stable environment, and prefer to follow established rules regardless of circumstances.

Quadrant C is the part of the model where interpersonal relationships are most important. Quadrant C individuals are intuitive, emotional, and people oriented. They have an outgoing nature and enjoy interacting with, supporting, and teaching other people. They are often verbally expressive. Public health leaders with this style of thinking are usually friendly, empathetic, and trusting of others. They put people ahead of projects and are concerned with the feelings of their followers.

Quadrant D is primarily associated with conceptual thinking, in which facts and patterns are integrated and synthesized for a holistic view. Quadrant

---

EXHIBIT 3.3

Herrmann's Whole Brain Thinking Model

Quadrant A	Quadrant B	Quadrant C	Quadrant D
• Logical	• Organized	• Interpersonal	• Holistic
• Analytical	• Sequential	• Feeling-based	• Intuitive
• Fact-based	• Planned	• Kinesthetic	• Integrating
• Quantitative	• Detailed	• Emotional	• Synthesizing

Source: Data from Herrmann, N. 1996. *The Whole Brain Business Book*. New York: McGraw-Hill.

D thinkers are intuitive by nature, and their curiosity may lead them to experiment, take risks, and pursue adventure. Public health leaders who favor this style tend to allow their followers a significant degree of freedom, because they themselves are quite flexible. Such leaders may also take risks as they experiment with changing processes.

The Whole Brain Thinking model does not propose that people will engage in cognitive processes strictly from one style. Reliance on only one quadrant would result in a stunted form of leadership and a limited breadth of options. Instead, the model assumes that an individual or leader will function using all four quadrants, even if one style tends to be dominant. Few individuals can ever be perfectly balanced in their cognitive approach, but leaders in public health should strive to develop aspects from all four quadrants for use in their day-to-day leadership. Efforts to develop and understand cognitive skills are especially important for public health leaders who are engaged in coalition building and collaborative enterprises; such leaders need to understand the thinking styles not only of followers but also of peers, constituents, and collaborators.

Myers-Briggs Type Indicator (MBTI)
A tool that identifies personality types through the assessment of individual preferences across four dimensions.

Carl Jung and the Myers-Briggs Type Indicator

A different approach to cognitive styles was introduced by psychologist Carl Jung[28] in the 1920s, and it held that differences in behavior were a result of individual preferences in dealing with information for evaluation and problem solving. Jung's model of personality encompassed three main dimensions: (1) extraversion and introversion, which describe the ways people interact with each other; (2) sensation and intuition, which describe the ways people gather information; and (3) thinking and feeling, which describe how people evaluate information.

Check It Out

The Myers-Briggs Type Indicator instrument is a psychometric questionnaire that measures people's psychological preferences based on their perception of the world and the way they make decisions. For more information, visit the Myers & Briggs Foundation site at www.myersbriggs.org/my-mbti-personality-type/mbti-basics/home.htm.

Jung had a powerful influence on Katharine Briggs and Isabel Briggs Myers, who developed the **Myers-Briggs Type Indicator (MBTI)** as an outgrowth of Jung's model.[29] In doing so, Briggs and Briggs Myers added a fourth dimension: judging and perceiving, which describes how people relate to the outside world.[30] A person's preferences across the four dimensions of the MBTI (shown in exhibit 3.4) can be used to identify that individual as one of 16 potential personality types. For instance, a person who prefers extraversion (E) over introversion (I), intuition (N) over sensing (S), thinking (T) over feeling (F), and judging (J) over perceiving (P) would have a personality type of extraversion + intuition + thinking + judging, or ENTJ.[29] Preferences are measured by the individual's answers to a questionnaire. A person's MBTI scores across the four dimensions may change over time

EXHIBIT 3.4
Myers-Briggs
Type Indicator
Dimensions

Extraverted vs. Introverted (E or I)

Whether a person tends to be outgoing and sociable or shy and quiet. Extraverts gain mental energy and interpersonal strength by interacting with other people, while introverts gain mental energy and interpersonal strength through their own thoughts and feelings.

Sensing vs. Intuitive (S or N)

Whether a person tends to focus on details or on the big picture when dealing with problems. Sensing individuals use their five senses to gather and absorb information, whereas intuitive people focus on relationships, hunches, and patterns instead of facts and details.

MBTI Dimensions

Thinking vs. Feeling (T or F)

Whether a person tends to rely on logic or emotions in dealing with problems. Feeling individuals rely on values and a sense of right and wrong, whereas thinking individuals rely on logic and are objective when making decisions.

Judging vs. Perceiving (J or P)

Whether a person prefers order and control or acts with flexibility and spontaneity. Judging individuals engage in certainty and closure and make decisions quickly based on data, whereas perceiving individuals do not like deadlines and prefer ambiguity while gathering information before making a decision.

Source: Data from Briggs Myers, I., M. H. McCaulley, N. L. Quenk, and A. L. Hammer. 1998. *MBTI Manual: A Guide to the Development and Use of the Myers-Briggs Type Indicator*, 3rd ed. Sunnyside, CA: Consulting Psychologists Press.

based on life experiences, education, and training; however, very high scores in certain dimensions generally indicate styles that will remain relatively stable. No personality type is considered the "right" one or better than the others, and each type can result in either positive or negative behavioral consequences.

Public health leaders should seek to understand both their own cognitive style and the styles of their followers, and they should strive to develop their ability to work with individuals who have styles different from their own. Leaders should also realize that growth occurs not by focusing on their own current style but by looking at the personality traits of the style directly opposite from their own, as shown in the diagram in exhibit 3.5. Doing so helps leaders recognize their need for balance and their dependence on others, while at the same time opening them up to fresh experiences.[31]

Leadership Application Case: To Change or Not to Change

The Leadership Application Case at the beginning of this book provides realistic scenarios for the application of key leadership concepts covered in the text. See the section marked "Chapter 3 Application" for the scenario and discussion questions that correspond with this chapter.

EXHIBIT 3.5
Complement-
arity Among
Personality
Types

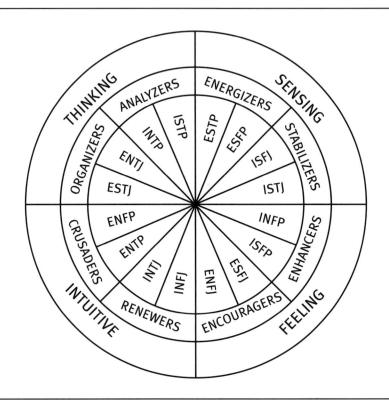

Source: Reprinted with permission from Johnson, R. 1999. *Your Personality and the Spiritual Life.* Gainesville, FL: Center for Applications of Personality Type, 163.

Social Appraisal Skills and Emotional Intelligence

social intelligence
The aptitude for
understanding the
thoughts, feelings,
and behaviors
of others, and
of oneself, in
social situations
and for acting
appropriately
based on that
understanding.

According to Zaccaro and his coauthors,[32,33,34,35,36] social appraisal skills are at the heart of effective leadership. Such skills represent **social intelligence**, which is the aptitude for understanding the thoughts, feelings, and behaviors of others, and of oneself, in social situations and for acting appropriately based on that understanding.[37] Zaccaro states that social intelligence consists of social awareness, social acumen, response selection, and response enactment.[34] These components are based on leaders' ability to understand the behaviors, thoughts, and feelings of other people within their social sphere and their ability to choose responses that appropriately match situations in that sphere.[4] Several studies have demonstrated that the self-monitoring aspect of social intelligence plays a major role in effective leadership.[38] Other studies have considered social intelligence in relation to leadership, controlling for other types of intelligence (general or emotional). These studies have demonstrated that social intelligence either predicted leader emergence[39] or reflected leadership experience.[40] Taken together, the various studies of social awareness and social intelligence provide strong evidence linking social awareness skills to effective leadership.

Understanding Emotional Intelligence

Because of the significant impact emotions can have on people's cognitive processes and behavior, **emotional intelligence** is a key attribute for effective leadership.[41] Daft[5(p146)] defines *emotional intelligence* as a "person's abilities to perceive, identify, understand, and successfully manage emotions in self and others." An understanding of emotions helps leaders to effectively manage themselves and their relationships. Many researchers accept eight categories or families of emotions: anger, sadness, fear, enjoyment, love, surprise, disgust, and shame. These eight families do not represent all emotions, but they include the four universally recognized emotions that are expressed through facial expressions: anger, fear, enjoyment, and sadness.

Caruso, Mayer, and Salovey[42] identify four distinct emotional intelligence skills: (1) emotion identification, which involves discerning and appraising one's feelings and the emotional expressions of others; (2) emotion use, which involves working with emotions to direct attention to important events and environmental cues; (3) emotion understanding, which involves assessing emotions within a larger network of causes and knowing how various emotions in oneself and others are connected; and (4) emotion management, which involves maintaining awareness of emotions and solving problems encumbered with emotional issues. Public health leaders who are in tune with their emotions as well as those of their followers can put this knowledge to use for the good of their organizations.

> **emotional intelligence**
> The ability to systematically review the emotions of oneself and other individuals, differentiating between various emotions, appropriately labeling them, and utilizing such information to guide behavior and thought.

Check It Out

For additional information about emotional intelligence, read Kendra Cherry's article "What Is Emotional Intelligence?" at www.verywell.com/what-is-emotional-intelligence-2795423.

The Emotional Competence Inventory

The Emotional Competence Inventory—developed by Goleman, Boyatzis, and Hay Group—is a framework for assessing specific competencies related to emotional intelligence.[43,44] The inventory is based on a two-by-two matrix, with *behavior* and *awareness* arranged opposite *self* and *others*. The four quadrants represent distinct areas of ability: (1) self-awareness, (2) self-management, (3) social awareness, and (4) relationship management (see exhibit 3.6). Emotional intelligence can be improved as individuals strengthen their abilities in all four areas.

Self-awareness, which depends on accurate self-assessment, is at the core of the emotional competency framework. Self-aware leaders can recognize and understand their emotions, assess their personal strengths and weaknesses, and project a sense of self-confidence. They trust their gut instincts and recognize that their feelings provide useful information. **Self-management** ability is essentially emotional self-control. Individuals with strong self-management tend to be trustworthy, conscientious, optimistic, and adaptable. They are

> **self-awareness**
> The ability associated with self-assessment, recognizing and understanding one's own emotions, and knowing one's personal strengths and weaknesses.

> **self-management**
> The ability to keep one's emotions in balance; emotional self-control.

EXHIBIT 3.6
The Emotional
Competence
Inventory

AWARENESS

Self-Awareness	**Social Awareness**
• Emotional self-awareness • Accurate self-assessment • Self-confidence	• Empathy • Organizational awareness • Service orientation
Self-Management	**Relationship Management**
• Emotional self-control • Trustworthiness • Conscientiousness • Adaptability • Optimism • Achievement orientation • Initiative	• Development of others • Change catalyst • Inspirational leadership • Conflict management • Influence • Bond building • Communication • Teamwork and collaboration

SELF   OTHERS

BEHAVIOR

Source: Data from Wolff, S. B. 2005. *The Emotional Competence Inventory—Technical Manual*. Boston, MA: Hay Group.

often achievement oriented and willing to take the initiative to accomplish the work at hand. They are also able to control negative emotions and desires, particularly those that are unproductive, disruptive, or harmful to themselves or others. Public health leaders can improve their self-management by learning to balance emotions such as desire, anxiety, worry, anger, and fear. By managing their emotions—rather than suppressing or denying them—leaders can think more clearly, increase their effectiveness, and proactively deal with any situations that arise.[5]

Social awareness and **relationship management** deal with others rather than the self. Leaders with high social awareness exhibit empathy, understand other people's points of view, and sense others' emotions. Frost[45] states that effective leaders learn to engage their followers with a "professional intimacy" that allows them to exhibit compassion and concern without becoming entangled in others' emotions in a way that would interfere with judgment. Socially aware leaders understand organizational dynamics, and this understanding produces a service orientation that assists the organization, peers, and followers. A key element of social awareness is the leader's ability to work effectively with a variety of individuals with different backgrounds and emotions, which

social awareness
The ability to understand the dynamics that occur in individual, group, and community relationships.

relationship management
The ability to relate to other individuals in a way that makes them feel understood and supported.

is essential for relationship management. Effective leaders are keen network builders, and they understand that networks help them achieve positive results. Habbel[46] found that leaders with strong relationship management skills treat other people with kindness, sensitivity, and compassion. Relationship management centers on the ability to connect with other people and build strong relationships, but it also includes developing people through inspirational leadership, building teamwork through collaboration, and resolving interpersonal conflicts. Leaders who excel in relationship management generally have good communication skills and are adept at using their influence to ensure positive results. Relationship management skills are particularly important for leaders in public health, given the highly collaborative nature of the field.

Research supports the idea that emotional intelligence serves as a strong base for public health leadership. Goleman[47] has found that effective leadership styles can arise from all four of the emotional intelligence quadrants, and Knight and colleagues[48] have observed that emotional intelligence among public health supervisors is related to conditions of trust among subordinates. Effective public health leaders learn to change or combine styles depending on the context or situation within which they are working. They are sensitive to emotions, both their own and those of others, and make adjustments to their leadership style accordingly.

The Behavioral Approach and Leadership Styles

During the 1950s, at a time when Stogdill and others were raising questions about the trait approach, many researchers shifted their attention to a behavioral approach, focusing on the behaviors used by effective leaders. Since behaviors are more readily learned than traits, this approach suggests that leadership skills can be developed by a broad array of people. Researchers soon identified two metacategories of effective leadership behavior—task-oriented behavior and people-oriented behavior—that were found to exist across time and situations.[49] In addition to examining leaders' behaviors, investigators also engaged in the study of **leadership styles**—the recurring patterns of behavior that leaders exhibit when dealing with followers. Researchers believed that, if one best style could be determined, effective leaders could be more easily trained.

leadership style
A pattern of behavior that a leader exhibits when dealing with followers.

Seminal studies of leadership styles were conducted by research teams at Ohio State University[50] and the University of Michigan.[51] They focused on two dimensions of leadership style: the task to be accomplished and the people doing the work. The Ohio State researchers termed these two dimensions "initiating structure" and "consideration," whereas the Michigan team labeled them "production-centered" and "employee-centered." Regardless of the terminology, the two dimensions represented leaders with a high concern for the task and leaders with a high concern for people. Task-oriented leaders define and plan the work to be accomplished, assign responsibilities, establish clear work standards, urge followers to complete the tasks, and monitor performance results. People-oriented leaders demonstrate a warm and supportive attitude, respect followers' feelings, and are sensitive to followers' needs. They maintain appropriate social relationships with followers, with trust as a key element. Although many initially believed that people-oriented leaders would be most effective, researchers over time concluded that effective leaders have high concern for both task and people.

The Leadership Grid

One of the most popular tools to emerge from behavioral leadership research has been the Managerial Grid developed by Blake and Mouton,[52] which was later restated as the Leadership Grid by Blake and McCanse.[53] The grid consists of two nine-point scales—concern for production (or task) and concern for people—and the combination of scores could point to five "pure" styles of leadership[54]:

1. *Team management*—high concern for both production and people (grid scores of 9, 9), with team members working together to complete a task; recommended for public health leaders
2. *Country club management*—low concern for production and high concern for people (1, 9)
3. *Authority-compliance management*—high concern for production and low concern for people (9, 1)
4. *Middle-of-the-road management*—moderate concern for both production and people (5, 5)
5. *Impoverished management*—the absence of a management philosophy, with little concern for interpersonal relationships or work accomplishment (1, 1)

Two additional leadership styles were later added to the framework, though they lack fixed points on the grid[53]:

1. *Paternalistic management*—an emphasis on reward and punishment
2. *Opportunistic management*—a tendency to shift styles for the leader's own benefit

 Check It Out

Visit www.12manage.com/methods_blake_mouton_managerial_grid.html for additional information on the Managerial/Leadership Grid.

The styles represented in the Leadership Grid correspond roughly with classic leadership approaches that have been observed for many years. As far back as 1938, Lewin and Lippitt[55] used the terms *autocratic* and *democratic* to describe leadership styles, and these terms remain in use today. Leaders described as autocratic typically function in a unilateral, command-and-control manner; such an approach aligns with the authority-compliance style from the Leadership Grid. Leaders with a democratic style place their emphasis on both people and task; such an approach corresponds with the grid's team management style. Another classic leadership style, known as a "human relations" approach, emphasizes people over task; it corresponds with the country club management style. Finally, the classic laissez-faire style of leadership shows little concern for the task and lets followers make decisions on their own; this approach corresponds with the impoverished management style, known for its careless "don't bother me" approach.

Research Findings

The early research on the classic leadership styles seemed to indicate that leaders were either autocratic or democratic in approach. However, in the 1950s, Tannenbaum and Schmidt[56] postulated that a continuum exists between the two styles of leadership and that leaders use a mix of autocratic and democratic actions (see exhibit 3.7). The particular style used by a leader is influenced by employee participation and organizational context. Heller and Yukl[57] found that leaders, regardless of style, could adjust their behaviors based on organizational circumstance or situational variables.

Leaders with high levels of concern for both tasks and people—often referred to as "high–high" leaders—have generally been assumed to be the most effective, and leadership training based on the Leadership Grid has aimed to develop leaders of this type. However, research has provided this position

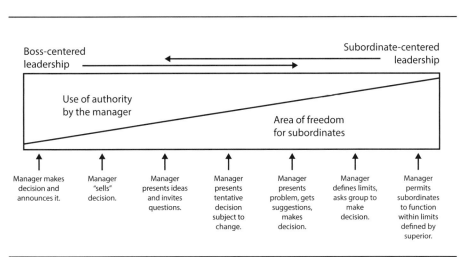

EXHIBIT 3.7
Leadership
Continuum

with only limited support. Yukl[6(p64–65)] writes that "research based on critical incidents and interviews strongly suggests that effective leaders guide and facilitate the work to accomplish task objectives while at the same time maintaining cooperative relationships and teamwork."

Case Study: New Jersey Ebola Quarantine

It was the fall of 2014, and an outbreak of the deadly Ebola virus in West Africa had the world on edge. American healthcare practitioners were on the ground helping address this frightening and, as yet, uncontrolled epidemic. The US Constitution empowers federal and state authorities in their handling of health matters, and ports and airports are governed by federal authority. Individual states have varying health laws, including laws governing the use of quarantine to control disease outbreaks. Many states had begun enacting quarantines to protect the public and dispel public fear.

In one widely publicized case, a Doctors Without Borders nurse, Kaci Hickox, returned to the United States after a month in Sierra Leone. Her flight entered the country in New Jersey, just days after New York Governor Andrew Cuomo and New Jersey Governor Chris Christie had issued a mandatory quarantine for healthcare workers who had been in West Africa and had contact with persons infected with Ebola. The quarantines exceeded federal standards and received backlash from the White House and medical practitioners. New York and New Jersey were two of the states (along with Maryland, Virginia, Pennsylvania, and Georgia) where more than 70 percent of air travelers from the hardest hit areas of West Africa (Liberia, Guinea, and Sierra Leone) were entering the United States.

Hickox was questioned for several hours upon landing at Newark Liberty International Airport, and despite having no symptoms of Ebola, she was placed under quarantine in a tent outside a New Jersey hospital. Hickox was released three days later after testing negative for Ebola, and she returned to her home state of Maine. She declined Maine's voluntary quarantine, but Maine officials subsequently pursued a court order for mandatory home quarantine for 21 days. A judge ultimately rejected that order, allowing Hickox to be free of quarantine as long as she submitted to active monitoring for 21 days and agreed to notify health officials in the event that symptoms appeared. Hickox never developed Ebola.

World Health Organization officials and US disease experts argued that the state quarantines were unnecessary and could potentially deter healthcare workers from helping with the outbreak in Africa. Hickox would later file a civil rights lawsuit against New Jersey Governor Christie, former New Jersey State Health Commissioner Mary O'Dowd, and other health department employees, claiming that she was illegally held against her will. She would also file suit against the state government of Maine and its health officials.

Discussion and Application Questions

1. In your opinion, were the quarantines warranted? Why or why not?
2. What circumstances complicated an effective public health leadership response to the Ebola outbreak?
3. How could government and public health leaders have responded more effectively in such circumstances?
4. What leadership traits would prove most effective in leading a community through the process of establishing a quarantine?

Summary

An individual's personal traits have long been regarded as a key factor determining a person's ability to lead. Empirical research on this topic was first conducted in 1904, when scientists sought to identify the qualities that differentiated leaders from nonleaders. Early studies advanced the idea that certain personal qualities are inherent in leaders and that these traits can be identified and assessed. This line of thinking became less prevalent after 1950, but research on the traits, skills, behaviors, and styles of effective leadership has continued and evolved. More recent research has examined a variety of behavioral and cognitive aspects spanning the breadth and depth of leadership practice.

Traits are the various attributes possessed by individuals, including personality, temperament, abilities, needs, motives, disposition, and values. They represent core elements of every leader, and they contribute to consistent leadership performance regardless of the organizational situation. Public health leaders are known to their followers, peers, collaborators, and constituents by their key personal traits. Leaders also possess skills, which reflect the ability to perform activities in an effective manner. The skills taxonomy consists of three broadly defined categories—technical skills, interpersonal skills, and conceptual skills—all of which are important for the effective practice of public health leadership.

The trait approach to leadership is based on the great man theory, which focused on the personal traits of individuals who were thought to be great men. However, the great diversity of traits represented by these individuals suggested that leadership was not simply genetic. Stogdill demonstrated that traits were based on specific situations and found no evidence for universal leadership traits—thus contributing to the demise of the great man theory. Still, some researchers determined that certain traits could distinguish leaders from nonleaders, and additional research suggested that leadership traits could be both inborn and learned. Over time, a lengthy list of leadership traits has developed. Such traits may not be universal in nature, but they at least suggest qualities that public health leaders can strive to possess.

Leadership skills are the competencies and knowledge that help leaders reach goals and objectives, and they fall under three categories: technical skills, interpersonal or human skills, and conceptual skills. Conceptual skills are the most important category for senior leaders and upper-level managers, whereas technical skills are more important for leaders in supervisory and middle management positions.

Personality—both the leader's own and the leader's ability to understand the personalities of others—strongly influences leadership effectiveness. Personality has many aspects, but researchers over time have identified a set of key dimensions known as the "big five": (1) extraversion (or surgency), (2) agreeableness, (3) conscientiousness (or dependability), (4) emotional stability (or neuroticism), and (5) openness (or intellectance).

Leaders also must understand cognitive style, which deals with the way individuals perceive, process, interpret, and use information. Herrmann's Whole Brain Thinking model is a four-quadrant approach to represent styles of thinking. Individuals may tend to have one style that is dominant, but effective leaders use all four styles. The Myers-Briggs Type Indicator is another tool for assessing cognitive styles and helping leaders understand themselves and others.

Another key attribute for effective leadership is emotional intelligence, which can be assessed using a framework called the Emotional Competence Inventory. The inventory presents four distinct areas of ability: (1) self-awareness, (2) self-management, (3) social awareness, and (4) relationship management. Socially aware leaders are adept at understanding the organizations in which they work.

The behavioral approach to the study of leadership focuses on behaviors rather than traits, and it distinguishes between two categories: task-oriented behaviors and people-oriented behaviors. One of the most popular tools in this area is the Leadership Grid, which uses two nine-point scales (representing concern for task and concern for people) to identify leadership styles. The styles represented in the grid correspond roughly with classic leadership approaches that have been observed for many years. The use of the terms *autocratic* and *democratic* to describe leadership behavior dates to the 1930s, and the terms are still used today.

Public health leaders may possess particular traits, skills, and styles, but their leadership actions should be appropriate to the organizational context or situation. Effective leadership is determined not by personality traits but by the leader's behavior.

Discussion Questions

1. Discuss the concept of leadership traits. How do such traits apply to public health leadership?
2. What traits do you think are the best predictors of effective public health leadership?
3. Describe how technical, interpersonal, and conceptual leadership skills are related to effective public health leadership.
4. Which types of skills are most important at the lower, middle, and higher levels of leadership?
5. Discuss social intelligence and how it is related to effective public health leadership.
6. Explain emotional intelligence. How does it relate to social intelligence and to the effective practice of public health leadership?
7. Consider the Myers-Briggs Type Indicator, and identify which two characteristics you believe would be most strongly associated with effective public health leadership. Support your opinion.
8. Review your own Myers-Briggs type, and explain how considering your complementary type might help your development as an effective public health leader.
9. How does the Leadership Grid assist public health leaders in understanding their own leadership style?
10. For deeper thought: Considering the importance of emotional intelligence to the effective practice of public health leadership, discuss how you can more fully develop your own emotional intelligence.

Web Resources

Cherry, K. 2016. "What Is Emotional Intelligence?" Verywell. Updated August 24. www.verywell.com/what-is-emotional-intelligence-2795423.

Myers & Briggs Foundation. 2017. "MBTI Basics." Accessed May 11. www.myersbriggs.org/my-mbti-personality-type/mbti-basics/home.htm.

Van Eersel, F. M. 2017. "Managerial Grid (Blake and Mouton) Knowledge Center." 12Manage. Accessed May 12. www.12manage.com/methods_blake_mouton_managerial_grid.html.

References

1. Bass, B. M. 1990. *Bass & Stogdill's Handbook of Leadership: Theory, Research, and Managerial Applications*, 3rd ed. New York: Free Press.

2. Hieder, J. 1985. *The Tao of Leadership*. Atlanta, GA: Humanics Limited.

3. Antonakis, J., A. T. Cianciolo, and R. J. Sternberg. 2004. *The Nature of Leadership*. Thousand Oaks, CA: Sage.

4. Stogdill, R. M. 1948. "Personal Factors Associated with Leadership: A Survey of the Literature." *Journal of Psychology* 25: 35–71.

5. Daft, R. L. 2015. *The Leadership Experience*, 6th ed. Mason, OH: South-Western.

6. Yukl, G. 2013. *Leadership in Organizations*, 8th ed. Upper Saddle River, NJ: Prentice Hall.

7. Arvey, R. D., Z. Zhang, B. J. Avolio, and R. F. Krueger. 2007. "Developmental and Genetic Determinants of Leadership Role Occupancy Among Women." *Journal of Applied Psychology* 92 (3): 693–706.

8. Katz, R. L. 1955. "Skills of an Effective Administrator." *Harvard Business Review* 33 (1): 33–42.

9. Mann, F. C. 1965. "Toward an Understanding of the Leadership Role in Formal Organizations." In *Leadership and Productivity*, edited by R. Dubin, G. C. Homans, F. C. Mann, and D. C. Miller, 68–103. San Francisco: Chandler.

10. Stogdill, R. M. 1974. *Handbook of Leadership: A Survey of Theory and Research*. New York: Free Press.

11. Mann, R. D. 1959. "A Review of the Relationships Between Personality and Performance in Small Groups." *Psychological Bulletin* 56 (4): 241–70.

12. Lord, R. G., C. L. DeVader, and G. M. Alliger. 1986. "A Meta-analysis of the Relation Between Personality Traits and Leadership Perceptions: An Application of Validity Generalization Procedures." *Journal of Applied Psychology* 71 (3): 402–10.

13. Kirkpatrick, S. A., and E. A. Locke. 1991. "Leadership: Do Traits Matter?" *The Executive* 5 (2): 48–60.

14. Zaccaro, S. J., C. Kemp, and P. Bader. 2004. "Leader Traits and Attributes." In *The Nature of Leadership*, edited by J. Antonakis, A. T. Cianciolo, and R. J. Sternberg, 101–24. Thousand Oaks, CA: Sage.

15. Northouse, P. G. 2016. *Leadership: Theory and Practice*, 7th ed. Los Angeles: Sage.

16. Kouzes, J. M., and B. Z. Posner. 2011. *Credibility: How Leaders Gain and Lose It, Why People Demand It*, 2nd ed. San Francisco: Jossey-Bass.

17. Gates, R. M. 2016. *A Passion for Leadership*. New York: Knopf.

18. Zaccaro, S. J., R. J. Foti, and D. A. Kenny. 1991. "Self-Monitoring and Trait-Based Variance in Leadership: An Investigation of Leader Flexibility Across Multiple Group Situations." *Journal of Applied Psychology* 76 (2): 308–15.

19. Harris, K. J., K. M. Kacmar, S. Zivnuska, and J. D. Shaw. "The Impact of Political Skill on Impression Management Effectiveness." *Journal of Applied Psychology* 92 (1): 278–85.

20. Lincoln, A. 1832. "First Political Announcement, New Salem, Illinois, March 9, 1832." Abraham Lincoln Online. Accessed May 10, 2017. www.abrahamlincolnonline.org/lincoln/speeches/1832.htm.

21. Simon, H. 1987. "Making Managerial Decisions: The Role of Intuition and Emotion." *Academy of Management Executive* 1: 57–64.

22. Digman, J. M. 1990. "Personality Structure: Emergence of the Five-Factor Model." *Annual Review of Psychology* 41 (1): 417–40.

23. Hough, L. M. 1992. "The 'Big Five' Personality Variables—Construct Confusion: Description Versus Prediction." *Human Performance* 5 (1–2): 139–55.

24. Jones, D. 2006. "Not All Successful CEOs Are Extroverts." *USA Today* June 6, B1.

25. Judge, T. A., J. E. Bono, R. Ilies, and M. W. Gerhardt. 2002. "Personality and Leadership: A Qualitative and Quantitative Review." *Journal of Applied Psychology* 87 (4): 765–80.

26. Hogan, R. T., G. J. Curphy, and J. Hogan. 1994. "What We Know About Leadership: Effectiveness and Personality." *American Psychologist* 49 (6): 493–504.

27. Herrmann, N. 1996. *The Whole Brain Business Book*. New York: McGraw-Hill.

28. Jung, C. 1923. *Psychological Types*. London, UK: Routledge and Kegan Paul.

29. Myers & Briggs Foundation. 2017. "MBTI Basics." Accessed May 11. www.myersbriggs.org/my-mbti-personality-type/mbti-basics/home.htm.

30. Briggs Myers, I. 1980. *Introduction to Type*. Palo Alto, CA: Consulting Psychologists Press.

31. Johnson, R. 1999. *Your Personality and the Spiritual Life*. Gainesville, FL: Center for Applications of Psychological Type.

32. Zaccaro, S. J. 1999. "Social Complexity and the Competencies Required for Effective Military Leadership." In *Out-of-the Box Leadership: Transforming the Twenty-First Century Army and Other Top-Performing*

Organizations, edited by J. G. Hunt, G. E. Dodge, and L. Wong, 131–51. Stamford, CT: JAI Press.

33. Zaccaro, S. J. 2001. *The Nature of Executive Leadership: A Conceptual and Empirical Analysis of Success*. Washington, DC: American Psychological Association.

34. Zaccaro, S. J. 2002. "Organizational Leadership and Social Intelligence." In *Multiple Intelligences and Leadership*, edited by R. E. Riggio, S. E. Murphy, and F. J. Pirozzolo, 29–54. Mahwah, NJ: Lawrence Erlbaum.

35. Zaccaro, S. J., R. J. Foti, and D. A. Kenny. 1991. "Self-Monitoring and Trait-Based Variance in Leadership: An Investigation of Leader Flexibility Across Multiple Group Situations." *Journal of Applied Psychology* 76 (2): 308–15.

36. Zaccaro, S. J., J. Gilbert, K. Thor, and M. Mumford. 1991. "Social Perceptiveness and Behavioral Flexibility as Characterological Bases for Leader Role Acquisition." *Leadership Quarterly* 2: 317–42.

37. Marlowe, H. A. 1986. "Social Intelligence: Evidence for Multidimensionality and Construct Independence." *Journal of Educational Psychology* 78 (1): 52–58.

38. Day, D. V., D. J. Schleicher, A. L. Unckless, and N. J. Hiller. 2002. "Self-Monitoring Personality at Work: A Meta-analytic Investigation of Construct Validity." *Journal of Applied Psychology* 87 (2): 390–401.

39. Ferentinos, C. H. 1996. "Linking Social Intelligence and Leadership: An Investigation of Leaders' Situational Responsiveness Under Conditions of Changing Group Tasks and Membership." *Dissertation Abstracts International: Section B: The Sciences & Engineering* 57: UMI No. 9625606.

40. Kobe, L. M., R. Reiter-Palmon, and J. D. Rickers. 2001. "Self-Reported Leadership Experiences in Relation to Inventoried Social and Emotional Intelligence." *Current Psychology: Developmental, Learning, Personality, Social* 20 (2): 154–63.

41. Goleman, D., R. Boyatzis, and A. McKee. 2002. *Primal Leadership: Realizing the Power of Emotional Intelligence*. Boston: Harvard Business School Press.

42. Caruso, D. R., J. D. Mayer, and P. Salovey. 2002. "Emotional Intelligence and Emotional Leadership." In *Multiple Intelligences and Leadership*, edited by R. E. Riggio, S. E. Murphy, and F. J. Pirozzolo, 55–74. Mahwah, NJ: Lawrence Erlbaum.

43. Hay Group. 2011. *Emotional and Social Competency Inventory (ESCI): A User Guide for Accredited Practitioners*. Published June. www.eiconsortium.org/pdf/ESCI_user_guide.pdf.

44. Wolff, S. B. 2005. *The Emotional Competence Inventory—Technical Manual*. Boston: Hay Group.

45. Frost, P. J. 2004. "Handling the Hurt: A Critical Skill for Leaders." *Ivey Business Journal* 68 (3): 1–6.

46. Habbel, R. W. 2002. "The Human(e) Factor: Nurturing a Leadership Culture." *Strategy + Business* 26: 83–89.

47. Goleman, D. 2000. "Leadership That Gets Results." *Harvard Business Review* 78 (2): 79–90.

48. Knight, J. R., H. M. Bush, W. A. Mase, M. C. Riddell, M. Liu, and J. W. Holsinger Jr. 2015. "The Impact of Emotional Intelligence on Conditions of Trust Among Leaders at the Kentucky Department for Public Health." *Frontiers in Public Health*. Published March 13. http://journal.frontiersin.org/article/10.3389/fpubh.2015.00033/full.

49. Yukl, G., A. Gordon, and T. Taber. 2002. "A Hierarchical Taxonomy of Leadership Behavior: Integrating a Half Century of Behavior Research." *Journal of Leadership and Organizational Studies* 9 (1): 13–32.

50. Stogdill, R. M., and A. E. Coons (eds.). 1951. *Leader Behavior: Its Description and Measurement*. Columbus, OH: Ohio State University Bureau of Business Research.

51. Kahn, R. L., and D. Katz. 1952. "Leadership Practices in Relation to Productivity and Morale." Published December. www.psc.isr.umich.edu/dis/infoserv/isrpub/pdf/Leadership_701_.PDF.

52. Blake, R. R., and J. S. Mouton. 1985. *The Managerial Grid III*. Houston, TX: Gulf Publishing Company.

53. Blake, R. R., and A. A. McCanse. 1991. *Leadership Dilemmas—Grid Solutions*. Houston, TX: Gulf Publishing Company.

54. Daft, R. L. 2016. *Management*, 12th ed. Mason, OH: South-Western.

55. Lewin, K., and R. Lippitt. 1938. "An Experimental Approach to the Study of Autocracy and Democracy: A Preliminary Note." *Sociometry* 1 (3–4): 292–300.

56. Tannenbaum, R., and W. H. Schmidt. 1958. "How to Choose a Leadership Pattern." *Harvard Business Review* 36 (2): 95–101.

57. Heller, F. A., and G. A. Yukl. 1969. "Participation, Managerial Decision-Making and Situational Variables." *Organizational Behavior and Human Performance* 4 (3): 227–41.

THE CONTINGENCY MODEL AND SITUATIONAL LEADERSHIP

James W. Holsinger Jr.

Learning Objectives

Upon completion of this chapter, you should be able to

- analyze contingency in terms of leadership theory;
- describe the importance of the follower in the contingency theories of leadership;
- discuss the role of individual behavior, including motivation, in the contingency theories;
- understand the situational focus of the contingency theories;
- analyze Fiedler's contingency model of leadership effectiveness, including the use of the least-preferred coworker scale;
- describe situational leadership and explain the importance of follower development and leader behaviors; and
- compare and contrast Fiedler's contingency model of leadership and situational leadership.

Focus on Leadership Competencies

This chapter emphasizes the following Association of Schools and Programs of Public Health (ASPPH) leadership competencies:

- Describe the attributes of leadership in public health.
- Describe alternative strategies for collaboration and partnership among organizations, focused on public health goals.
- Develop strategies to motivate others for collaborative problem solving, decision-making, and evaluation.

(continued)

- Influence others to achieve high standards of performance and accountability.
- Create a shared vision.

It also addresses the following Council on Linkages public health leadership competency:

- Analyzes internal and external facilitators and barriers that may affect the delivery of the 10 Essential Public Health Services.

Note: See the appendix at the end of the book for complete lists of competencies.

Introduction

contingency theories of leadership
Theories that consider the influence of intervening situational variables on leadership behavior and outcomes; such theories focus on leaders, followers, and the situation.

contingency
A fact or event that is incidental to or dependent on something else.

In chapter 3, we studied leadership traits, skills, behaviors, and styles. We now approach the next major wave in leadership models, the **contingency theories of leadership**. Such theories build on the idea, noted in the last chapter, that effective leadership varies from one situation to another. Past research has been unable to identify universal traits that produce effective leadership in every instance, and some leadership styles have been found to be effective in certain situations but not in others. Since the 1960s, researchers have shifted their attention to the ways that effective leadership depends on—or is contingent on—the specific organizational situations encountered by the leader.[1] A **contingency** is a fact or event that is incidental to or dependent on something else, and the contingency theories are built on the basic understanding that one thing depends on another. Under the contingency approach, leadership is not one-size-fits-all. The leader's behavior must fit with the particular situation in order to be effective.

The contingency theories of leadership focus on three key elements—the leader, the followers, and the situation—and each of these elements interacts with and influences the other two. The contingency theories thus present greater complexity than the trait-based universal approach. Under the universal approach, the leader's traits, skills, and behaviors were seen to produce outcomes, such as performance or satisfaction, among the followers. Under the contingency approach, on the other hand, the leader's traits, skills, and behaviors interact with the followers' needs, training, maturity, and cohesion, as well as the situation's task, structure, environment, and organizational system, to produce the outcomes.

 Effective Public Health Leaders . . .

. . . recognize the importance of the situation or context in which they are leading.[2]

This chapter will examine the ways that effective public health leadership is molded through close consideration of the leader's leadership style, the attributes of followers, and organizational characteristics. A key point that we will encounter repeatedly in this discussion is that the most effective approach in a given situation depends on numerous interconnected factors. Effective public health leaders learn to adapt through experience and practice, as well as by understanding the nature of various contingencies.

Situational Moderator Variables

Empirical research has focused on the ways that various aspects of a situation can enhance or negate a leader's traits, skills, and behaviors. These aspects are known as **situational moderator variables**, and their application is central to the contingency theories. Situational moderator variables affect the relationship between two other variables—for our purposes, leader behavior and outcome criteria—without correlating with either one of them. Virtually all leadership theories have at least one moderator, and many have several or more. Leadership moderators can be identified and classified based on the influence they have on leader behaviors and outcome criteria variables. A typology advanced by Howell, Dorfman, and Kerr[3] distinguishes between neutralizers/enhancers, substitutes/supplements, and mediators.

situational moderator variable An aspect of a particular situation that might enhance or negate a leader's skills, traits, and behaviors.

Neutralizer variables are moderators that block or weaken leader influence on follower outcomes, and they can make relationship- or task-oriented leadership virtually impossible.[4] For example, a supportive leadership style has little or no impact on followers who respond to a highly authoritarian leadership style, but it has a significant impact on followers who respond to a less authoritarian leadership style. **Enhancer variables**, on the other hand, are moderators that strengthen relationships between leader behaviors and outcome criteria. For instance, if followers are highly experienced in their work, that quality can make a leader's ambiguous direction more effective than it otherwise would have been. A leader's ability to reward followers can also have an enhancing impact on outcomes, particularly if followers recognize that rewards are contingent on performance or behavior. Enhancer variables are seen as a positive moderating influence, whereas neutralizers are seen as a negative moderating influence. However, some moderator variables may act either to enhance or to neutralize the actions of leaders. Consider group cohesiveness, for instance. If a group's norms operate in opposition to the leader's goals, cohesiveness within the work group can serve as a neutralizer, impeding the leader's ability to make an impact. However, if the organization and the work group have common goals and act in a cooperative fashion, cohesiveness can serve as an enhancer, potentially even rescuing weak leaders. A leader's expertise can also serve as either an enhancer or a neutralizer: Typically, low expertise will function as a neutralizer, whereas high expertise will enhance effectiveness.

neutralizer variable A variable that blocks or weakens leader influence on follower outcomes.

enhancer variable A variable that strengthens relationships between leader behaviors and outcome criteria.

leadership substitute
A characteristic of a task, organization, or followers that makes relationship- or task-oriented leadership impossible or unnecessary.

Some moderator variables may substitute for or supplement leadership. **Leadership substitutes** are characteristics of tasks, organizations, or followers that essentially take the place of active leadership behaviors, thereby making relationship- or task-oriented leadership impossible or unnecessary.[4] A variable must meet three criteria to be considered a leadership substitute: (1) A logical reason must explain why the leader's behavior and the potential substitute for it provide the appropriate guidance or positive feeling indicated by the criterion measure[5]; (2) the potential substitute must act as a neutralizer to weaken the influence of the leader's behavior on the criterion measure[3]; and (3) the potential substitute must have a significant influence on the criterion, such that increasing amounts of the substitute result in higher levels of the criterion. Leadership substitutes have a positive influence, so they are clearly distinguishable from neutralizers. Kerr and Jermier[4] found that satisfying tasks in and of themselves are a substitute for relationship-oriented behaviors of leaders. Similarly, followers' ability and professionalism can be a substitute for certain task-oriented leadership behaviors. In public health, for instance, practitioners' expertise reduces the need for task-oriented data and information, and their need for autonomy makes them less receptive to leaders who provide such information. In some situations, a moderator variable may serve to supplement, rather than neutralize or replace, a leader's ability to influence a follower's performance.[6] A moderator variable that does not specifically inhibit a leader's behavior to the extent of affecting a criterion is not a leadership substitute in this sense.

mediator variable
A variable that represents an intermediate step between independent and dependent variables.

Howell, Dorfman, and Kerr[3] identify **mediator variables** that represent an intermediate step between independent and dependent variables. They interact with the managerial and situational variables to determine the work unit's performance. The authors use the example of behavioral uncertainty—defined as "the degree of uncertainty an individual possesses that a particular work behavior will yield a certain outcome"—to demonstrate how a mediator variable functions in the causal chain[3(p94)]:

Task-oriented leadership (the independent variable) reduces a subordinate's behavioral uncertainty by clarifying appropriate behaviors and rewards for attaining work goals. This reduced behavioral uncertainty, in turn, is related to higher motivation, satisfaction, and it is hoped, performance. Here the leader behavior affects the criteria through its relationship with the mediator.

 Spotlight

Baron and Kenny[7(pp1174,1176)] explain the distinction between moderator variables and mediator variables:

> In general terms, a moderator is a qualitative (e.g., sex, race, class) or quantitative (e.g., level of reward) variable that affects the direction and/or strength of the relation between an independent or predictor variable and a dependent or criterion variable. . . . A given variable may be said to function as a mediator to the extent that it accounts for the relation between the predictor and the criterion. Mediators explain how external physical events take on internal psychological significance. Whereas moderator variables specify when certain effects will hold, mediators speak to how or why such effects occur.

Yukl[8] also includes mediators, which he calls *intervening variables*, as one of the four types of variables that play a role in leadership and group effectiveness: managerial behaviors, intervening variables, criterion variables, and situational variables.

Howell, Dorfman, and Kerr[3] have assembled the major elements of their typology into the model shown in exhibit 4.1. The model—with arrows representing direct effects and moderating influences—illustrates the way that the behaviors of the leader and the actions of the moderators influence followers as well as organizational outcomes. The leader's behaviors have usually been thought to serve as independent variables, but some investigators have also classified them as criteria measures. For the purposes of this model, leadership can be both a causal variable and a dependent variable. For instance, a leader who has high-performing followers may feel confident that the group has role clarity, adequate task structure, and positive expectancies; the leader may therefore feel that these followers require little or no instrumental leader behavior and instead focus on providing supportive and participative leadership.[3]

Effective Public Health Leaders . . .

. . . "are almost never as much in charge as they are pictured to be, and followers almost never are as submissive as one might imagine."

—John W. Gardner[9(p4)]

Focus on Followers

The contingency theories of leadership place a strong emphasis on the role of followers, who themselves serve as a moderator variable. Leadership is a relationship, and leaders, by definition, must interact with other individuals. And if leaders interacted only with other leaders, then leadership would lose

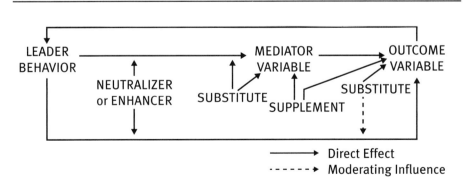

EXHIBIT 4.1
A Causal Model of Leader Behavior, Moderators, and Mediators

its meaning and make little sense.[9] Followers play such an important role that some have argued that the word *follower* itself, with its notion of passivity, is not appropriate for the concept[10]; however, no better term has been forthcoming.

Most individuals spend the majority of their lives as followers. Even when they hold leadership positions, they are usually in a subordinate position to someone and therefore function as followers. Furthermore, the distinction between leaders and followers has evolved as the study of leadership has advanced. Just as leaders can no longer be assumed to be managers, followers cannot be expected to be subordinates. Followers and leaders can be anyone within the organization.

The relationship between leaders and followers is a two-way conversation that is greatly influenced by followers' expectations. Leaders and their followers make up social groups, and social groups share a variety of attributes (e.g., needs, values, aspirations, fears) and develop their own norms. These norms, in turn, control the group's behavior, producing a social order. Effective public health leaders must function within this context while understanding that many of the needs, hopes, symbols, and ideals held by followers are partly buried and partly conscious.[9] Organizations rise and fall depending on two things—how well their leaders lead and how well their followers follow.

Rost's[10] concept of the follower incorporates several key points:

- Followership is an active concept. Passive followers are not part of the relationship because they have chosen not to be involved and are therefore without influence.
- Followers decide how active they are going to be, and this decision determines their influence in the leadership equation. (Individual followers may shift from minimal to full activity over time.)
- Leaders and followers may exchange roles within the leadership relationship. This ability to change roles without changing organizational positions results in significant influence for followers.
- Depending on the group or organization, people at all levels can be either followers or leaders.
- Most importantly, both leaders and followers are engaged in leadership, forming one relationship together.

Kelley[11] developed a model for categorizing followership patterns based on two dimensions—the follower's use of independent critical thinking and the degree to which the follower is passive or active. The model identifies five followership patterns:

1. *Sheep* are followers who are passive in nature and dependent and uncritical in their thinking.

2. *Yes people* are more active, but they are nonetheless dependent and uncritical in their thinking. They are often dependent on others for inspiration, aggressively deferential, and potentially servile in character.

3. *Alienated followers* are passive yet independent in nature. They think critically but are often cynical, disengaged, or opposed to the leader's efforts.

4. *Survivors* rank in the middle for both dimensions, hunkered down and surviving.

5. *Effective followers* think for themselves and function with energy and assertiveness.

Obviously, the key to effective organizations is effective followers—people who take risks, are self-starters, solve problems independently, and find their work to be a source of accomplishment and pride. Kelley[11] writes that effective followers share four essential qualities: (1) self-management, (2) commitment, (3) competence and focus, and (4) courage. They can think for themselves and also manage themselves. They are individuals to whom leaders can safely delegate responsibility. Whereas ineffective followers feel subservient, effective followers see themselves as the equal of their leaders. Insightful followers take a certain pride in being candid and fearless, and they work diligently to keep their leaders and coworkers informed as well as honest. Certainly, public health leaders would like the practitioners on their staffs to be effective followers—honest, loyal, candid, and credible.

Leader Behavior

Leader behavior plays an important role in the contingency theories, and such behavior must be rooted in a firm understanding of **motivation**—the internal or external impetus that produces enthusiasm and persistence in followers to carry out a course of action. Lewin[12] defined *individual behavior* as a function of the person and the environment or situation, suggesting that such behavior depends on factors both inside the person and outside in the environment or specific situation.[2] The person and the environment (or situation) influence one another, and this interdependence is crucial to the contingency theories of leadership.

A leader's behavior is goal oriented; however, leaders are not always conscious of the goals they are seeking, and the reasons for their actions are not always apparent. A leader's personality is made up of individual behavioral patterns that are often subconscious and not easily accessible to be evaluated or examined.[1] An activity is the basic unit of a leader's individual behavior, and leaders are always engaged in one or more activities. In considering leader

motivation
The internal or external impetus that produces enthusiasm and persistence in followers to carry out a course of action.

behavior for contingency theories, key questions emerge: Why do leaders engage in a particular activity rather than a different one? And how do leaders direct or control the activities of the individuals being led?

Motives and needs are at the core of individual behavior and action. A motive, as discussed in chapter 3, is a need or desire for doing something, which causes a person to act, whether consciously or unconsciously.[1] Motives instigate and sustain activity and decide the direction of individual behavior for both leaders and followers. When leaders consider their own behavior or that of their followers, motives answer the "why" question. Motivation, or the willingness of followers to do something, is just as important as their ability to do it. Needs are similar to motives in that they occur within individuals and stimulate individuals to take action. A goal is an aim or a purpose usually found outside the person, and it serves as the intangible incentive or reward that engages the individual's motives. Leaders need to understand which motives or needs will produce a definite follower action at a specific time.

Consider This

"As we look ahead into the next century, leaders will be those who empower others."

—Bill Gates[13]

What is required of effective public health leaders to empower their followers?

Effective public health leaders can use motivation theory to meet the needs and motives of their followers, while at the same time encouraging high-performing individuals and teams. Such leaders understand that follower motivation has a significant impact on productivity, and they direct their efforts toward motivating followers to reach the vision and goals of the organization. They know what influences their followers to choose, initiate, and maintain a particular course of action, and they provide an environment in which the followers are enabled to reach goals that satisfy their needs.

Leaders who understand motivation can effectively use reward systems to encourage behaviors that are positive and productive. Follower motivation is often rooted in such needs as recognition, achievement, friendship, or money.[1] These needs produce internal tensions that result in individual behaviors. If the person's behaviors are successful and the need or motive is satisfied, the individual reaps a reward. The reward serves as feedback to the individual, indicating that the behavior was appropriate and should be used again in the future. Rewards can be either intrinsic or extrinsic, and either individual or systemwide. Intrinsic rewards come from the action itself and provide inner satisfaction to the follower. Extrinsic rewards are given by the leader. Individual rewards are different for individual followers, even within the same work unit, whereas systemwide rewards apply to all members of the organization or work unit. These attributes of the reward system can be arranged in a two-by-two matrix to form four categories: (1) intrinsic individual rewards, such as a feeling of self-fulfillment; (2) extrinsic individual rewards, such as a significant pay increase; (3) intrinsic systemwide rewards, such as pride in being a part of a high-performing organization; and (4) extrinsic systemwide rewards, such as valuable fringe benefits for all of the members of the organization.

Situational Focus

While many researchers have exhaustively studied the traits, skills, and behaviors of leaders, others have examined the situation or social context of leadership. This **situational focus** centers on the strong influence that elements of the situation, independent of the individual, have on the emergence and behavior of leaders. Chemers[14] identifies three major areas on which situational researchers have concentrated: (1) the impact of group communication on the emergence of leaders; (2) the relationship between leadership and spatial relationships, such as seating arrangements; and (3) the effects of support and feedback on the emergence of leaders.

situational focus An emphasis on the strong influence that elements of the situation, independent of the individual, have on the emergence and behavior of leaders.

The study of group communication patterns has demonstrated that different levels of information accessibility can affect the emergence of leaders. Leavitt[15] compared four communication patterns—a chain, a wheel, a Y shape, and a circle. In patterns that had one individual positioned at the center, such as the Y and the wheel, that central person was most often the leader. In communication patterns that allowed for more interaction between the group members, such as the circle, communication flowed more freely, and every member of the group had an equal opportunity to be identified as the leader. Interestingly, researchers found that the emergence of leaders was not based on the members' personal characteristics or behavior but rather on the flow of information reaching them.[16]

Researchers studying space and seating arrangements found similar connections to leadership. In studies of seating arrangements, the person who sat at the head of the table and was able to obtain the most eye contact with the other team members tended to have the most control of the situation and was the designated team leader.[17,18] As a consequence, leaders normally choose the most visible seating location, to maximize their access to all team members. Similarly, Sommer[19] reported that leaders often reinforce their high status by occupying the most favored seating location.

Various other situational elements have been shown to affect leader emergence and behavior. Certain events can lead groups to convey their confidence in a person, which can result in leadership being bestowed.[20] Individuals who feel supported and endorsed by team members will contribute in a positive manner and thus be recognized as leaders. Organizational culture and workplace norms are also important determinants of how leaders behave. Shartle[21] found that the behavior of a leader's supervisor, not the leader's personality, is the best predictor of the leader's behavior.

The situational focus reflected in these and other studies contributed to the emergence of the contingency theories of leadership in the 1960s.

Fiedler's Contingency Model of Leadership Effectiveness

Fiedler's contingency model of leadership effectiveness, formulated by Fred Fiedler[22] in 1964, was the first contingency model of leadership to be derived empirically. He would ultimately propose that effective leadership depends on matching situational demands and leadership style.[23]

Fiedler's model measures people's leadership styles using the **least-preferred coworker (LPC) scale**. Leaders receive LPC scores based on their answers to questions about people with whom they had difficulty working; these scores, in turn, indicate their leadership style. Under Fiedler's model, leaders can have either a **task-motivated leadership style** (marked by a low LPC score) or a **relationship-motivated leadership style** (marked by a high LPC score). The word *or* is key, as the model functions on an either/or basis. Task-motivated leaders are most concerned with reaching a goal, whereas relationship-oriented leaders are most concerned with developing close interpersonal relationships. Fiedler maintained that leadership style is personality driven, and thus it is difficult to change and essentially enduring in nature. Under Fiedler's model, a task-motivated leader has little ability to change to a relationship-motivated approach, and vice versa, even with leadership training. Fiedler found that leadership success occurs when leaders use their existing leadership styles to work in situations where they fit best.[24]

The model predicts that relationship-oriented leaders will be more effective in moderate-control situations, whereas task-oriented leaders will be more effective in both high- and low-control situations.[16] Leaders in situations in which the model predicts successful leadership are considered to be in match; those in situations where the model predicts less success are considered to be out of match. Because of its emphasis on matching the leader to the situation, Fiedler's contingency model of leadership is also known as the *leader-match model*. The model is discussed in greater detail in the following sections.

The LPC Score and Leadership Styles

Fiedler's contingency model is based on the moderating influence of the situation on the relationship between the LPC trait measure and leadership effectiveness. To determine a leader's LPC score, the leader is asked to identify the coworker with whom the leader worked *least* well. The person the leader chooses is not necessarily the coworker the leader likes the least; rather, the

Fiedler's contingency model of leadership effectiveness
A model, developed by Fred Fiedler, based on the idea that effective leadership depends on matching situational demands and leadership style; also known as the *leader-match model.*

least-preferred coworker scale (LPC)
A scale used in Fiedler's contingency model to measure leadership style and distinguish between task-motivated leaders (low LPC score) and relationship-motivated (high LPC score) leaders.

task-motivated leadership style
The style of leadership most concerned with reaching a goal.

relationship-motivated leadership style
The style of leadership most concerned with the development of close interpersonal relationships.

individual selected should be the coworker with whom the leader has the most difficulty getting required work accomplished. Once the coworker has been selected, the measure's instructions ask that the leader rate the coworker on a set of 18 bipolar adjective scales—such as *pleasant/unpleasant, gloomy/cheer-ful*, and *supportive/hostile*—each of which is on an eight-point scale. After the ratings have been completed, the sum of the eighteen ratings becomes the leader's total LPC score. Even though the questions focus on the coworker's attributes, the LPC score is intended to depict something about the leader, not the coworker.[25] A highly critical leader will generally receive a low LPC score, whereas a more lenient leader will receive a higher LPC score.[8]

Fiedler's model uses the LPC score to categorize leaders as either task motivated or relationship motivated. A leader who scores 57 or below is said to have a low LPC, suggesting task-motivated leadership. A score between 58 and 63 represents a middle LPC, suggesting that the leader is independent. Leaders scoring 64 and above possess a high LPC, meaning they are more motivated by relationships.

Since the LPC is a personality measure, a leader's score is thought to be relatively stable over time. Fiedler and Garcia[26] demonstrated that test–retest reliability was strong. Fiedler stated that the LPC score explained the leader's motive hierarchy. Rice,[27] however, reviewed 25 years of LPC score research and came to a somewhat different interpretation—namely, that the data suggested the leader's "value-attitude" instead of a motive hierarchy. Rice concluded that low-LPC leaders place their emphasis on task success, whereas high-LPC leaders emphasize interpersonal success. The two interpretations are in basic accord, but Rice's interpretation is more sparing and supported by more diverse research.

Situational Favorability

Situational favorability, or situational control, is the degree to which a particular situation provides leaders with control over followers or subordinates, and it has a significant impact on the relationship between a leader's LPC and effectiveness. Under Fiedler's model, situational favorability is based on three main variables: (1) leader–member relations, (2) task structure, and (3) position power.[28]

The first variable, leader–member relations, is based on the atmosphere of the group, the degree to which members are loyal and confident, and the feelings members have for the leader. When the atmosphere is positive, members are friendly and cooperative, and followers trust and like the leader, leader–member relations can be considered good. When friction exists within the group and the atmosphere is unfriendly, relations can be considered poor.

The second situational variable is **task structure**, which can be defined as the degree to which task requirements are clearly spelled out. It involves pro-mulgating standard operating procedures for accomplishing the task, developing a detailed description of the product or service provided, and having clear and

situational favorability
The degree to which a particular situation provides leaders with control over followers or subordinates.

task structure
A situational variable based on the degree to which task requirements are clearly spelled out.

objective indicators of how well the task is being accomplished. Completely structured tasks provide greater control to the leader, whereas unclear tasks reduce the leader's influence.[28] A well-structured task is defined by (1) clearly stated task requirements that are understood by the individuals who must perform them; (2) few alternatives to the direction required to accomplish the task; and (3) availability of only a few correct solutions to the task.

The third situational variable in Fiedler's model is position power, which, as noted in chapter 1, is the legitimate power granted to leaders as a result of the position to which they have been appointed. It reflects the extent to which leaders can evaluate subordinates and reward or punish them accordingly. Position power is obviously strong if the leader has the ability to hire and fire, promote, and give pay raises. Without this level of authority, the leader's control is relatively weak.

These three situational variables determine the degree of favorability in various situations within organizations. Northouse[28(p113)] summarizes: "Situations that are rated most favorable are those having good leader–follower relations, defined tasks, and strong leader-position power. Situations that are rated least favorable have poor leader–follower relations, unstructured tasks, and weak leader-position power. Situations that are rated moderately favorable fall between these two extremes."

To effectively utilize Fiedler's model, leaders must know two things. First, they need to know whether their style is task-motivated or relationship-motivated. Second, they need to know, through analysis of the situation, the favorability of leader–member relations, task structure, and position power. According to the model, leaders with low LPC scores, who are task motivated, will be effective in situations that are extremely favorable or unfavorable—in other words, in situations that either are going very well or are simply out of control. Leaders with high LPC scores, who are relationship motivated, are most effective in moderately favorable conditions, where the situation is neither fully under their control nor completely out of control. However, the reasoning behind these aspects of the model can be difficult to understand.[28] In 1995, Fiedler[29] sought to clarify certain aspects of his model and further explain why a leader in a mismatched situation is ineffective. He reasoned that leaders become stressed and anxious when their LPC style does not match the situation, and they revert to immature coping skills learned in early development. These skills, in turn, result in inadequate decision making and poor outcomes.

Matching the Style to the Situation

Exhibit 4.2 shows how Fiedler's[30] contingency model predicts the effectiveness of leaders by matching their LPC scores with the organizational context. This context is based on the three situational variables, and the possible combinations of these variables result in eight categories, which correspond with LPC scores. The key predictions are as follows:

- Leaders with high LPC scores, who are relationship oriented, are well matched when they have good leader–member relations, low task structure, and weak position power. They also function well when leader–member relations are poor and structure is high, regardless of the strength of their position power.
- Leaders with low LPC scores, who are task oriented, function well in situations with poor leader–member relations, low structure, and weak position power. These leaders, as well as leaders with middle LPC scores, also function well when leader–member relations are good and structure is high, regardless of their position power. If leader–member relations are good and structure is low, they function well when their position power is strong.

Leaders whose style matches their work situation will likely succeed; if the style does not match the situation, failure may ensue.[28] However, the model recognizes that leaders can be successful in all situations. Fiedler found that leadership training aimed at changing a leader's style tended to be ineffective, because leaders have personal motivation hierarchies and behavioral tendencies that are deeply rooted in their personalities and experiences. Leadership training is more effective when it helps leaders modify key situational variables to improve the fit with their style.[25] Thus, training should focus on situational engineering instead of developing leaders' behavioral flexibility. The assignment of leaders is best served by matching their characteristics to the demands of the situation rather than attempting to change their behavior.

Strengths and Weaknesses of Fiedler's Model

Like any leadership theory, Fiedler's model has both strengths and weaknesses. Its major strength is its understanding of the impact that situations have on leaders. Fiedler helped move the field of leadership study beyond the notion of a single best style of leadership, and he shifted the emphasis to the context of leadership—specifically, the link between leaders and situations. Another

Leader–member relations	Good				Poor			
Task structure	High structure		Low structure		High structure		Low structure	
Position power	Strong power	Weak power	Strong power	Weak power	Strong power	Weak power	Strong power	Weak power
Situational category	1	2	3	4	5	6	7	8
Preferred leadership style	Low LPC; middle LPC				High LPC			Low LPC

EXHIBIT 4.2
Fiedler's Contingency Model of Leadership

Source: Data from Fiedler, F. E. 1967. *A Theory of Leadership Effectiveness*. New York: McGraw-Hill.

strength is that the model is research based and supported by a significant body of empirical evidence.[31] Out of all the leadership theories, it is one of the most extensively researched and validated.[25] Fiedler's model, unlike most leadership theories, is predictive in nature, thus indicating the type of leadership to use in a particular situation. It does not require leaders to be effective in every situation, and it demonstrates the importance of matching LPC scores to specific situations. Individuals' LPC scores can be used to create leadership profiles within organizations, so that the organizations can more effectively match leaders to appropriate situations.

One of the chief criticisms of the model is that certain aspects are unclear or difficult to understand. Even Fiedler himself has been unable to explain why certain leadership styles are linked to certain categories of situations. Some critics have found fault with the LPC system itself, questioning why a leader's description of another person would determine the leader's own style of leadership. Similarly, some have difficulty understanding why the scale is based on the least *preferred* coworker rather than the least *liked* coworker. Perhaps the most significant weakness is the limited guidance the model offers for organizations that discover they have assigned a mismatched leader. Situational engineering is not as simple as it might sound, particularly in the public health system, where leaders tend to be matched to positions based on required technical skills. The model simply does not address this issue.

Situational Leadership

situational leadership
The idea that there is no one best way to influence other people and that the readiness of the people being influenced determines the style that a leader should use.

The concept of **situational leadership** is based on the premise that there is no one best way to influence other people and that the readiness of the people being influenced determines the style that a leader should use. Situational leadership theory falls generally within the contingency model of leadership pioneered by Fiedler, though it diverges from Fiedler's positions at certain points. It was developed by Hersey and Blanchard,[32] though it has roots in the Ohio State University studies and the Blake and Mouton Leadership Grid (both discussed in chapter 3). The key to situational leadership is that it places the needs of the followers, not the ego needs of the leader, at the center of the model. In this sense, *leadership style* refers to the behavior employed by leaders as perceived by the followers.

Situational leadership breaks significantly from Fiedler's model in that it is based on effective leaders adjusting their styles. Under this approach, leaders focus a great deal of attention on the characteristics of the followers, and they use this information to determine which leadership behavior is appropriate. Followers in different situations require different styles of leadership; thus, to be effective, leaders must adapt their style to the requirements of the situation. The situation itself is influenced by a complex variety of conditions, which will be discussed later. Hersey and Blanchard are quick to point out that the situational leadership approach can be used in any number of settings, whether in the workplace, school, the family, or peer relationships. In this theory, the leader and follower are not necessarily in a hierarchical manager–employee relationship.

As situational leadership has evolved, its two creators, Hersey and Blanchard, have developed somewhat different approaches to it. Hersey and his colleagues at the Center for Leadership Studies call their approach *Situational Leadership*, whereas Blanchard and colleagues have developed a slightly different model termed *Situational Leadership II* (SLII).[32,33] In this discussion, we will focus primarily on SLII, which is somewhat less complex than Hersey's model, particularly with regard to the development of followers.

> ### Check It Out
>
> The Ken Blanchard Companies offer Situational Leadership II training at www.kenblanchard.com/Products-Services/Leadership-Fundamentals/Situational-Leadership-II.
>
> The Center for Leadership Studies, founded by Paul Hersey, offers a variety of resources at http://situational.com/the-cls-difference/situational-leadership-who-we-are/.

> ### Consider This
>
> "The key to successful leadership today is influence, not authority."
>
> —Ken Blanchard[34]
>
> As the director of a local county health department, do you have more influence or more authority? Why or why not?

Task and Relationship Behavior

The Ohio State studies identified two broad dimensions of leader behavior— "initiating structure" and "consideration." As Hersey and Blanchard developed their situational leadership approach, these dimensions were termed *task behavior* and *relationship behavior*. Hersey, Blanchard, and Johnson[2(p104-5)] explain that **task behavior** is "the extent to which the leader engages in spelling out the duties and responsibilities of an individual or group. These behaviors include telling people what to do, how to do it, when to do it, where to do it, and who to do it." A key element of task behavior is one-way communication that occurs between the leader and the follower. With task behavior, leaders are not overly concerned with the follower's feelings; they are primarily concerned with assisting the follower to achieve the goal. The authors explain that **relationship behavior** is "the extent to which the leader engages in two-way or multiway communication. The behaviors include listening, facilitating, and explaining the whys of something while offering supportive behavior to others." Task behavior is sometimes called *directive behavior*, whereas relationship behavior is sometimes called *supportive behavior*.

Under situational leadership, task behavior and relationship behavior are separate and distinct dimensions that can be represented in a two-by-two matrix. Relationship behavior is plotted on the vertical axis and task behavior is

task behavior
Behavior through which a leader spells out duties and responsibilities to followers; providing direction on what to do, who to do it, when to do it, where to do it, and how to do it.

relationship behavior
Two-way communication in the relationship between leader and follower, including such actions as encouraging, listening, clarifying, and facilitating.

on the horizontal axis. Both axes run from "low" to "high"; they do not begin at zero, because all leaders, regardless of whether they are effective or ineffective, will always use at least some level of both relationship and task behavior. The arrangement of the dimensions on the matrix produces four quadrants that represent four distinct leadership styles: Style 1, with high task behavior and low relationship behavior; Style 2, with high amounts of both task and relationship behavior; Style 3, with high relationship behavior and low task behavior; and Style 4, with low amounts of both relationship and task behavior.[12] All four leadership styles—which will be discussed in more detail in the sections ahead—can be effective and appropriate depending on the situation. The styles combine with the continuum of follower developmental level or readiness to complete the model.

Follower Developmental Levels

The developmental level of followers is the degree to which followers have the competence and commitment necessary to accomplish a given task or activity, and it largely determines the follower's performance or achievement.[35] The ability of followers to accomplish a task is determined by their knowledge, skill, and experience. However, sometimes followers simply lack interest and motivation in doing a job. Thus, both mastery of the skills to accomplish a given task and a positive attitude toward the task's accomplishment are significant attributes of follower development.[32] Followers with a high level of development possess all the necessary skills and knowledge to accomplish the assigned task.

Followers with a low level of development, in all likelihood, do not possess the skills to accomplish the task, though they may have sufficient motivation or confidence. When used to describe a follower's development level, competence and commitment are task specific; they pertain strictly to the task at hand and do not reflect the follower's overall level of development.

Under the SLII approach to situational leadership, followers can be divided into four categories based on developmental level: D1, D2, D3, or D4. D1 followers are low in competence but high in commitment for the specific task assigned. At the D1 level, the followers are developing and must focus on their knowledge, skill, and experience to build competence for the assigned task. Individuals who are new to a particular task often bring transferable skills and knowledge that they developed while working on other

Spotlight

Hersey, Blanchard, and Johnson[2(p136)] describe the keys to follower development:

Knowledge is demonstrated understanding of a task. *Skill* is demonstrated proficiency in a task. *Experience* is demonstrated ability gained from performing a task. *Competence* is a function of *knowledge* and *skills*, which can be gained from education, training, and/or experience. *Commitment* is a combination of confidence and motivation. *Confidence* is a measure of a person's self-assurance—a feeling of being able to do a task well without much supervision—whereas *motivation* is a person's interest in and enthusiasm for doing a task well.

tasks. Although they do not know exactly how to accomplish the task at hand, they bring a level of excitement. Followers at the D2 level are continuing to develop, and their level of competence pertaining to the task grows. However, their commitment drops at this stage of development, because their initial motivation subsides and they lose momentum. Followers at the D3 level continue to build competence for the task, but their commitment has not yet returned to the original level. They have developed the skills required for the task, but they continue to have doubts about their ability to accomplish it. Finally, followers at the D4 level are fully developed. They have a high degree of competence for the task, as well as a high degree of commitment. They both possess the skills to accomplish the task and are highly motivated to complete it.

Hersey's model of situational leadership differs somewhat from the SLII approach in that it uses follower readiness level (R1–R4) rather than developmental level (D1–D4).[2]

Leadership Styles

Under situational leadership, the leadership styles are based on the behaviors used to influence other people, and they include both directive (task) behavior and supportive (relationship) behavior. The four styles of leadership can be summarized as follows:

- **Style 1 (S1) leadership**, often called the "directing" style, is high in directive behaviors and low in supportive behaviors. It involves telling followers what to do, how to do it, when to do it, and where to do it. Leaders using this style focus their communication on achieving goals and on meeting followers' socioeconomic requirements or needs. (Note that a leader using *low* supportive behavior still does show *some* supportive behavior.)
- **Style 2 (S2) leadership**, called "coaching," combines highly directive and highly supportive behaviors. Leaders using the S2 approach continue the directive behavior of S1 but add more supportive behaviors, such as giving followers encouragement and soliciting their input. Such leaders will often discuss with followers why a task is important, but the leaders themselves remain responsible for making final decisions about what is to be accomplished and how it is to be done.
- **Style 3 (S3) leadership** is termed the "supporting" style because the leader's behaviors are high in supportive behavior and low in directing behavior. This style places less emphasis on goals and greater emphasis on social support and recognition. Leaders using the S3 approach listen to their followers, offer praise, provide feedback, and request the followers' input. This style requires leaders to assist followers with problem solving, while giving them day-to-day decision-making authority.

Style 1 (S1) leadership The situational leadership style that involves telling followers what to do, how to do it, when to do it, and where to do it; the "directing" style of leadership.

Style 2 (S2) leadership The situational leadership style that combines highly directive and highly supportive behaviors; the "coaching" style of leadership.

Style 3 (S3) leadership The situational leadership style that is high in supportive behavior and low in directing behavior; the "supporting" style of leadership.

Leadership Application Case: A New Leadership Model

The Leadership Application Case at the beginning of this book provides realistic scenarios for the application of key leadership concepts covered in the text. See the section marked "Chapter 4 Application" for the scenario and discussion questions that correspond with this chapter.

Style 4 (S4) leadership
The situational leadership style that is low in both supportive and directive behavior; the "delegating" style of leadership.

- **Style 4 (S4) leadership**, the "delegating" style, is low in both supportive behavior and directive behavior. Leaders using this style provide less task input and less social support. Under S4 leadership, followers are charged with the responsibility to accomplish the task as they see fit. The leader shifts control to the followers and no longer needs to intervene with unnecessary social support.

Using the Situational Leadership Model

Exhibit 4.3 shows how the situational leadership model can be constructed using the various leadership styles (S1–S4) and follower developmental levels (D1–D4). The key concepts of the model are that the leader is attuned to the developmental level of each follower for the task each is accomplishing and that the leader is prepared to change leadership styles to match the developmental level. Followers may move back and forth along the developmental continuum, and the same follower might have different developmental levels for different tasks. Leaders therefore must ask themselves questions that will explicate the nature of each situation. They need to know the specific tasks that each follower has been assigned, understand the complexity of those tasks, and determine whether the follower has the requisite skills and commitment to carry them out. Once the follower's developmental level has been properly assessed, leaders adjust their leadership style accordingly. Then, further adjustment is needed as the follower progresses from one developmental level to the next. Leaders must be constantly aware of the developmental levels of their followers, and they must have the flexibility to shift their leadership style quickly and effectively.

For a D1 follower (low competence but high commitment), an S1 leadership style (the "directing" style) is appropriate. Leaders must recognize when a follower moves from the D1 level to D2, because at this point the follower's commitment has plummeted; the S2 leadership style (the "coaching" style), with its increased supportive behavior, then becomes appropriate. Coaching comes at a critical point in the process. If a leader fails to recognize key points in the follower's development, leadership style and follower developmental level become mismatched,

Effective Public Health Leaders . . .

. . . place the needs of their followers ahead of their own ego needs.

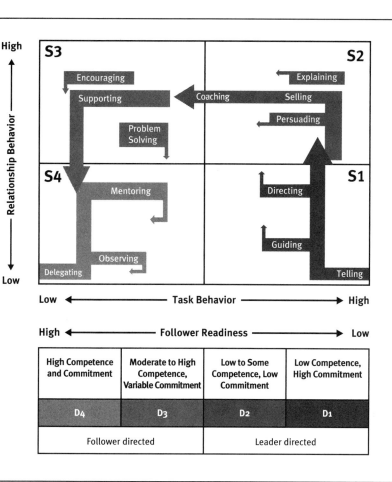

EXHIBIT 4.3
Situational
Leadership
Model

Source: Adapted from Rabarison, K., R. C. Ingram, and J. W. Holsinger Jr. 2013. "Application of Situational Leadership to the National Voluntary Public Health Accreditation Process." *Frontiers in Public Health* 1: 26.

causing a failure in leadership. All too often, leaders make the mistake of attempting to delegate to followers who are not yet developmentally ready to accept such a style. Also, if leaders fail to maintain at least *some* directive behavior and *some* supportive behavior while delegating, they are abrogating their responsibility to their followers.

For decades, many practitioners have found the situational leadership model to be practical, intuitive, effective, and easy to apply across a variety of situations. The approach has proved useful in a variety of settings, whether in the workplace, family, or education. Holsinger[36] has applied situational leadership to the dissertation process; Pawlina and colleagues[37] have used it in teaching gross anatomy; and Rabarison, Ingram, and Holsinger[38] have applied it to the public health department accreditation process. Northouse[28] points out that, whereas many other models of leadership are descriptive, situational leadership offers prescriptive value, telling leaders what they should do in various situations. Yukl[8] writes that the model's emphasis on adaptive, flexible behavior has been a significant contribution to leadership theory. The model is particularly well suited to public health, where the leader's ability to adapt to changing situations and follower behaviors is key.

Despite its widespread use in training and development situations, the lack of published research studies supporting the model has led some to question its validity. Vecchio and his coauthors[39,40,41] have raised questions about the model's theoretical basis, and Graeff[42] points out that follower developmental levels, based on commitment and competence, can be difficult to establish. As the model has changed over time, Hersey and Blanchard have failed to explain the theoretical bases for making the changes. In their 25-year review of situational leadership, Blanchard and his coauthors[32] noted that additional research was needed to determine how competence and commitment are understood for each of the four follower developmental levels. The prescriptive nature of the model is based on the idea that the follower developmental level determines the appropriate style of leadership, yet the reasons for the follower's progression through the four developmental stages is not clearly understood. Vecchio and his coauthors have studied high school teachers and principals,[39] university employees,[43] and United States Military Academy cadets,[41] and they have failed to find strong evidence supporting the prescribed leadership styles when applied to follower developmental level. Vecchio and Boatwright,[40] in an effort to determine the influence of certain demographic variables relating to the prescribed leadership style, found differences based on age, gender, level of education, and job experience; their findings may suggest that follower preference for leadership style is influenced by characteristics not considered in the model.[28] Furthermore, Graeff[42] has suggested that the format of the leadership questionnaire used in the model is biased in favor of situational leadership. Some have criticized the model for not addressing differences between prescription of leadership styles for an individual and for a group[28]; however, the practice of situational leadership clearly calls for leaders to consider each individual's developmental level for the task at hand, as well as the group's developmental stage.[44] Finally, the model has been found to have a conceptual weakness in that the four quadrants of leadership behavior have not been clearly and consistently defined.

Regardless of the criticism, situational leadership can be highly useful in training leaders to consider the needs of followers and develop a flexible leadership style. Daft[1] points out that situational leadership is more easily understood than Fiedler's contingency model because its focus is not on the larger situation but rather on the followers' characteristics. Thus, the leader's style is subordinated to the follower's developmental level. Under this model, effective public health leadership occurs through the selection of an appropriate leadership style, with both directive and supportive behaviors, based on the developmental level of the followers.

Case Study: Situational Leadership and Local Health Agency Accreditation[38]

The movement toward public health agency accreditation received a significant boost from the Institute of Medicine's 2002 report titled *The Future of the Public's Health in the 21st Century*, which led to the creation of the Public Health Accreditation Board (PHAB)[45] and the development of standards and measures for voluntary national accreditation in 2011. The accreditation process is based on setting standards for public health services and evaluating performance against those standards, and it has proved to be a useful tool for improving the quality of services provided to the public. The PHAB accreditation process has seven steps: (1) preapplication, (2) application, (3) documentation selection and submission, (4) site visit, (5) accreditation decision, (6) reports, and (7) reaccreditation.

A local public health agency was serving as a beta test site for the accreditation program. The agency director determined that leadership was a key element for accreditation success and that commitment to the process—both from employees and from members of the local board of health—was essential. The agency decided to apply situational leadership principles to the process.

Early on, agency staff members were unfamiliar with the accreditation process and occupied the D1 follower developmental level, which necessitated that the director engage in leader-directed activities of the S1 approach. The director informed agency staff of the requirements and processes of accreditation and used task behaviors to answer the question, What is public health accreditation?

As agency staff learned the value of accreditation, understood their roles in the process, and became familiar with the documents necessary for review, they transitioned to the D2 level of development. In response, the director shifted to the S2 style of leadership. Highly directive behavior continued, but relationship behavior increased. Taking on a coaching role, the director raised the question, Why is accreditation important to our agency?

By the time the agency reached the beta test site-visit phase, the staff had reached a D3 level of development. As a result, the director shifted to the more follower-directed activities of the S3 leadership style, which is high in supportive behavior but lower in directive behavior. Leadership behaviors revolved around encouraging and championing the efforts of a highly participatory agency staff.

(continued)

By the conclusion of the beta test, when mock accreditation feedback was provided, the agency staff members had reached a D4 level of development. The staff members were able, willing, and confident with respect to accreditation. As a result, the leader's style shifted to the low task and low relationship approach of S4. The director successfully delegated tasks to an accreditation coordinator, thus becoming an engaged mentor. As a result of the commitment and preparation exhibited by the staff, the agency was awarded five-year accreditation status in 2013.

Discussion and Application Questions
1. How did the agency director demonstrate effective public health leadership?
2. How can situational leadership be applied to other issues faced by local public health agencies?
3. Are there personal and professional issues that you face where the application of situational leadership might be useful or effective?

Summary

The contingency theories of leadership are based on the idea that effective leadership is *contingent* on specific organizational situations, meaning that leaders must adjust their leadership styles from one situation to another. A contingency is a fact or event that is incidental to or dependent on something else, and the contingency theories are built on the basic understanding that one thing depends on another. The theories focus on three key elements—the leader, the followers, and the situation—each of which interacts with and influences the other two.

The contingency approach focuses on the relationship between leadership styles—whether task-oriented and directive or relationship-oriented and supportive—and their effectiveness in specific situations. Situational moderator variables are aspects of the situation that can neutralize, enhance, or even replace leadership behaviors. The application of such variables is central to the contingency theories.

The contingency theories place significant emphasis on the role of the follower. The relationship between leaders and followers is a two-way conversation, and followership is an active concept. Passive followers are not part of the leadership equation because they have chosen not to be involved. For an organization to succeed, it must have leaders who lead and followers who follow. Leaders should understand followers' motivation and strive to meet followers' needs. They also must consider other aspects of the situational context, such as communication patterns and physical arrangement of the workplace.

Fiedler's contingency model of leadership effectiveness, formulated in 1964, was the first contingency model of leadership to be derived empirically. The model measures leadership styles using the least-preferred coworker (LPC) scale, which uses the leader's assessment of a coworker as a source of information about the leader's own style. Low LPC scores suggest task-motivated leadership, and high LPC scores suggest relationship-motivated leadership. Under Fiedler's model, task-motivated leaders have little ability to change to a relationship-motivated approach, and vice versa. Leadership success occurs when leaders are matched with situations in which their styles fit best.

Situational leadership differs from Fiedler's model in that leaders are expected to shift their style of leadership based on the situation and the developmental needs of the follower. Under situational leadership, task behavior and relationship behavior are distinct dimensions that can be placed in a two-by-two matrix to produce four leadership styles: S1 (directing), S2 (coaching), S3 (supporting), and S4 (delegating). These leadership styles are paired with four levels of follower development (D1–D4), which are based on each follower's commitment and competence with regard to the task at hand.

Discussion Questions

1. How do the contingency theories of leadership compare with theories based on the skills, behaviors, and traits of leaders?
2. Compare and contrast moderators and mediators within the contingency theory of leadership.
3. Why do the contingency theories of leadership place so much emphasis on the role of the follower?
4. Identify the four essential qualities of effective followers, and explain how those qualities function within the leader–follower relationship.
5. Assess the importance of motivation in the role of followers.
6. How does the situational focus affect the leader–follower relationship?
7. Explain Fiedler's contingency model of leadership effectiveness. Why is the least-preferred coworker scale important for the model?
8. Explain the situational leadership model, and discuss the importance of both leadership style and follower developmental level.
9. What contribution has situational leadership made to leadership theory in general?
10. For deeper thought: Imagine you are a newly trained epidemiologist, anxious to move ahead in your profession. Which contingency

leadership model do you select—Fiedler's contingency model or situational leadership? Justify your selection.

Web Resources

Center for Leadership Studies. 2017. "Who We Are." Accessed May 15. http://situational. com/the-cls-difference/situational-leadership-who-we-are/.

Graeff, C. L. 1997. "Evolution of Situational Leadership Theory: A Critical Review." *Leadership Quarterly*. Accessed May 15. http://crossculturalleadership.yolasite. com/resources/Graeff%20(1997)%20Evolution%20of%20Situational%20 Leadership%20-%20%20A%20Critical%20Review.pdf.

Ken Blanchard Companies. 2017. "Situational Leadership II." Accessed May 15. www.kenblanchard.com/Products-Services/Leadership-Fundamentals/ Situational-Leadership-II.

References

1. Daft, R. L. 2015. *The Leadership Experience*, 6th ed. Mason, OH: South-Western.

2. Hersey, P., K. H. Blanchard, and D. E. Johnson. 2008. *Management of Organizational Behavior: Leading Human Resources*, 9th ed. Upper Saddle River, NJ: Pearson Prentice Hall.

3. Howell, J. P., P. W. Dorfman, and S. Kerr. 1986. "Moderator Variables in Leadership Research." *Academy of Management Review* 11 (1): 88–102.

4. Kerr, S., and J. M. Jermier. 1978. "Substitutes for Leadership: Their Meaning and Measurement." *Organizational Behavior and Human Performance* 22 (3): 375–403.

5. Howell, J. P., and P. W. Dorfman. 1981. "Substitutes for Leadership: Test of a Construct." *Academy of Management Journal* 24 (4): 714–28.

6. Kerr, S., and J. W. Slocum. 1981. "Controlling the Performances of People in Organizations." In *Handbook of Organizational Design*, vol. 2, *Remodeling Organizations and Their Environments*, edited by P. C. Nystrom and W. H. Starbuck, 116–34. New York: Oxford University Press.

7. Baron, R. M., and D. A. Kenny. 1986. "The Moderator-Mediator Variable Distinction in Social Psychological Research: Conceptual, Strategic, and Statistical Considerations." *Journal of Personality and Social Psychology* 51 (6): 1173–82.

8. Yukl, G. 2013. *Leadership in Organizations*, 8th ed. Upper Saddle River, NJ: Prentice Hall.

9. Gardner, J. W. 1987. "Leaders and Followers." *Liberal Education* 73 (2): 4–6.

10. Rost, J. C. 1993. *Leadership for the Twenty-First Century*. Westport, CT: Praeger.

11. Kelley, R. 1988. "In Praise of Followers." *Harvard Business Review* 66 (6): 142–48.

12. Lewin, K. 1951. "Behavior and Development as a Function of the Total Situation." In *Field Theory in Social Science*, edited by D. Cartwright, 239–40. New York: Harper & Brothers.

13. Kruse, K. 2013. "What Is Leadership?" *Forbes*. Published April 9. www.forbes.com/sites/kevinkruse/2013/04/09/what-is-leadership/.

14. Chemers, M. M. 1997. *An Integrative Theory of Leadership*. Mahwah, NJ: Lawrence Erlbaum.

15. Leavitt, H. J. 1951. "Some Effects of Certain Communication Patterns on Group Performance." *Journal of Abnormal and Social Psychology* 46 (1): 38–50.

16. Day, D. V., and J. Antonakis. 2012. *The Nature of Leadership*, 2nd ed. Thousand Oaks, CA: Sage.

17. Howells, L. T., and S. W. Becker. 1962. "Seating Arrangement and Leadership Emergence." *Journal of Abnormal and Social Psychology* 64 (2): 148–50.

18. Shaw, M. E. 1981. *Group Dynamics: The Psychology of Small Group Behavior*, 3rd ed. New York: McGraw-Hill.

19. Sommer, R. 1967. "Leadership and Group Geography." *Sociometry* 24 (1): 99–110.

20. Gruenfeld, L. W., D. E. Rance, and P. Weissenberg. 1969. "The Behavior of Task Oriented (Low LPC) and Socially Oriented (High LPC) Leaders Under Several Conditions of Social Support." *Journal of Social Psychology* 79: 99–107.

21. Shartle, C. L. 1951. "Studies of Naval Leadership, Part I." In *Groups, Leadership and Men*, edited by H. Guetzkow, 119–33. Pittsburgh, PA: Carnegie Press.

22. Fiedler, F. E. 1964. "A Contingency Model of Leadership Effectiveness." In *Advances in Experimental Social Psychology*, vol. 1, edited by L. Berkowitz, 149–90. New York: Academic Press.

23. Fiedler, F. E., M. M. Chemers, and L. Mahar. 1978. *The Leadership Match Concept*. New York: Wiley.

24. Schermerhorn, J. R. 2014. *Management*, 13th ed. Hoboken, NJ: Wiley & Sons.

25. Hughes, R. L., R. C. Ginnett, and G. J. Curphy. 2010. "Contingency Theories of Leadership." In *Leading Organizations: Perspectives for a New Era*, 2nd ed., edited by G. R. Hickman, 101–21. Thousand Oaks, CA: Sage.

26. Fiedler, F. E., and J. E. Garcia. 1987. *New Approaches to Effective Leadership: Cognitive Resources and Organizational Performance*. New York: Wiley.

27. Rice, R. W. 1978. "Construct Validity of the Least Preferred Coworker Score." *Psychological Bulletin* 85 (6): 1199–214.

28. Northouse, P. G. 2013. *Leadership: Theory and Practice*, 6th ed. Los Angeles: Sage.

29. Fiedler, F. E. 1995. "Reflections by an Accidental Theorist." *Leadership Quarterly* 6 (4): 453–61.

30. Fiedler, F. E. 1967. *A Theory of Leadership Effectiveness*. New York: McGraw-Hill.

31. Peters, L. H., D. D. Hartke, and J. T. Pohlman. 1985. "Fiedler's Contingency Theory of Leadership: An Application of the Meta-analysis Procedures of Schmidt and Hunter." *Psychological Bulletin* 97 (2): 274–85.

32. Blanchard, K. H., D. Zigarmi, and R. Nelson. 1985. "Situational Leadership After 25 Years: A Retrospective." *Journal of Leadership Studies* 1 (1): 22–36.

33. Blanchard, K. H. 1985. *SLII: A Situational Approach to Managing People*. Escondido, CA: Blanchard Training and Development.

34. Ken Blanchard Company. 2017. "How We Help." Accessed May 19. www.kenblanchard.com/government/How-We-Help.

35. Blanchard, K. H., P. Zigarmi, and D. Zigarmi. 1985. *Leadership and the One Minute Manager: Increasing Effectiveness Through Situational Leadership*. New York: William Morrow.

36. Holsinger, J. W., Jr. 2008. "Situational Leadership Applied to the Dissertation Process." *Anatomical Sciences Education* 1 (5): 194–98.

37. Pawlina, W., M. J. Hromanik, T. R. Milanese, R. Dierkhising, T. R. Viggiano, and S. W. Carmichael. 2006. "Leadership and Professionalism Curriculum in the Gross Anatomy Course." *Annals of the Academy of Medicine of Singapore* 35 (9): 609–14.

38. Rabarison, K., R. C. Ingram, and J. W. Holsinger Jr. 2013. "Application of Situational Leadership to the National Voluntary Public Health Accreditation Process." *Frontiers in Public Health Reports* 1: 26.

39. Vecchio, R. P. 1987. "Situational Leadership Theory: An Examination of a Prescriptive Theory." *Journal of Applied Psychology* 72 (3): 444–51.

40. Vecchio, R. P., and K. Boatwright. 2002. "Preferences for Idealized Styles of Supervision." *Leadership Quarterly* 13 (4): 327–42.

41. Vecchio, R. P., R. C. Bullis, and D. M. Brazil. 2006. "The Utility of Situational Leadership Theory: A Replication in a Military Setting." *Small Group Leadership* 37 (5): 407–24.

42. Graeff, C. L. 1997. "Evolution of Situational Leadership Theory: A Critical Approach." *Leadership Quarterly* 8 (2): 153–70.

43. Fernandez, C. F., and R. P. Vecchio. 1997. "Situational Leadership Theory Revisited: A Test of an Across-Jobs Perspective." *Leadership Quarterly* 81 (1): 67–84.

44. Blanchard, K. H., D. Carew, and E. Parisi-Carew. 1990. *The One Minute Manager Builds High Performing Teams.* Escondido, CA: Blanchard Training and Development.

45. Public Health Accreditation Board (PHAB). 2017. "The Seven Steps of Public Health Department Accreditation." Accessed May 22. www.phaboard.org/accreditation-process/seven-steps-of-public-health-accreditation/.

PATH–GOAL THEORY AND THE VROOM-JAGO MODEL OF LEADERSHIP

James W. Holsinger Jr.

Learning Objectives

Upon completion of this chapter, you should be able to

- summarize the expectancy theory of motivation and explain its importance to the contingency theories of leadership,
- describe the roles of the leader in the path–goal theory of leadership,
- analyze the four leader behaviors of the path–goal theory and evaluate their importance to the theory,
- assess the personal characteristics of followers and explain their importance to the path–goal theory,
- explain the task structure of the path–goal theory,
- discuss the overall structure and use of the path–goal theory,
- analyze how the Vroom-Jago model of leadership relates to the contingency theories of leadership,
- identify the five decision procedures of the Vroom-Jago model and understand their importance to the model,
- explain the use of the seven diagnostic questions of the Vroom-Jago model,
- discuss the role of the situational variables in the Vroom-Jago model, and
- summarize the decision rules underlying the Vroom-Jago model and discuss their use in the decision tree.

Focus on Leadership Competencies

This chapter emphasizes the following Association of Schools and Programs of Public Health (ASPPH) leadership competencies:

(continued)

- Describe the attributes of leadership in public.
- Develop strategies to motivate others for collaborative problem solving, decision-making, and evaluation.
- Describe alternative strategies for collaboration and partnership among organizations, focused on public health goals.
- Create a shared vision.

It also addresses the following Council on Linkages public health leadership competency:

- Analyzes internal and external facilitators and barriers that may affect the delivery of the 10 Essential Public Health Services.

Note: See the appendix at the end of the book for complete lists of competencies.

Introduction

This chapter continues our study of the contingency theories of leadership, focusing specifically on the path–goal theory and, later, on the Vroom-Jago model of leadership. The path–goal theory was put forth initially by Georgopoulos, Mahoney, and Jones[1] in 1957 and further developed by Evans[2] and House[3] in the 1970s. It also has roots in the Ohio State leader-behavior approach[4] (discussed in chapter 4) and Vroom's expectancy theory of motivation.[5] It may be the most comprehensive and sophisticated of all the contingency theories.

The path–goal theory provides a mechanism for explaining the influence of leaders' behaviors on the performance and satisfaction of their followers. Unlike situational leadership, in which the leader adapts to the developmental level of the follower, or Fiedler's contingency model, which matches the leader's style and certain situational variables, the path–goal theory emphasizes the interaction between three elements: (1) the leader's style, (2) the follower's characteristics, and (3) the work setting within which the leader and follower relate. The path–goal theory is considered a contingency theory of leadership because of its focus on these groups of contingencies, as well as on the rewards that meet followers' needs.[6] Under the path–goal theory, leaders change their behavior to match the situation, and they seek to increase followers' motivation for reaching organizational and personal goals.

In laying the foundation for the theory, House[3] found that, by reducing pitfalls and roadblocks and by clarifying subordinates' direction for attaining work goals,

Effective Public Health Leaders . . .

. . . have their egos under control.

leaders were able to provide motivation that led to positive results. Later, he determined that subordinates will accept their leaders' behaviors when they determine that the behaviors will provide them with immediate satisfaction or are important to future satisfaction.[7] The path–goal theory's underlying assumption is that followers will be motivated if they believe they are capable of accomplishing their assigned work, conclude that their efforts will produce a specific outcome, and feel that the rewards for their work are beneficial. Thus, leaders can assist subordinates in meeting goals by using specific behaviors that best meet the subordinates' needs and match their work situations. When leaders select the appropriate style, the subordinates' expectations for satisfaction and success significantly increase.[8]

The Expectancy Theory of Motivation

The path–goal theory of leadership is based on Vroom's expectancy theory of motivation, which explains the means by which leaders are able to influence their followers' performance and satisfaction.[1,5] In 1964, Vroom introduced his expectancy theory, which combines the processes of leadership and motivation.

According to the expectancy theory, follower actions and behaviors are the result of conscious decisions made by the follower from among various options (e.g., a reward or no reward). In making these decisions, the follower determines the amount of effort to devote to a particular task at a certain point in time. A follower choosing between a minimal, moderate, or maximal effort must determine if a certain level of effort will produce a desirable outcome or an undesirable one. Desirable outcomes might include, for instance, a promotion, increased pay, recognition, or a sense of achievement. Undesirable outcomes might include heightened stress, termination, reprimand, or rejection. **Expectancy** is the probability of a certain outcome as perceived by the follower, whereas **valence** is the outcome's desirability.[9] Ledlow and Coppola[10(p52)] further explain that valence involves "the affective/emotional orientations that subordinates have regarding rewards based on outcomes" and the extent to which subordinates' motivation is extrinsic (e.g., money, promotion, time off) or intrinsic (e.g., satisfaction, self-esteem). Under the expectancy theory, leadership behavior seeks to influence the follower's perceptions in order to direct performance. Leaders must understand each follower's needs and wants well enough to know what rewards will best motivate each individual.

The key to the expectancy theory is that leaders have the responsibility to

expectancy
The perceived probability that a certain behavior will lead to a certain outcome.

valence
The perceived desirability of an outcome associated with a behavior.

Leadership Application Case: Making a Decision

The Leadership Application Case at the beginning of this book provides realistic scenarios for the application of key leadership concepts covered in the text. See the section marked "Chapter 5 Application" for the scenario and discussion questions that correspond with this chapter.

smooth the path for their followers by removing obstacles that might impede success. They are also expected to provide the appropriate resources to enable followers to perform at maximum capability. Leaders must fulfill the promises they make to followers and ensure that followers are appropriately rewarded for their performance. Followers will commit to pursuing prized outcomes only if they perceive that the outcomes can be obtained through honest effort and that they will succeed through such effort. Expectancy theory forms the substrate upon which the path–goal theory of leadership is constructed.

The Path–Goal Theory of Leadership

path–goal theory
An exchange theory of leadership that explains how contingent rewards function and how such rewards influence subordinates' satisfaction and motivation.

The **path–goal theory** is an exchange theory of leadership that explains how contingent rewards function and how such rewards influence subordinates' satisfaction and motivation.[11] Under the path–goal theory, the leader takes responsibility for increasing followers' motivation to reach organizational as well as personal goals. Leaders increase their followers' motivation through two means: (1) by clarifying their followers' path to reach the rewards that are available or (2) by augmenting the rewards valued and desired by their followers.[12] Clarifying the followers' path involves defining the requirements that each follower must meet in order to attain work outcomes. Followers must clearly understand their work roles, and the leader is responsible for clarifying them. As followers' knowledge increases, so too does the followers' confidence to achieve outcomes. Augmentation of the rewards involves efforts by the leader to learn the needs of the follower and match those needs to appropriate rewards. Leaders can make rewards contingent on satisfactory performance by the follower, and they have the ability to increase the value and size of the rewards.[2]

If a leader effectively clarifies the follower's path and augments the rewards, the follower will show increased motivation and will exert effort that results in the accomplishment of assigned work outcomes.[12] As such, the path–goal theory is based on the same assumptions as the expectancy theory of motivation: Fundamentally, the goal is a valued reward made available to followers by the leader, and the path is the best means by which the leader assists the follower to reach it.[13] The effective leader assists the follower both by removing obstacles to the follower's efforts and by providing the appropriate emotional support—applying both task and relationship behaviors as discussed in chapter 4. The leader's behavior strengthens the follower's expectations that, for a certain degree of effort, the follower will be able to complete the assigned tasks and thus gain a valued outcome. The result is an increase in the probability that the follower will meet the performance requirements.

In the next sections, we will address the three types of variables—leader behaviors, follower characteristics, and the situation—that conceptually make up the theory.

Leader Behaviors

Leaders influence followers' efforts through specific behaviors that contribute to the ability of followers to attain certain goals. Such supportive efforts include working to reduce follower boredom and work frustration, particularly during stressful periods; coaching; providing direction; and encouraging expectations that followers' efforts at task completion will be successful.[14] The use of path–goal leadership behaviors varies depending on the follower and the situation, and the behaviors are not needed in all cases.[15] In specific instances, one of the elements necessary for follower performance, satisfaction, and motivation may be missing, and the leader will have to provide that missing element. For instance, if the means and ends of a work situation are unclear or missing, the leader can enhance the follower's productivity by providing structure and delineating roles.[11] Alternatively, if the tasks and roles are clear, the leader can provide support and attention to meet the follower's needs for fulfilling relationships.[14]

The path–goal leadership theory identifies four types of leader behaviors: directive, supportive, participative, and achievement oriented.[13] **Directive leadership** behaviors involve telling followers what is to be accomplished, who is to accomplish it, where and when it should be done, and how the leader wants the task to be performed. Setting expectations, norms, and schedules are examples of directive leader behaviors. **Supportive leadership** behaviors demonstrate concern for the followers' well-being and for each individual's needs. They include being open and approachable, showing courtesy, and maintaining friendly interactions. **Participative leadership** behaviors involve sharing work problems with followers while soliciting recommendations, concerns, and suggestions to be considered in the decision-making process. These behaviors are similar to the group and consultative behaviors described by Vroom and Yetton.[16] **Achievement-oriented leadership** behaviors are both supporting and demanding. They set challenging goals for followers and seek to inspire confidence that followers can achieve desired results and assume additional responsibility in the future.[13]

The four types of leader behaviors are not personality traits but rather behavioral approaches that any leader can adopt and use as situations warrant. A leader might use each of the four behaviors with a single follower, or different behaviors with different followers. The behaviors, when properly suited to the motivational needs of the followers and to the situation, can improve the followers' acceptance of the leader, enhance the followers' satisfaction, and raise the followers' expectations that effective performance will result in valuable rewards.[13] In path–goal theory, as in situational leadership, the needs that motivate the followers are important, and the leader's impact is contingent on the followers' characteristics and their tasks.

directive leadership
A type of leadership behavior that involves telling followers what is to be accomplished, who is to accomplish it, where and when it should be done, and how the leader wants the task to be performed.

supportive leadership
A type of leadership behavior that involves demonstrating concern for the followers' well-being and for each individual's needs.

participative leadership
A type of leadership behavior that involves sharing work problems with followers and soliciting their input in the decision-making process.

achievement-oriented leadership
A type of leadership behavior that involves setting challenging goals for followers and interactions that are both supporting and demanding.

Follower Characteristics

The needs and personal characteristics of followers—including personality traits, skills and abilities, and expectations and perceptions about the work group's abilities—determine how they interpret the leader's behavior in a specific context and whether they find the leader's behavior to be a source of immediate or future satisfaction. These variables generally belong to two groups: (1) variables related to follower satisfaction and (2) variables related to followers' perception of their own abilities to complete a task.

Followers are more likely to actively support their leader if they perceive that the leader's actions will increase their own level of satisfaction. Follower characteristics related to satisfaction include preferences for structure in the work situation and need for affiliation. Under the path–goal theory, followers who have affiliation needs are more likely to derive satisfaction from supportive leadership, with its elements of friendliness and concern for others. Desire or need for control is another follower characteristic closely linked to satisfaction. People who desire to be in control of their life situations are said to have an internal locus of control, whereas people who believe they are at the mercy of chance or other people's actions have an external locus of control. Research has demonstrated a contingency relationship between followers' locus of control and the satisfaction they receive from participatory and directive leadership behaviors.[18] According to path–goal theory, followers who have an internal locus of control tend to prefer participative leadership, because it makes them feel that they are participating in decision making and are in charge of their work. Meanwhile, followers with an external locus of control respond well to directive leadership, because it is consistent with their belief that forces outside themselves are in control of their circumstances.

Followers' perceptions about their own skills and abilities to perform work tasks also influence how they interpret and respond to leadership behaviors. Followers who feel that their abilities are insufficient tend to respond best to directive leadership. This preference for directive leadership decreases for followers who have higher perceptions of their skills, abilities, and competence. For followers who feel they are fully capable of carrying out an assigned task, directive leadership can become superfluous and be perceived as overly controlling.[8] Such followers are likely to prefer a more participatory style.

The Situation

Under path–goal theory, the effects of a leader's behavior on the attitudes and behaviors of followers can be impacted or moderated by three variables

Consider This

"The task of leadership is not to put greatness into people, but to elicit it, for the greatness is there already."

—John Buchan[17]

What actions can leaders take that will help elicit their followers' greatness?

of the situation: (1) the design of the follower's task, (2) the formal authority structure of the organization, and (3) the characteristics of the primary work group. Each of these variables can influence the leadership situation by serving as a reward, acting as an independent motivational factor, or being a constraint on follower behavior.

The first variable, the design of the task, is based on the extent to which the task is defined for the followers. It is similar to the concept of task structure in Fiedler's contingency model (discussed chapter 4). Followers expect to have job descriptions that define their roles and outline their work procedures. If tasks are unclear or ambiguous, leaders must provide structure. If tasks are repetitive, leaders must provide support that maintains the followers' motivation. The second variable, the formal authority structure of the organization, is based on the degree to which leaders possess and use legitimate power, as well as the degree to which formal rules and policies constrict followers' behavior. When formal organizational authority is weak, effective leadership assists followers by establishing clear rules and work requirements. Finally, the characteristics of the primary work group, the third variable, include the levels of education possessed by the followers and the relationships and norms that exist within the group. In situations where work group norms are weak or followers do not support one another, effective leadership helps build group cohesiveness and role responsibility.

Linking the Path and the Goal

The path–goal theory links the follower's path to the goal to be reached. Although complex, the theory is remarkably pragmatic in nature. The exchange occurs when followers find that high productivity is a relatively easy path to attaining their personal goals. As a direct result, they become productive. When leaders assess the work situation and select an effective leadership behavior, they are able to influence the followers' effort-to-performance and performance-to-reward expectancies, as well as the outcome valences.[13] The result is an increase in the followers' levels of effort and, therefore, in the rewards they attain. In the end, the followers' performance and satisfaction increase, along with the followers' satisfaction with their leaders.

The path–goal theory suggests that leaders should choose a leadership style that fits the needs of the followers and their work. By using the appropriate style, leaders can help followers gain the confidence and skills they need to per-form their tasks and thereby attain the rewards that are available to them. When task characteristics are complex or ambiguous and work rules are unclear, and when follower characteristics are authoritarian or dogmatic in nature, leadership behavior should be directive, providing guidance and psychological support to the followers. Directive leadership behavior can clarify the path to the followers' reward, leading to increased effort and improvement in follower satisfaction and performance. Supportive leadership behavior can produce similar positive

Check It Out

For more information on the path–goal theory, read the summary by Donald Clark at www.nwlink. com/~donclark/leader/lead_path_goal.html.

outcomes in situations where tasks are repetitive, mundane, or unchallenging. In these situations, followers who are unsatisfied by their work may require affiliation, which can be accomplished through a human touch. Supportive leadership behavior can nurture followers and increase their confidence for achieving required work outcomes. In many cases, helping followers build confidence can be more important than urging them to develop more drive. When challenging work is unavailable, positive outcomes may be produced when the leader establishes challenging and complex goals, that may even be ambiguous, to be met by the followers. In such situations, followers may be characterized as needing to excel in order to meet their own high expectations. Participative leadership behavior can provide the type of leader involvement appropriate for followers who desire control and autonomy, particularly when they are dealing with tasks that are ambiguous, unclear, or even unstructured. Participative behavior can help provide clarity and, in turn, improve follower satisfaction and performance.

The use of rewards is a key component of the path–goal theory. Leaders are responsible for clarifying the path to the rewards that followers can expect, as well as for working to increase the quantity of rewards to enhance follower job satisfaction and performance. They also must assist followers to acquire the confidence and skills to perform their work-related tasks and thereby attain the rewards that are available to them. In some situations, leaders must design or acquire new rewards to meet the needs of certain followers.

Strengths and Weaknesses of the Theory

Although research dealing with the precepts of path–goal theory has been varied, some investigators have provided encouraging results.[19,20] The model provides leaders with a means for matching leadership behavior to situational contingencies and using that behavior to motivate followers, even though accurately predicting follower outcomes has proved difficult.[12]

The path–goal theory has a number of strengths. It gives leaders a useful behavioral framework for working with and coaching followers in an effort to affect the followers' satisfaction and performance in the workplace. Conceptually, it provides four types of leadership, moving the theory of leadership beyond simple relationship-oriented and task-oriented leadership behaviors.[21] Another key element in the theory is the understanding of how task characteristics and follower characteristics influence the effect that leadership behavior has on the performance of followers. This understanding helps leaders select a type of leadership behavior based on the needs of the follower and the work task at hand. Perhaps the greatest strength of the path–goal theory is its practical nature, in that it demonstrates specific behaviors by which leaders can assist their followers. The theory requires leaders to establish a clear path by which followers can reach their goals and to smooth the path by removing obstacles and by providing direction and coaching. The name of the theory states its purpose well.

The expectancy theory resides at the core of the path—goal theory, and it has been considered by some to be a strength[8] and by others a weakness.[9] Those considering it a strength note that no other leadership model deals so directly with the issue of follower motivation. Leaders who use the path—goal theory must focus on what is motivating their followers in order to choose the appropriate leadership behavior that will have the greatest effect on the followers. However, some people have criticized the path—goal theory for not explicitly describing how leadership is related to the requirements of the expectancy theory. The expectancy theory proposes that followers who feel competent and who trust that their work will produce results will be highly motivated, but the path—goal theory does not clearly establish how the various leader behaviors increase follower motivation. As a consequence, leaders using the path—goal theory may have difficulty understanding how their leadership will produce an effect on the work expectations of the followers.[8]

Although the path—goal theory was initially supported empirically,[15,22] including in a meta-analysis by Indvik,[23] later research has produced somewhat mixed results. A meta-analysis of the results for task and relationship behavior[24] and a review of the moderator variables[25] were inconclusive. When considering situational moderators, directive leadership was not supported, although followers with low ability appeared to be more highly satisfied with this form of leadership than were followers with high ability. The use of supportive behavior did not seem to correlate with follower satisfaction with the leader. For participatory and achievement-oriented leadership behaviors, research has been insufficient for drawing meaningful conclusions about the impact on follower performance. Some investigators have argued that research design limitations—as well as selectivity in the variables being studied—have made adequate testing of the theory nearly impossible.[9] Virtually no study has been inclusive in its design, and surrogates have been studied in place of the theory's specified situational variables. Thus, claims concerning the usefulness of the theory remain somewhat tentative. Research efforts have failed to demonstrate consistency among the theory's core assumptions.[21,26,27]

The theory's breadth and complexity, with its reliance on many variables, also present a weakness. Northouse[8(p123)] explains: "For example, path—goal theory makes predictions about which of four different leadership styles is appropriate for tasks with different degrees of structure, for goals with different levels of clarity, for workers at different levels of ability, and for organizations with different degrees of formal authority. To say the least, it is a daunting task to incorporate all of these factors simultaneously into one's selection of a preferred leadership style."

An important final criticism of the path–goal theory centers on the one-way nature of its use. Leaders are expected to coach, guide, and direct their followers to assist them in following a path to their goals. In this view, leaders are the most important factor in the equation and hold most of the responsibility for the leader–follower relationship, creating a significant imbalance. Such an arrangement can quickly become counterproductive if followers become dependent on the leader for the accomplishment of work, ultimately preventing them from becoming fully capable of completing the assigned tasks on their own.

Application of the Path–Goal Theory

The path–goal theory has played an important role in the continued study of leadership. Its conceptual framework has been useful to researchers looking to examine and explain situational variables relevant to the workplace, as well as to practitioners of leadership seeking insight into their behaviors and the effects of those behaviors on followers.

The path–goal theory, like other contingency theories of leadership, is based on the leader–follower–situation framework. Of the theory's key variables, only the primary work group fails to fit neatly into this approach. The theory's four types of leadership behavior and its approach to matching them with situational contingencies have proved useful for motivating followers. In general, the theory suggests that leaders should be directive when they assign complex tasks and supportive when they assign dull tasks. At the same time, it suggests that leaders use achievement-oriented behaviors when followers need to excel and participative behaviors when followers need control.[8] Leaders are responsible for building confidence in followers and for making sure that followers know that their efforts will be appropriately recognized by meaningful rewards. To the extent that it works to improve followers' satisfaction and work performance, the path–goal theory can be said to provide a pathway to follower success.

Effective Public Health Leaders . . .

. . . are responsible for building confidence in insecure followers.

The path–goal theory is considered useful even though it has limited research support and has received mixed reviews from a theoretical point of view. Yukl[9(p233)] writes, "Despite its limitations, path–goal theory has made an important contribution to the study of leadership by providing a conceptual framework to guide researchers in identifying potentially relevant situational variables." As Hughes, Ginnett, and Curphy[13] point out, effective public health leaders will look for a model of leadership that is practical and understandable and that can be easily applied in their own situations.

The Vroom-Jago Model of Leadership

Victor H. Vroom, who introduced the expectancy theory of motivation in the 1960s, later developed the **Vroom-Jago model of leadership**, another contingency theory of leadership. The Vroom-Jago model focuses on the degree to which a leader takes a participatory approach to leadership (i.e., involving followers in the decision-making process) or an autocratic approach (i.e., making the decision alone). The model begins with the need for the leader to make a decision based on a problem, and the use of a participatory or autocratic style is determined by the situation or context.

Earlier leadership research had demonstrated that the way a leader chooses to make decisions reflects forces within the leader, the subordinates, and the situation[28] and that, in selecting a decision-making procedure, the leader should consider not only the decision's quality requirements but also how likely the followers will be to accept it.[29] In 1973, Vroom and Yetton[16] developed a model that was based on this earlier work but also designated which decision-making procedures would be most effective in various situations. In 1988, Vroom and Jago revised the Vroom-Yetton model to create the Vroom-Jago model, which included additional decision rules and variables.[30] A key to understanding the Vroom-Jago model is recognizing that it was designed to assist leaders in making more effective decisions as well as in obtaining follower support for the decisions once the decisions are made.

Although the Vroom-Jago model is typically grouped in the contingency theory arena, Vroom has argued that it should not be included in the same category as Fiedler's model.[30] Fiedler's model is based on the characteristics of leaders and the ways that leaders interact with the situation, whereas the Vroom-Jago model is directed toward the situation at hand and the way leaders respond to it.[31] However, Vroom and Jago have stated that their model shares a similar perspective on behavioral contingencies with the path–goal theory.[32] Regardless of how the model is categorized, it does suggest that the leader's decision-making style is bound by the situation.

The Vroom-Jago model is normative in nature, because it prescribes the decision-making process of the leader. It informs the leader of the exact amount of follower participation that should be a part of a specific leader decision. As a result, it is narrower in focus than the other contingency models of leadership. The Vroom-Jago model has three components—(1) leader participation styles, (2) diagnostic questions used to analyze the decision, and (3) a set of decision rules—which will be discussed in the upcoming sections.

> **Vroom-Jago model of leadership**
> A contingency model of leadership that identifies various levels of participative leadership, with each level having an impact on the quality and accountability of the decision being made.

Consider This

"Leadership depends on the situation."
— Victor H. Vroom and Arthur G. Jago[32(p17)]

In the practice of effective public health leadership, how would you define the situation or context in which you practice?

Leader Participation Styles

The Vroom-Jago model identifies five decision procedures, or participation styles, with which leaders can make decisions involving followers. They include two autocratic styles, labeled Autocratic I (AI) and Autocratic II (AII); two consultative styles, labeled Consultative I (CI) and Consultative II (CII); and one group style, labeled Group II (GII). The five leader participation styles exist on a continuum, running from highly autocratic on one end (AI) to highly democratic on the other (GII). They range from a solo decision made by the leader (*decide*), to the inclusion of followers at some level (*consult individually* or *consult group*), to the complete engagement of the followers in the decision-making process or the decision itself (*facilitate* or *delegate*).[12] The leader chooses the appropriate style based on the situation at hand. Exhibit 5.1 provides more detailed descriptions of the decision procedures, and exhibit 5.2 depicts the styles on a continuum (based on Vroom's adaptation of Tannenbaum and Schmidt's taxonomy[33]).

EXHIBIT 5.1
Five Decision Procedures of the Vroom-Jago Model

Autocratic I (AI)	Using available information, leaders make the decision or solve the problem themselves.
Autocratic II (AII)	After obtaining the necessary information from individual followers, leaders make the decision to solve the problem themselves. In obtaining information, leaders may or may not tell the followers the nature of the problem. The followers' role is simply to provide the necessary information to the leader, not to develop solutions to the problem.
Consultative I (CI)	The leaders share the problem with the followers individually, obtaining both suggestions and ideas, but without convening the followers as a group. Leaders make the decision, and they do not have to use the followers' ideas or influence.
Consultative II (CII)	Leaders share the problem with the followers as a group, requesting their ideas and suggestions as a group. Leaders then make the decision, and they do not have to use the followers' ideas or influence.
Group II (GII)	Leaders share the problem with the followers as a group, and together they develop and evaluate alternative solutions to the problem. This action generates a consensus solution, with the leader serving as group chair. The leader makes no effort to influence the group to reach a preferred solution. The leader is willing to implement any solution supported by the group as a whole.

Source: Data from Vroom, V. H., and P. W. Yetton. 1973. *Leadership and Decision-Making*. Pittsburgh, PA: University of Pittsburgh Press.

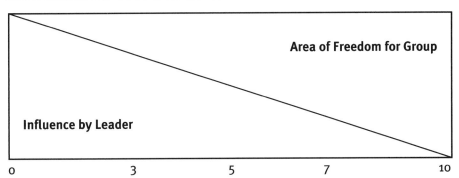

EXHIBIT 5.2

Vroom's Adaptation of Tannenbaum and Schmidt's Taxonomy

Decide	**Consult Individually**	**Consult Group**	**Facilitate**	**Delegate**
You make the decision alone and either announce or "sell" it to the group. You may use your expertise in collecting information that you deem relevant to the problem from the group or others.	You present the problem to the group members individually, get their suggestions, and then make the decision.	You present the problem to the group members in a meeting, get their suggestions, and then make the decision.	You present the problem to the group in a meeting. You act as facilitator, defining the problem to be solved and the boundaries within which the decision must be made. Your objective is to get concurrence on a decision. Above all, you take care to ensure that your ideas are not given any greater weight than those of others simply because of your position.	You permit the group to make the decision within prescribed limits. The group undertakes the identification and diagnosis of the problem, developing alternative procedures for solving it, and deciding on one or more alternative solutions. While you play no direct role in the group's deliberations unless explicitly asked, your role is an important one behind the scenes, providing needed resources and encouragement.

Source: Reprinted with permission from Vroom, V. 2000. "Leadership and the Decision-Making Process." *Organizational Dynamics* 28 (4): 82–94.

Diagnostic Questions

Under the Vroom-Jago model, the leader answers seven diagnostic questions to determine which decision-making process to use. The questions, which were developed from the situational factors in Vroom's earlier normative model,[33] are listed in exhibit 5.3. Although the seven diagnostic questions seem detailed, their use can quickly narrow the possibilities and direct the leader to the appropriate degree of follower participation in decision making.

The first diagnostic question deals with decision significance, which is the level of importance of the decision to the organization and the level of quality that the decision requires for a successful outcome. The central issue is, Does the decision require the active involvement of the leader? The second diagnostic question deals with the importance of the followers' commitment to carrying out the decision. If their engagement in the process is of high importance, more consultative decision making may be beneficial. The third question addresses the leader's level of expertise. If the leader's expertise on a matter is low, appropriate input from knowledgeable followers may be helpful in the decision-making process. The fourth question, about whether the followers would be committed to a decision made solely by the leader, can have a significant impact on the success of the decision. The fifth question deals with the group's support for the organization's goals. If this support is low, the leader should not allow the group to make the decision by itself. The sixth question focuses on the followers' level of knowledge and expertise about the problem being solved, and it helps determine the level of responsibility the followers should be granted. The seventh and final diagnostic question addresses the followers' level of competence in working together as a team. If this competence is high, the group can be granted greater responsibility in decision making.

In approaching the diagnostic questions, the leader should assess the situation with four aims in mind: (1) to improve the decision quality, (2) to improve follower involvement, (3) to reduce the time required to make the decision, and (4) to develop followers.[34] These same four points can be used as criteria for measuring the effectiveness of the decision.

Check It Out

For more information on the Vroom-Jago model of leadership, go to the Mind Tools summary at www.mindtools.com/pages/article/newTED_91.htm.

EXHIBIT 5.3
Seven Diagnostic Questions of the Vroom-Jago Model

1. Decision significance	What is the decision's level of significance for the organization or project?
2. Importance of commitment	What is the level of importance of the followers' commitment to carrying out the decision?
3. Leader expertise	What is the leader's level of expertise in relation to the problem?
4. Likelihood of commitment	If the leader made the decision alone, would the followers have a high or low commitment to the decision?
5. Group support for goals	How strong is the followers' support for the organization or team objectives at stake in the decision?
6. Goal expertise	What is the level of knowledge and expertise among the followers in relation to the problem?
7. Team competence	What is the group's level of skill and commitment to working as a team to solve the problem?

Source: Data from Daft, R. L. 2015. *The Leadership Experience*, 6th ed., 82–83. Stamford, CT: Cengage Learning.

Situational Variables

The Vroom-Jago model is one of the contingency models of leadership, so situational variables play a significant role. Key variables include (1) the quantity of pertinent information possessed by leaders and followers, (2) the probability that followers will accept an autocratic decision by their leaders, (3) the probability that followers will cooperate if their leaders allow them to participate, (4) the level of disagreement among the followers based on their preferred alternatives, and (5) the degree to which the problem requiring a decision is unstructured and creativity is required to solve it. Vroom and Jago[34(p174)] write that a leader "will be more participative when the problem is important, when subordinate commitment is required, when the leader lacks certain relevant information or expertise, when the problem is unstructured, when it is unlikely that subordinates will commit to a decision made autocratically, when subordinates share the organization's goals, when subordinate conflict is unlikely, and when subordinate information is high." Some studies have demonstrated that followers prefer variability in the leader's style rather than the consistent use of a single style.[35]

Decision Acceptance

The acceptance of a decision is based on the commitment of the leader and the followers to effectively implement it. Acceptance is a critical issue if the success of a decision depends on followers' actions and their motivation in the workplace. Followers' acceptance of a decision can be increased if the leader effectively uses personal influence or if the decision is known to be beneficial to the followers. Followers are less likely to accept an autocratic decision if they resent being excluded from the decision-making process or if the decision is considered inimical to their interests. Typically, we can assume that decision acceptance will increase with follower participation and that followers will be more motivated to implement decisions as their influence in the process increases. The model predicts that a consultative process will produce greater acceptance than an autocratic process but that joint decision making will produce greater acceptance than consultation.[9]

Decision Rules

Underlying the Vroom-Jago model is a set of seven decision rules, initially put forth by Vroom and Yetton[16(pp32–34)]:

1. The Leader Information Rule: "If the quality of the decision is important and if [leaders do] not possess enough information or expertise to solve the problem by [themselves], AI is eliminated from the feasible set."

2. The Trust Rule: "If the quality of the decision is important and if subordinates cannot be trusted to base their efforts to solve the problem on organizational goals, GII is eliminated from the feasible set."

3. The Unstructured Problem Rule: "When the quality of the decision is important, if [leaders] lack the necessary information or expertise to solve the problem [themselves], and if the problem is unstructured, . . . the method used must provide not only for [them] to collect the information but to do so in an efficient manner . . . with interaction among all subordinates with a full knowledge of the problem. . . . Under these conditions, AI, AII, and CI are eliminated from the feasible set."

4. The Acceptance Rule: "If the acceptance of the decision by subordinates is critical to effective implementation, and if it is not certain that an autocratic decision made by the leader would receive that acceptance, AI and AII are eliminated from the feasible set."

5. The Conflict Rule: "If the acceptance of the decision is critical, an autocratic decision is not certain to be accepted, and subordinates are likely to be in conflict or disagreement over the appropriate decision . . . AI, AII, and CI are eliminated from the feasible set."

6. The Fairness Rule: "If the quality of decision is unimportant, and if acceptance is critical and not certain to result from an autocratic decision, AI, AII, CI, and CII are eliminated from the feasible set."

7. The Acceptance Priority Rule: "If acceptance is critical, not assured by an autocratic decision, and if subordinates can be trusted, AI, AII, CI, and CII are eliminated from the feasible set."

Putting the Model Together

When the decision rules are applied in conjunction with the seven diagnostic questions, a decision tree develops, as shown in exhibit 5.4.[36] The seven questions are at the top of the matrix, and the answers to the questions, guided by the rules, create a pathway that determines the decision-making style to be used. All five styles appear at the right side of the matrix.

Significant refinement of the Vroom-Jago model has occurred in the decades since it was first introduced. As a result, two approaches to the model have emerged—one based on time constraints in the decision-making process and the other based on the development of the followers. In applying the model, the leader initially considers the organization's need for timeliness in making the required decision compared to the organization's need for follower development.

With a Focus on Time Constraints

A time-based decision matrix is used when the leader is dealing with a crisis or another situation in which the timeliness of the decision is of high importance.

EXHIBIT 5.4

Vroom-Jago
Decision Model
(Emergency
Situations)

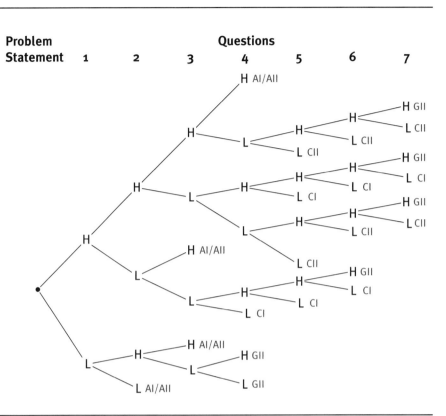

Problem Statement   **Questions**   1   2   3   4   5   6   7

Note: H = high; L = low; AI/AII = decide; CI = consult (individually); CII = consult (group); GII = facilitate/delegate.

Source: Data from Vroom, V. H., and P. W. Yetton. 1973. *Leadership and Decision-Making*. Pittsburgh, PA: University of Pittsburgh Press.

For instance, this approach would be used if a public health leader is faced with a major natural disaster and needs to make a decision about mobilization of emergency personnel. To begin the process, the leader engages on the left side of the model—with the first diagnostic question—and considers the problem to be addressed. The leader then moves through the model from left to right, answering the diagnostic questions in sequence to arrive at a leadership style. The answer to each question is either "high" or "low."

    In an emergency situation, the leader's answer to the first diagnostic question (What is the decision's level of significance for the organization or project?) would be expected to be "high." If the answer to the second question (What is the level of importance of the followers' commitment to carrying out the decision?) is "high" as well, the leader moves to the third question (What is the leader's level of expertise in relation to the problem?). At this point, a leader who possesses the expertise to deal with the emergency would answer "high," whereas a leader who lacks expertise would answer "low." If the answer is "high," the leader then considers the fourth question (If the leader made the decision alone, what is the likelihood that the followers would be committed to the decision?). If the answer is once again "high," the leader chooses an autocratic style (AI or AII), making the decision unilaterally and announcing it to the followers for implementation.

In the same scenario, if the answer to question 4 is "low," the leader moves on to the next question. If the answer to the fifth question (How strong is the followers' support for the organization or team objectives at stake in the decision?) is "low," the leader chooses to consult (CII) with the group as a whole. Should the answer to the fifth question be "high," the leader moves to the sixth question (What is the level of knowledge and expertise among the followers in relation to the problem?). If the group's expertise is "low," the leader moves immediately to consult with the group as a whole. But if the group's expertise is "high," the leader moves to the seventh question (What is the group's level of skill and commitment to working as a team to solve the problem?), about team competence. If team competence is "high," the leader chooses to delegate to the group (GII); if team competence is considered "low," the leader consults with the group as a whole.

Returning to the third question, if the leader's expertise is considered "low," the decision tree directs us down a different pathway. The leader next goes to the fourth question, dealing with the likelihood of follower commitment. If that likelihood is deemed "high," the leader moves to the fifth question, dealing with the group's support for the goals. If group support is "low," the leader consults (CI) with the group members individually to engage them in the process. The leader also consults individually if the answers to the sixth and seventh questions are low. Should the answer to the fifth, sixth, and seventh questions all be "high," the leader facilitates the group in solving the problem. The decision tree offers additional pathways if the answers to the first and second questions are "low."

With a Focus on Follower Development

In other instances that are less time sensitive and have a greater emphasis on follower development—for instance, when a public health leader is looking to develop a new program—the leader uses a development-driven model. Again, the leader begins at the left side of the model and answers the first question, about the decision's level of significance. If the significance is "high," the leader moves to the second question, about the importance of follower commitment. If the focus is on follower development, leader expertise is not an issue, so the third question can be skipped. If the answer to the fourth question, concerning the likelihood of follower commitment, is "high" and the answers to the fifth, sixth, and seventh questions are likewise "high," the leader delegates the work, within certain limits, to the group of followers, thereby using the problem for follower developmental purposes. If the answers to the fifth, sixth, and seventh questions are "low," the leader facilitates the group to continue follower development. If the answer to the fourth question is "low," and if the answers to the fifth, sixth, and seventh questions are "high," the leader delegates the work. The decision tree presents different courses if the answer to the second question is "low."

Leadership styles in the development-driven model are generally delegating, facilitating, or group consulting. If the emphasis is on developing followers, the only time an autocratic leadership style is used is when the answer to the first question, about decision significance, is "low." If the answer to the second question, concerning the importance of follower commitment, is also "low," no follower development is possible, and the leader simply makes the decision. Similarly, if the answer to the fourth question, about the likelihood of follower commitment to the leader's decision, is "high," follower development is unlikely, since the followers would be just as happy if the leader made the decision; in such an instance, the leader simply makes the decision. If the answer to the fourth question indicates that the followers would be less likely to accept a decision made by the leader, the leader allows the followers to make the decision, within certain limits.

Strengths and Weaknesses of the Model

The strengths of the Vroom-Jago model are borne in several directions. The model clearly stresses that decisions are made within a situation or context, and it recognizes the aspects of the situation or context that temper the relationship between outcomes and behavior.[9] The model encompasses a broad range of leadership styles for making decisions, and it includes both leaders and followers in the decision-making process.[10] The accuracy and quality of decisions increase with follower involvement, and the Vroom-Jago model calls for such involvement consistently, except when strict time constraints intervene. Since the model is prescriptive in nature, it can help leaders learn how to address specific situations, and it can guide leaders to appropriate leadership styles for difficult decisions. Among the contingency theories of leadership, the Vroom-Jago model, with its focus on specific characteristics of follower behavior, is the best supported empirically.

However, the model also has conceptual weaknesses. First, it treats a decision as a single circumstance, even though, in reality, tough decisions usually involve a number of people and meetings over an extended period. The chance that leaders will have to deal with revisions to solutions for major problems means that they may have to engage the model multiple times within a sequential decision-making episode. In addition, Yukl[9] criticizes the model for having five leadership styles and finds little difference between AI and AII and between CI and CII. As an alternative, Yukl suggests distinguishing instead between the three core categories of autocratic, consultative, and joint decision procedures. Another potential weakness is that the model assumes that leaders possess the skills to use the various processes, even though certain aspects may not be valid for unskilled leaders.[37] Finally, the Vroom-Jago model involves only a relatively small part of leadership.[9]

In short, the Vroom-Jago model, like other leadership theories, has both positive and negative aspects. Still, if effective public health leaders engage the model to assist with decision making, they will likely find that the benefits justify the time spent developing the skills needed for its use. The model provides an opportunity to develop followers, particularly as they work in groups, into effective problem-solving teams, and it lends itself well to efforts to provide training to new and emerging leaders in public health. Owing to its emphasis on the situational aspects of leadership, the Vroom-Jago model may be integrated with situational leadership to produce an effective approach for leaders. Training is readily available for both models, and such training is frequently offered within organizations.

Case Study: Comprehensive Community Health Needs Assessments in Kane County, Illinois

To meet Internal Revenue Service requirements, nonprofit hospitals must conduct regular community health needs assessments and implement community health improvement plans. At the same time, health departments also must conduct these assessments to meet many of their mandated functions, as well as to achieve accreditation. Such requirements, if not well coordinated, can create excessive duplication and waste, which can make citizens and leaders hesitant to participate and thus less fully engaged in health assessment and improvement. To remedy these concerns, many localities are developing more collaborative approaches to community health needs assessment and improvement planning. One such place is Kane County, an Illinois county just west of Chicago with more than half a million residents. In addition to the local health department, Kane County has five hospitals and a number of civic organizations vested in health improvement efforts.

Dr. Paul Kuehnert is a former Kane County Health Department executive director and county health officer who currently serves as an assistant vice president with the Robert Wood Johnson Foundation. He learned that the county's hospitals were spending in excess of $60,000 on their needs assessments and that the county's two largest United Way organizations, as well as the health department and the local community mental health board, were spending similar amounts. Recognizing an opportunity for greater interorganizational collaboration and sharing of resources, Kuehnert worked to align the resources of the health department with those of each of the local hospitals, the United Way organizations, and the mental health board. In doing so, the county was able to produce a much more comprehensive, meaningful, and informative assessment, with each organization investing approximately $20,000. In addition to saving significant human and financial resources, the collaborative assessment also helped health and civic leaders to discern and address health problems that they had not previously identified, such as high rates of smoking among low-income Latino men.

Discussion and Application Questions

1. How did effective public health leadership improve community health needs assessments and planning in Kane County?
2. What characteristics of effective public health leaders were demonstrated in this case?
3. How might the style of leadership shown in this case be effectively leveraged toward other collaborative activities?
4. Imagine you are leading your community through a health needs assessment. Which of the contingency theories of leadership would you use to accomplish the task?

Summary

The contingency theories of leadership practice are based on the leader's need to understand the context or situation in the workplace. Like other contingency theories, the two examined in this chapter—the path–goal theory and the Vroom-Jago model—are based on the leader–follower–situation framework.

The path–goal theory of leadership has roots in Vroom's expectancy theory of motivation, which explains the means by which leaders can influence followers' performance and satisfaction. Under the expectancy theory, leaders have the responsibility to smooth the path for their followers by removing obstacles that might impede success and by providing resources to enable followers to perform at maximum capability. The path–goal theory builds on the expectancy theory and explains how contingent rewards function and how such rewards influence subordinates' satisfaction and motivation.

The path–goal theory centers on the interaction between leader behaviors, follower characteristics, and the situation. It identifies four types of leader behaviors: directive leadership, supportive leadership, participative leadership, and achievement-oriented leadership. These four types are not personality traits but rather behavioral approaches that any leader can adopt as needed.

Follower characteristic variables generally belong to two groups: those related to follower satisfaction and those related to followers' perception of their own abilities to complete a task. Key variables of the situation include the design of the task, the formal authority structure of the organization, and the characteristics of the primary work group. The path–goal theory suggests that leaders should choose a leadership style that fits the needs of the followers and their work situation. By using the appropriate style, leaders can help followers gain the confidence and skills they need to perform their tasks and thereby attain the rewards that are available to them. Clearly, this theory is useful for public health leaders not only in the workplace but also in their engagement with constituents and collaborators.

The Vroom-Jago model of leadership is also useful for public health leaders, specifically as a means for making decisions. The model begins with the need for the leader to make a decision based on a problem, and the situation or context determines the degree to which the leader uses a participatory or autocratic decision-making style. The Vroom-Jago model identifies five leader participation styles—Autocratic I (AI), Autocratic II (AII), Consultative I (CI), Consultative II (CII), and Group II (GII)—that range from highly autocratic to highly democratic. The leader uses a series of diagnostic questions and a set of decision rules to determine which of the participation styles best suits the situation and the followers' needs. Different approaches are available depending on whether the focus is on time constraints or follower development.

Discussion Questions

1. What is the basis for including the path–goal theory and the Vroom-Jago model in the contingency family of leadership theories?
2. Define the terms *valence* and *expectancy*, and explain their use in the expectancy theory of motivation.
3. In implementing the path–goal theory of leadership, what is the role of the situation or context?
4. Explain the use and importance of the leader behaviors in the path–goal theory.
5. Identify the key personal characteristics of followers in the path–goal theory. What role do they play in the use of the theory by effective public health leaders?
6. Describe the decision procedures in the Vroom-Jago model and explain their use.
7. What purpose do the diagnostic questions serve in the Vroom-Jago model?

8. How do the various parts of the Vroom-Jago model interact in the decision tree?

9. Give examples of how effective leaders can use the Vroom-Jago model in the practice of public health.

10. For deeper thought: As the commissioner of health of a mid-sized Southern city, you are faced with an outbreak of the Zika virus. Describe how you could use the path–goal theory of leadership in providing leadership to your director of epidemiology.

Web Resources

Clark, D. 2015. "Path–Goal Leadership Theory." Updated September 9. www.nwlink. com/~donclark/leader/lead_path_goal.html.

Decision Making Confidence. 2016. "Vroom-Jago Decision Model." Accessed May 15, 2017. www.decision-making-confidence.com/vroom-jago-decision-model.html.

References

1. Georgopoulos, B. S., G. M. Mahoney, and N. W. Jones. 1957. "A Path–Goal Approach to Productivity." *Journal of Applied Psychology* 41 (6): 345–53.

2. Evans, M. G. 1970. "The Effects of Supervisory Behavior on the Path–Goal Relationship." *Organizational Behavior and Human Performance* 5 (3): 277–98.

3. House, R. J. 1971. "A Path–Goal Theory of Leader Effectiveness." *Administrative Science Quarterly* 16 (3): 321–39.

4. Stogdill, R. M., and A. E. Coons (eds.). 1951. *Leader Behavior: Its Description and Measurement*. Columbus, OH: Ohio State University Bureau of Business Research.

5. Vroom, V. H. 1964. *Work and Motivation*. New York: John Wiley.

6. Evans, M. G. 1974. "Leadership." In *Organizational Behavior*, edited by S. Kerr, 230–33. Columbus, OH: Grid.

7. House, R. J., and G. Dessler. 1974. "The Path–Goal Theory of Leadership: Some Post Hoc and A Priori Tests." In *Contingency Approaches to Leadership*, edited by J. Hunt and L. Larson, 29–55. Carbondale, IL: Southern Illinois University Press.

8. Northouse, P. G. 2016. *Leadership: Theory and Practice*, 7th ed. Los Angeles: Sage.

9. Yukl, G. 2013. *Leadership in Organizations*, 8th ed. Upper Saddle River, NJ: Prentice Hall.

10. Ledlow, G. R., and M. N. Coppola. 2014. *Leadership for Health Professionals: Theory, Skills, and Applications*, 2nd ed. Sudbury, MA: Jones & Bartlett Learning.

11. Bass, B. M. 2008. *The Bass Handbook of Leadership: Theory, Research, and Managerial Applications*, 4th ed. New York: Free Press.

12. Daft, R. L. 2015. *The Leadership Experience*, 6th ed. Mason, OH: South-Western.

13. Hughes, R. L., R. C. Ginnett, and G. J. Curphy. 2010. "Contingency Theories of Leadership." In *Leading Organizations: Perspectives for a New Era*, 2nd ed., edited by G. R. Hickman, 101–21. Thousand Oaks, CA: Sage.

14. Fiedler, F. E., and R. J. House. 1988. "Leadership: A Report of Progress." In *International Review of Industrial and Organizational Psychology*, edited by C. Cooper, 73–92. Greenwich, CT: JAI Press.

15. House, R. J., and T. R. Mitchell. 1974. "Path–Goal Theory of Leadership." *Journal of Contemporary Business* 3: 81–97.

16. Vroom, V. H., and P. W. Yetton. 1973. *Leadership and Decision-Making*. Pittsburgh, PA: University of Pittsburgh Press.

17. Edberg, H. 2017. "50 Inspiring Leadership Quotes." *Positivity Blog*. Accessed February 6. www.positivityblog.com/index.php/2007/07/06/25-great-quotes-on-leadership/.

18. Mitchell, T. R., C. M. Smyser, and S. E. Weed. 1975. "Locus of Control: Supervision and Work Satisfaction." *Academy of Management Journal* 18 (3): 623–31.

19. Greene, C. 1979. "Questions of Causation in the Path–Goal Theory of Leadership." *Academy of Management Journal* 22 (1): 22–41.

20. Schriesheim, C., and M. A. Von Glinow. 1977. "The Path–Goal Theory of Leadership: A Theoretical and Empirical Analysis." *Academy of Management Journal* 20 (3): 398–405.

21. Jermier, J. M. 1996. "The Path–Goal Theory of Leadership: A Subtextual Analysis." *Leadership Quarterly* 7 (3): 311–16.

22. Schriesheim, C. A., and S. Kerr. 1974. "Psychometric Properties of the Ohio State Leadership Scales." *Psychological Bulletin* 81 (11): 756–65.

23. Indvik, J. 1986. "Path–Goal Theory of Leadership: A Meta-analysis." In *Proceedings of the 46th Annual Meeting of the Academy of Management*, edited by J. A. Pearce and R. B. Robinson, 189–92. Chicago: Academy of Management.

24. Wofford, J., and L. Z. Liska. "Path–Goal Theories of Leadership: A Meta-analysis." *Journal of Management* 19 (4): 857–76.

25. Podsakoff, P. M., S. B. MacKenzie, M. Ahearne, and W. H. Bommer. 1995. "Searching for a Needle in a Haystack: Trying to Identify the Illusive Moderators of Leadership Behaviors." *Journal of Management* 21 (3): 423–70.

26. Evans, M. G. 1996. "R. J. House's 'A Path–Goal Theory of Leader Effectiveness.'" *Leadership Quarterly* 7 (3): 305–9.

27. Schriesheim, C. A., and L. L. Neider. 1996. "Path–Goal Leadership Theory: The Long and Winding Road." *Leadership Quarterly* 7 (3): 317–21.

28. Tannenbaum, R., and W. H. Schmidt. 1958. "How to Choose a Leadership Pattern." *Harvard Business Review* 36 (2): 95–101.

29. Maier, N. R. F. 1963. *Problem-Solving Discussions and Conferences: Leadership Methods and Skills.* New York: McGraw-Hill.

30. Sternberg, R. J., and V. H. Vroom. 2002. "The Person Versus Situation in Leadership." *Leadership Quarterly* 13 (3): 301–23.

31. Day, D. V., and J. Antonakis. 2012. *The Nature of Leadership*, 2nd ed. Thousand Oaks, CA: Sage.

32. Vroom, V. H., and A. G. Jago. 2007. "The Role of the Situation in Leadership." *American Psychologist* 62 (1): 17–24.

33. Vroom, V. H. 2000. "Leadership and the Decision-Making Process." *Organizational Dynamics* 28 (4): 82–94.

34. Vroom, V. H., and A. G. Jago. 1995. "Situation Effects and Levels of Analysis in the Study of Leader Participation." *Leadership Quarterly* 6 (2): 169–81.

35. Schuller, J. J. 1982. "Follower Acceptance of Variability of Leadership Style in Decision-Making." PhD diss., Michigan State University.

36. McDermott, D. 2017. "Vroom-Jago Decision Model." Decision Making Confidence. Accessed May 15. www.decision-making-confidence.com/vroom-jago-decision-model.html.

37. Crouch, A., and P. W. Yetton. 1988. "The Management Team: An Equilibrium Model for Management Performance and Behavior." In *Emerging Leadership Vistas*, edited by J. G. Hunt, B. R. Baliga, and C. A. Schriesheim, 107–28. Lexington, MA: Lexington Books.

6

THE LEADER–MEMBER EXCHANGE THEORY

William A. Mase and James W. Holsinger Jr.

Learning Objectives

Upon completion of this chapter, you should be able to

- employ the leader–member exchange (LMX) theory of organizational leadership,
- interpret trust as it relates to public health practice,
- explain the importance of dyadic pairs in public health practice,
- discuss the measurement of trust,
- describe the Conditions of Trust Inventory (CTI) measurement tool,
- compare and contrast the in-group and out-group concepts,
- explain how the in-group and out-group concepts affect individuals,
- describe the stages in the development of LMX theory,
- discuss the impact of organizational citizenship behavior on the mission of a public health organization, and
- summarize the impact of job tension on public health practitioners and organizations.

Focus on Leadership Competencies

This chapter emphasizes the following Association of Schools and Programs of Public Health (ASPPH) leadership competencies:

- Describe the attributes of leadership in public health.
- Develop strategies to motivate others for collaborative problem solving, decision-making, and evaluation.
- Create a shared vision.
- Describe alternative strategies for collaboration and partnership among organizations, focused on public health goals.

(continued)

It also addresses the following Council on Linkages public health leadership competency:

- Analyzes internal and external facilitators and barriers that may affect the delivery of the 10 Essential Public Health Services.

Note: See the appendix at the end of the book for complete lists of competencies.

leader–member exchange (LMX) theory
A leadership model in which the leader develops exchange agreements with each follower and the quality of each exchange relationship influences the follower's performance, decisions, responsibilities, and access to resources; also called *vertical dyad linkage theory.*

trust
Belief or faith in another individual; a fundamental and foundational tenet of human relationships.

dyadic pair
A unit of analysis consisting of a leader (manager) and a follower (subordinate) within the work environment.

sponsorship
The degree to which the leader supports or backs a follower.

Introduction

The contingency theories of leadership, as discussed in chapters 4 and 5, approach the study of leadership with an emphasis on the behavioral interactions among the individuals within the work situation. In this chapter, we turn our attention to the **leader–member exchange (LMX) theory** (also called *vertical dyad linkage theory*). LMX theory, like the contingency theories, considers the interactional aspects of actors within organizations; however, it also introduces organizational structure as a determinant of how leadership should be practiced. At the center of LMX theory are the leader and follower roles, the exchange relationship that develops between them, and the **trust** that exists between pairs of people within the work situation.[1,2] Many leadership theories have examined leadership from the vantage point of the leader or the followers, and some have implied that "leadership" is simply what leaders do to followers. LMX theory, however, shifts attention toward the interactions that occur between the leader and each of the leader's followers, and it provides a rubric by which organizational relationships, specifically those between leaders (managers) and followers (subordinates), can be analyzed and understood. The unit of analysis for the theory is the **dyadic pair**, which consists of a leader and a follower within the work environment.

Under LMX theory, the network of trust relationships in the work setting is key to the successful accomplishment of work. Trust can be measured using a validated tool such as the Conditions of Trust Inventory, which considers the dimensions of availability, competence, consistency, discreetness, fairness, integrity, loyalty, openness, promise fulfillment, and receptivity. Related to trust is the concept of **sponsorship**, which refers to an outward manifestation of support provided by a leader toward the efforts of a follower. Stated simply, it is the degree to which the leader supports or backs the follower.

LMX theory first began to appear in the leadership literature in the mid-1970s.[3] Since that time, a growing body of research has added depth to the theory through higher-level analysis of interactions, expansion to a variety of workplace settings, and multidimensional explanations of relationship patterns. A number of researchers during the 1990s conducted workforce analysis, typically in manufacturing organizations and the for-profit workforce sector, to advance the application of LMX theory.

Given its focus on the network of trust relationships within organizations, LMX theory is especially applicable to the field of public health. Public health organizations vary in size and scope, but each organization's environment consists of numerous vertical dyadic pairs of leaders (managers) and followers (subordinates). These dyads are the building blocks of the public health organization and the basis on which public health goals are accomplished. At the primary public health organizational level, dyadic pairs can consist of a leader and such individuals as a sanitarian, a nurse, an area director, an epidemiologist, a health commissioner, or a health educator. In addition, dyads in public health organizations extend beyond traditional employees to include such constituents and collaborators as members of boards of health, volunteers, and affiliated health and human services practitioners. In providing a unit of analysis for LMX theory, the leader–follower dyads transcend the individual and serve as proxy measures for the trust that exists within the larger organization and community. LMX theory may also be used with the public health organization serving as the unit of analysis.

In LMX theory, the leader does not use a common leadership style for all members of the group. Rather, the leader practices **individualized leadership**, based on the individual needs of followers in relationship to the leader. Every follower is part of a unique leader–follower relationship, and this dyadic relationship determines the behavior of the leader with the follower and the follower's response to the leader. Within each relationship, an exchange occurs, with the leader and the follower providing something to one another.[5,6]

Individualized Leadership

As LMX theory has been refined over the years, distinct stages in the development of individualized leadership have been identified (see exhibit 6.1). The first stage is **vertical dyad linkage (VDL)**, marked by an awareness that

---

Effective Public Health Leaders . . .

. . . understand that their relationships with followers are important for the creation of effective work environments.

Consider This

"Virtually every study of human happiness reveals that satisfying close relationships constitute the very best thing in life; there is nothing people consider more meaningful and essential to their mental and physical well-being than their close relationships with other people."

—Ellen Berscheid[4(p260)]

How do you think this kind of relationship can be established between public health leaders and their followers?

---

individualized leadership
Use of leadership styles appropriate for each follower, rather than a style that is common for all members of the group.

vertical dyad linkage (VDL)
The pairing of leader (manager) and each follower (subordinate) in an individual relationship.

EXHIBIT 6.1
Stages of
Individualized
Leadership

Stage 1
Vertical Dyad Linkage

Followers are impacted differently by the behavior and traits of leaders resulting in out-groups and in-groups.

Stage 2
Leader–Member Exchange

Leaders develop individualized leadership styles for each subordinate, and for each dyad relationship a unique exchange occurs that is independent of other leader–follower dyads.

Stage 3
Partnership Building

A positive exchange is created for each follower by the leader with a resulting increase in performance.

Source: Data from Graen, G. B., and M. Uhl-Bien. 1995. "Relationship-Based Approach to Leadership: Development of Leader–Member Exchange (LMX) Theory of Leadership over 25 Years: Applying a Multi-Level Multi-Domain Approach." *Leadership Quarterly* 6 (2): 219–47.

partnership building
A stage in individualized management marked by a positive exchange between the leader and each follower, with a resulting increase in follower performance.

in-group
A category of vertical dyad linkage in which the follower has a high degree of exchange with the leader and takes on extra roles and responsibilities in the work setting.

out-group
A category of vertical dyad linkage in which the follower has a low degree of exchange with the leader and takes on defined roles according to a formal employment arrangement.

individual relationships exist between the leader and each follower, rather than just between the leader and the group of followers as a whole. The next stage occurs when individualized leadership for each follower is based on the unique exchange that develops between the two members of the dyad, independent of other pairs. The final stage, **partnership building**, is based on the leader's purposeful efforts to develop partnerships with each individual follower in the group.[7] When partnership building has occurred, a positive exchange occurs between the leader and each follower, with a resulting increase in follower performance.

Vertical Dyad Linkage, In-Groups, and Out-Groups

The initial version of LMX theory was based on Graen and Cashman's[2] vertical dyad linkage theory, in which a vertical linkage is developed between the leader and each individual follower.[6] Each member of the work group is related to the leader through a vertical dyad, and each relationship has its own characteristics, based on both positive and negative interactions.[8] These relationships result in assignment of each follower either to an **in-group** or to an **out-group** within the work setting. Individuals with in-group status are understood to have high LMX, and they are likely to be offered better work assignments, to have more input in decision making, and to receive greater compensation for their work efforts. Conversely, individuals with out-group status tend to be lower in LMX and have more limited opportunities in the workplace.

The followers in in-group and out-group relationships have different experiences with the same leader. In-group followers tend to describe relationships based on a high level of trust and respect, with the leader and follower sharing a mutual obligation to the relationship. Out-group followers, meanwhile, often feel a low level of trust and respect and little in the way of mutual obligation. In-group followers find their relationships to be high in both task and people orientation, whereas out-group followers experience lower levels of both. Leaders typically use a more participatory leadership style with in-group followers and a more directive approach with out-group followers.[9]

A study by Manzoni and Barsoux[10] highlighted a number of significant differences between in-group and out-group relationships. In-group followers reported that their leaders discussed the objectives to be obtained and then allowed the followers to create their own approaches to achieving those objectives. They also found that the leaders listened to their suggestions, strongly considered their opinions, and allowed them to choose interesting work assignments. In-group followers also noted that the leaders praised their results and treated their mistakes as learning opportunities. Out-group followers reported that their leaders gave them specific directions for completing assigned tasks and that, as a consequence, the leaders had little interest in their suggestions. Out-group followers were usually assigned routine task assignments, and the leaders closely monitored their progress toward completing these tasks. The out-group followers were more likely to be punished or criticized for making mistakes.

The followers in the in-group receive a disproportionate amount of the leader's time and attention. Many serve as lieutenants, assistants, or advisers, with a high-exchange relationship with the leader.[11] In their early research on vertical dyads, Dansereau, Graen, and Haga[1] determined that personal characteristics, such as personality, play a key role in the way followers work with leaders, and vice versa, and that these characteristics affect one's assignment to the in-group or the out-group. The follower's willingness to become involved in expanding roles is an especially important attribute.[12] By negotiating with the leader for work activities that go beyond the regularly assigned duties and formal tasks, followers can become part of the in-group. They do more for the leader, who in turn does more for them. Out-group followers, on the other hand, are usually content with their defined roles and uninterested in taking on additional responsibilities.[13] They are less involved in the work situation and less communicative.[1] Some leaders will categorize followers into the out-group as early as five days into the leader–follower relationship.[10]

The vertical dyad linkage concept is based on social exchange theory. If the follower puts forth additional or improved performance, the leader is expected to offer something in return.[9] High-exchange relationships develop gradually when complementary behaviors are repeated and reinforced. Through repetition, cycles of positive exchanges produce loyalty, support, and mutual dependence between the leader and the follower.[11]

Advancement of LMX Research

As LMX theory developed, research began to move beyond simply studying dyadic pairs and the differences between in-groups and out-groups and toward examining the relationship between leadership exchange and organizational effectiveness. Researchers such as Graen and Uhl-Bien,[6] as well as Liden, Wayne, and Stilwell,[14] helped focus attention on ways that aspects of the theory positively affected the leader, the followers and groups, and the organization itself. Northouse[13(p140)] writes that "high-quality leader–member exchanges produced less employee turnover, more positive performance evaluations, high frequency of promotions, greater organizational commitment, more desirable work assignments, better job attitudes, more attention and support from the leader, greater participation, and faster career progress over 25 years."

Some investigators have linked the use of the LMX approach with energy and creativity.[15] Followers who have perceived the use of LMX theory by leaders have shown an increase in energy and engagement in creative processes—likely the result of the followers' feelings being effectively nurtured. Other researchers have examined the relationship between LMX and the empowerment of followers. The quality of the exchange between a leader and follower has been found to have a heightened impact on followers who sense less empowerment, suggesting that high-quality exchange can help offset negative aspects of not being empowered.[16]

The exchanges between leaders and followers are important for the creation of effective work environments. When followers feel valued, important, and capable of accomplishing organizational goals, both members of the exchange—in addition to the organization as a whole—prosper.[13] The higher the quality of the exchange relationships, the more positive are the outcomes produced. In a high-quality exchange, the follower will have more interesting assignments and greater responsibility, and the leader will benefit through the increased productivity, initiative, and effort of the follower.

Leadership Making

leadership-making model
A model of leader, follower, and organizational development based on the leader's characteristics, the characteristics of the follower, and the level of maturity of the relationship between them.

In furthering the development of LMX theory, Graen and his coauthors[6,17,18] introduced a **leadership-making model** that takes a life-cycle approach to the leadership–follower relationship. The model is based on three components: (1) the leader's characteristics, (2) the characteristics of the follower, and (3) the level of maturity of the relationship between them. The influence process between these components is shown in exhibit 6.2. The follower and the leader each provide core, or base, contributions to teamwork effectiveness. At the same time, the interaction between the leader and the follower contributes to a level of maturity in the leadership relationship, which itself has an incremental influence on teamwork effectiveness. The higher the level of maturity within the team, the greater will be the incremental influence. The maturity of the leader–follower relationship leads to a transformation when team internalization occurs.

Under the leadership-making theory, the leader–follower relationship is social/emotional in nature, and it progresses from being a relationship between

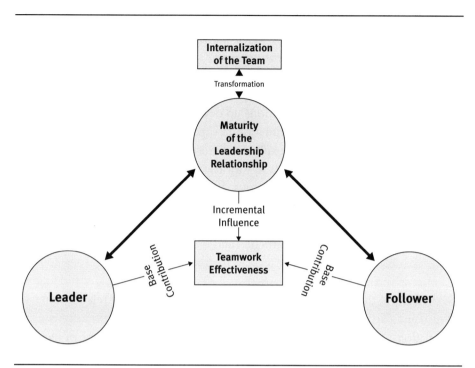

Source: Data from Graen, G. B., and M. Uhl-Bien. 1991. "The Transformation of Professionals into Self-Managing and Partially Self-Designing Contributors: Toward a Theory of Leadership-Making." *Journal of Management Systems* 3 (3): 25–39.

EXHIBIT 6.2
Three-Component Model of Leadership

two strangers, to a relationship between two acquaintances, and to, eventually, a mature relationship. Graen and his coauthors[18,19,20] identified four key features, all of which must be integrated for leadership making to occur:

1. *Growth*. Effective public health leaders will engage followers who desire to outgrow their formally defined organizational roles and expand their responsibilities.

2. *Investment*. Leaders invest in followers who want to grow; they provide career advancement opportunities and seek to build on the followers' personal motivations.

3. *Focus*. Leaders focus their limited resources specifically toward followers who have the ability and motivation to outgrow their current job requirements.

4. *Integration*. The leader and the follower who has been targeted integrate to form a cohesive work team that can effectively collaborate with other units within the organization.

Graen and Uhl-Bien[17] propose that the leadership-making process occurs in three phases: (1) **role finding**, (2) **role making**, and (3) **role implementation**. Role finding, also called *team finding*, is the phase during which the leader and

role finding
The first phase of the leadership-making process, in which the leader and the follower evaluate the other's abilities and motivations; also called *team finding*.

role making
The second phase of the leadership-making process, in which the dyadic relationship develops and both members come to understand how the other will function in specific situations; also called *team making*.

role implementation
The third phase of the leadership-making process, in which the behaviors of the leader and follower become interlocked; also called *team implementation*.

the follower evaluate the other's abilities and motivations. A form of sampling occurs as the leader and the follower learn about each other. If the sampling process results in a negative view on either side, the relationship is likely to remain at a relatively low level; if the sampling process is positive, the relationship will continue to grow and develop. Role making, also called *team making*, is the phase where the dyadic relationship develops and both members come to understand how the other will function in specific situations. At this point, the leader and follower tend not to explicitly discuss the nature of their relationship; instead, they test their approaches to various tasks by working together. Mutual trust grows as the relationship develops. Role implementation, or *team implementation*, is the phase at which the behaviors of the leader and follower become interlocked. They refine the exchange relationship and coordinate their work so that positive behaviors are strengthened and ineffective behaviors are weakened.

Exhibit 6.3 takes a closer look at the progression of the leader–follower relationship through the three phases of its life cycle. When the leader and follower are strangers in the role-finding phase, the reciprocity within the relationship takes a "cash and carry" approach, emphasizing immediate gratification of needs. As the relationship becomes more mature, an indefinite, "in-kind" type of reciprocity develops. The level of exchange between the members of the dyad shows a similar shift, starting low when the leader and follower are strangers and growing higher as the relationship becomes more mature. Likewise, incremental influence moves from none to almost unlimited as the leadership-making process unfolds.

EXHIBIT 6.3
Life Cycle of Leadership Making

	Time →		
Stage	**Stranger →**	**Acquaintance →**	**Mature**
Characteristic			
A. Relationship-building phase	Role finding	Role making	Role implementation
B. Type of reciprocity	Cash and carry	Mixed	In kind
C. Time span of reciprocity	Immediate	Some delay	Indefinite
D. Leader–member exchange	Low	Medium	High
E. Incremental influence	None	Limited	Almost unlimited
F. Type of leadership 1) Transactional	Behavioral management	→	Reciprocal favors
2) Transformational	Self-interest	→	Team interest

Source: Adapted with permission from Graen, G. B., and M. Uhl-Bien. 1991. "The Transformation of Professionals into Self-Managing and Partially Self-Designing Contributors: Toward a Theory of Leadership-Making." *Journal of Management Systems* 3 (3): 25–39.

Integrating the three components of leadership with the three-phase life cycle, Graen and Uhl-Bien[17] propose that no leadership component exists when the leader and the follower are strangers. At the acquaintance level, the leader and the follower develop a transactional relationship based on mutual self-interest. Under certain conditions, this transactional relationship may develop over time into a transformational relationship, based on the mutual interest of both the leader and the follower. Graen and Uhl-Bien believe their approach is compatible with Burns's[21] idea of transformational leadership (discussed in the next chapter). In exhibit 6.3, when a transactional style of leadership is implemented, a focus on behavioral management is gradually subsumed by an emphasis on the exchange of reciprocal favors. When a transformational style is used, self-interest during the early phase gives way to team interest in the mature stage.[17]

Northouse[13] approaches the phases of leadership making by considering the roles of the leader and the follower. When the leader and the follower are strangers, roles are scripted and prescribed within the organization; when they are acquaintances, roles are being tested; and when the relationship is mature, roles are negotiated between the two. Similarly, during the stranger phase, influence is directed in one way, from the leader to the follower; during the acquaintance phase, influences become mixed; and during the mature phase, influences are reciprocal in nature. As would be expected, leader–follower exchanges improve in quality as the dyad moves from the stranger phase to the acquaintance phase to the partnership phase. Strangers, naturally, consider their own self-interest first, whereas acquaintances are concerned both with themselves and the other member of the dyad. When relationships mature to a partnership level, the interests of the group become paramount. Thus, the ultimate goal in a leader–follower relationship is a mature partnership.

Research by Graen[19,22] demonstrated that greater leader investment in the follower has occurred in mature leader–follower relationships. In these mature relationships, 75 percent of leaders provided special information to the followers, allowing them to better understand how the organization functioned. In 83 percent of instances, the leader gave challenging assignments to the follower. Also in 83 percent of instances, the leader delegated sufficient authority to the follower to complete the assignments. In mature relationships, the leader included input from the follower in 78 percent of instances where the leader alone was responsible for the decision. Graen and Uhl-Bien[17(p35)] add: "Furthermore, followers in mature relationships with their leaders do more than their less fortunate colleagues of the following: (a) take the initiative, (b) attempt to exercise leadership to make the unit more effective, (c) take risks to accomplish missions, (d) build networks to extend capabilities, (e) influence others by doing something extra, and (f) work to get one's leader promoted."

As the leader–follower relationship matures through leadership making, the team orientation that develops between the leader and follower may become generalized to include other team members. Effective teamwork is cultivated, and teams become self-managing. Followers feel assured of the leader's support and are therefore willing to take risks, ask for direction, and outgrow their usual roles.

Graen's approach to the development of the LMX theory is summarized in exhibit 6.4. Stage 1 encompasses the vertical dyad linkages discussed earlier, and it includes a validation of differences within work units. Stage 2 focuses on the leader–member exchange, and it considers the implications of the differentiated dyadic relationships for organizational outcomes. Stage 3 is the leadership-making stage, which explores the development of the dyadic relationship as it matures (see exhibit 6.1). Stage 4 produces the team-making competence network, in which effective dyadic relationships are assembled in larger groups or teams.[6] According to Graen, leaders have a primary responsibility for developing a group of followers into a team through the process of team making.[23]

Consider This

"To predict a relationship's future, we also have to predict the nature of the environments the relationship will inhabit as it moves through time."
—Ellen Berscheid[4(p265)]

Why do you think that the environment or context of the situation is so important?

EXHIBIT 6.4
Graen's Four Stages in the Development of LMX Theory

> **Stage 1 VDL**
> Validation of Differentiation Within Work Units
> (Level of Analysis: Dyads with Work Unit)

> **Stage 2 LMX**
> Validation of Differentiated Relationship for Organizational Outcomes
> (Level of Analysis: Dyad)

> **Stage 3 Leadership-Making**
> Theory and Exploration of Dyadic Relationship Development
> (Level of Analysis: Dyad)

> **Stage 4 Team-Making Competence Network**
> Investigation of Assembling Dyads into Larger Collectivities
> (Level of Analysis: Collectivities as Aggregations of Dyads)

Source: Graen, G. B., and M. Uhl-Bien. 1995. "Relationship-Based Approach to Leadership: Development of Leader–Member Exchange (LMX) Theory of Leadership over 25 years: Applying a Multi-Level Multi-Domain Perspective." *Leadership Quarterly* 6 (2): 219–47. Reprinted with permission from *Leadership Quarterly* by International Leadership Association.

Partnership Building

After vertical dyad linkages have been developed and unique exchange relationships between the members of the dyad have been established, partnership building becomes a priority. In partnership building, leaders try to develop and maintain mature relationships with all of their followers, treating each person individually but positively. When the leader strives to treat each follower in a positive manner and followers respond accordingly, followers improve their performance, enhancing the output of the professional work group.[7] Doing so can be a challenge, however, as relationships develop differently with in-group members and out-group members.

LMX theory functions both prescriptively and descriptively. It prescribes how leaders can engage their followers, and it describes followers and the nature of their relationships with leaders. As discussed previously, in-group followers do more than their jobs require and strive to reach the group's goals in an effective and innovative manner; in return, leaders provide them with increased attention, opportunities, and responsibilities. Their extra effort is tangibly rewarded by the leader. Out-group followers, on the other hand, simply do what is required of them by their position in the organization. They are treated fairly, receiving the standard benefits they expect from their job, but their leaders often provide nothing more.[13] McClane[24] has pointed out that sharp differentiation between the in-group and out-group (and the groups' relationships with the leader) can lead to resentment among members of the out-group, which can hamper partnership building.

Individualized leadership anticipates that leaders will develop special relationships with all of their followers. The leader should make every effort to provide each follower with high-quality, mature exchanges—essentially striving to make every member part of the in-group. As trust and respect grow, partnerships with likeminded leaders and groups enhance the efforts of the entire organization. Even out-group followers are likely to improve their performance, thereby increasing the group's productivity.

Analysis of LMX

Investigators have identified a wide variety of elements that can influence LMX—including mutual trust and respect, support and loyalty, affection, influence, shared values, and personal attributes[25]—and this complexity has made the measurement of LMX a challenge. According to Yukl,[11] more than 15 measures have been proposed for the study of LMX theory. However, the most commonly used is a scale called the LMX-7, which is based on a seven-item questionnaire. The LMX-7 measures three key dimensions of the relationship: trust, respect, and obligation. Thus, it reflects the degree to which leaders and followers reciprocate trust, the level of respect they have for one another's capabilities, and their sense of obligation. Research has thus far not demonstrated that other multidimensional scales are more effective than the LMX-7.

Several studies have sought to measure LMX from both the leader perspective and the follower perspective.[26,27,28,29] However, the findings have generally shown low correlation between the leader and follower ratings of the quality of a relationship. As a result, Gerstner and Day[30], as well as others, have questioned the validity of a scale in which either the leader or follower is the source. Yukl[11(p124)] explains: "Subordinate ratings of LMX appear to be strongly influenced by the perception that the leader is supportive and fair, whereas leader ratings of LMX appear to be strongly influenced by the perception that the subordinate is competent and dependable." Nonetheless, Uhl-Bien and Graen[23] have found LMX-7 to be a reliable and valid measure.

Trust

To a large extent, LMX theory is based on the concept of trust. Interpersonal trust is vital to the successful accomplishment of work, and in public health, it effectively serves as the foundation upon which the organizational mission is attained.

Individuals first develop trust at an early age within the family, and trust develops further as children engage in relationships outside the home, such as at school or in the community. Within the professional work setting, trust can be observed at the dyadic pair and group levels. The trust that exists in dyadic pairs throughout an organization has a direct impact on the organizational culture (discussed in greater detail in chapter 9). Many organizational cultures hold trust as a core value; in others, however, trust is fragmented and broken. Leadership behavior for building trust unites social exchange theory and the concept of **organizational citizenship behavior (OCB)**—that is, behavior that demonstrates commitment to the organization and its goals. Such behavior typically reflects civic virtue and altruism, and it represents an individual's ongoing contributions to the workplace. Under LMX theory, dyadic pairs function organizationally in relationship to personal OCB. High levels of trust and followers' perception of fairness are essential for the development of rewarding and satisfying relationships.[31]

Quantifying the trust relationship among dyadic pairs is of particular importance for developing a thorough understanding of an organization and its operational features. One way to measure trust is by using a validated trust inventory such as the **Conditions of Trust Inventory (CTI)**. The CTI, developed by Butler,[32] measures the dimensions of trust across 11 scales: availability, competence, consistency,

---

organizational citizenship behavior (OCB)
Behavior that demonstrates an individual's commitment to the organization and its goals, typically through civic virtue and altruism.

Conditions of Trust Inventory (CTI)
A validated trust inventory with 11 dimensions: availability, competence, consistency, discreetness, fairness, integrity, loyalty, openness, promise fulfillment, receptivity, and overall trust.

 Check It Out

To further explore the concept of trust and its measurement, see the paper by Marcia L. Watson at www.instituteforpr.org/wp-content/uploads/2004_Watson.pdf.

discreetness, fairness, integrity, loyalty, openness, promise fulfillment, receptivity, and overall trust.

Extra-Role Behavior

Some researchers have demonstrated differences in the ways that leaders evaluate high- and low-LMX followers, particularly with regard to the tasks required of their roles. Duarte, Goodson, and Klich[33] found that many leaders seem to ignore task completion when rating high-LMX followers who are performing poorly, even when completion of the task is considered critical for defining the organization's effectiveness. Such findings demonstrate that the importance that leaders place on certain aspects of a follower's performance may not always match the importance typically assigned to those aspects by the organization.

Liden and Graen[34] point out that high-quality leader–follower relationships provide a means for moving followers past their formal organizational roles. High-LMX followers are more likely to engage in **extra-role behavior (ERB)**—that is, work-related activities that are not included as part of the employee's formal position description. The concept of ERB is especially applicable to public health. Given the field's evolving work demands and multidisciplinary nature (where core competencies include environmental health, biostatistics, epidemiology, health behaviors, and management), effective leader–follower relationships and the expansion of responsibilities are essential for carrying out organizational operations. Public health offers a wide range of career paths leading to middle- and upper-level leadership positions, even though formal education in leadership and management skills is often lacking.

> **extra-role behavior (ERB)**
> Work-related activities that are not included in the formal description of the employee's role.

Tierney and Bauer[35(p299)] state: "Relevant to the concept of ERB is the notion that the nature of exchange on the part of the employee is likely to move from in-role behavior to extra-role as the quality of the supervisor–employee relationship enhances over time." Managerial efficacy and concomitant mission accomplishment are of vital importance to dyadic relationships between managers and direct reports.

Communication

As the adage says, "Information is power." Leader–follower relationships and workforce performance are strongly influenced by access to information, the communication networks within the workplace, and the in-group or out-group status of individuals. Continuous two-way communication is essential for effective leader–follower relationships, and it should be built into the exchange process throughout the year.

One of the most important communication tools is the employee performance evaluation, and leaders should be aware of the ways that high or low LMX can influence their assessments. For instance, the use of vague or unmeasurable descriptions (e.g., "dependable," "able to get along with others," "takes initiative") in an evaluation may create inconsistencies and allow for biases to more easily enter the process. As noted by Duarte, Goodson, and Klich,[33] many leaders have a tendency, often without their knowledge, to favor high-LMX followers in the rating process. High-LMX followers also have the advantage of having greater day-to-day interaction with the leader, which improves their ability to adjust their performance as needed. Many out-group followers, on the other hand, receive little or no feedback between annual performance evaluations. Effective leaders understand the need to treat in-group and out-group followers equally in order to improve the workforce.

Leaders also must understand the way that LMX structure is lodged into the organization's larger network of informal relationships.[36] Communication networks are complex and involve relationships both within and outside the work environment. Whether at the formal or informal level, access to information has a direct effect on job performance and organizational mobility.

Job Satisfaction

Job satisfaction is a complex issue, involving employee perceptions related to a number of internal and external variables, but it can have a significant impact on productivity and organizational success. Stringer[37] has shown a positive correlation between follower job satisfaction and strong leader–follower relationships. Such relationships thrive when leadership is focused on the follower with thoughtful attention, continued support (i.e., sponsorship), and responsiveness toward the psychosocial impact of work. Positive follower-centered relationships can foster trust and organizational citizenship, reduce the impact of negative job-related tension, encourage extra role behavior, promote continuous individual-level quality improvement, and improve access to information for all followers. Functional and productive relationships are vital for job satisfaction and key to the success of any organization, particularly those in public health.

Effective Public Health Leaders . . .

. . . promote work-centered job design, building strong trust relationships with all employees.

Job Tension

job tension
Emotional or mental strain resulting from job stress.

Job tension—the emotional or mental strain that results from job stress—has a differential effect on follower performance and productivity. Some followers thrive under pressure and become more productive as workplace tension increases, whereas others become uncomfortable or less productive. Leaders should assess how each member of the team responds to tension and pay close attention to the effects of tension on employee productivity specific to the LMX relationship. In general, Hochwarter[8] has found that job tension is lowest when the LMX is highest and highest when the LMX is lowest.

Tension exists within all workplace environments, and leadership has the responsibility to design work arrangements to capitalize on it. Effective leaders can and do use tension within the work setting to foster a healthy level of competitiveness, which can result in increased productivity. However, ineffective application of competition can result in tension that damages relationships and adversely affects the achievement of the organization's goals. A key challenge for leaders is striking a healthy balance between tension and slack, or ease, within the workplace. Such balance can be especially difficult to achieve in public health settings, where work varies from consumer-driven clinical service delivery to assurance functions such as community inspections.

Research by Harris and Kacmar[38] suggests that a U-shaped pattern exists with regard to LMX relationships and tension. When LMX is low, followers may experience high levels of tension and anxiety. Leaders can reduce the adverse effects of this tension by increasing their support, leading to a higher level of LMX. However, when LMX reaches the higher levels, the new duties and expectations placed on the follower may exceed the level of support provided by the leader, which can cause tension to increase. Ultimately, the key to successful leadership with regard to tension is to promote appropriate individual-level tension that achieves organizational objectives. Tension that results from interpersonal conflict and does not add value toward achieving the desired outcome must be eliminated from the LMX relationship.

> ### Leadership Application Case: A Leadership Study
>
> The Leadership Application Case at the beginning of this book provides realistic scenarios for the application of key leadership concepts covered in the text. See the section marked "Chapter 6 Application" for the scenario and discussion questions that correspond with this chapter.

Application of LMX Theory to Public Health

As noted throughout the chapter, LMX theory is highly applicable to the field of public health. Mase,[39] for instance, invited employees of two health departments to complete the Conditions of Trust Inventory to establish the levels of trust in each workforce as a basis for implementing LMX theory. The CTI's 11 domains allowed for the identification of patterns and themes related to leader–follower trust within categorical subgroupings of health department employees. The resulting data indicated areas where trust was high and areas where trust was waning or low, enabling public health leaders to take appropriate action in specific areas. Where trust indicators were high, leaders sought to reinforce positive relationships; where they were low, leaders implemented new strategies to boost trust and, ultimately, organizational productivity. Measures such as the CTI are highly valuable both for public health organizations seeking to evaluate the effectiveness of initiatives to promote trust and for public health leaders practicing individualized leadership approaches such as LMX theory. Workforce assessment tools can help leaders better understand trust within their organizations and make data-driven decisions at the organizational level.

Leaders applying LMX theory to the field of public health should be aware of issues associated with gender and ethnicity. The published literature lacks studies that directly investigate how LMX level correlates with gender and racial/ethnic disparities in the workplace, but one could logically argue that such correlations exist. Of particular concern is the lack of racial/ethnic minorities in middle- and upper-level management positions in US public health organizations. In 2010, National Association of County and City Health Officials (NACCHO)[40] reported that less than 4 percent of top agency executives were black. NACCHO also found that 58 percent of top executives were women, which is a relatively low figure given that women represent up to 80 percent of the local health department workforce.

Shortell and Kaluzny[41(pp124–25)] write:

> While issues related to gender and leadership are not necessarily distinctive to health services organizations, they are certainly very important. Several reviews of the literature suggest that, while females may demonstrate different patterns of leadership behaviors than males, gender is not a particularly good predictor of leadership effectiveness and success. However, there does appear to be some evidence that individuals who ranked higher in male sex role orientation (describing themselves as having more masculine characteristics) were perceived to be better leaders than those with feminine, androgynous, or undifferentiated gender roles.

Effective mentoring and relationship building with women and minorities can help public health organizations to achieve appropriate representation in management and to address concerns about bias and discrimination.

Successful achievement of a public health organization's mission is contingent upon its ability to achieve work-related tasks in an effective and informed manner, and LMX theory offers a useful method for public health leaders to lead their followers and constituents.[32] However, like other approaches, it has both strengths and weaknesses.

Strengths of LMX Theory

LMX theory is a useful approach for public health leaders in that it intuitively distinguishes between followers who are strong contributors to the organization and those who are not. The theory is strongly descriptive, dividing followers into in-groups and out-groups. Such categorization can be seen in every public health organizational setting, where in-group followers seem to not only do more but also receive more in return. The advantages provided to the in-group may suggest an inherent unfairness, but the theory simply validates what we already know about leader–follower relationships in public health.

LMX has certain similarities to situational leadership, particularly in that it deals specifically with the relationship between two individuals, the leader and the follower. However, whereas situational leadership suggests that leaders tailor their leadership style to the follower's developmental level, LMX theory places the leader–follower dyadic relationship at the core of the leadership process. Each follower is expected to have a different and unique relationship with the leader. A major strength of LMX theory is its emphasis on effective communication between the leader and follower, without which high-quality exchanges are impossible. The three key elements examined by the LMX-7—trust, respect, and obligation—characterize effective communication between the members of the dyad. Public health leaders utilizing LMX theory must become skilled communicators.

Northouse[13] notes that LMX theory urges leaders not to allow their personal biases—whether based on race, ethnicity, age, gender, sexual orientation, or religion, and whether conscious or subconscious—to influence which followers are invited into the in-group. LMX theory is based on fair and equal treatment of followers, and partnership building is rooted in an effort to treat each follower in a positive manner.

Finally, LMX theory is closely tied to a number of important organizational variables, and Graen and Uhl-Bien[6] have demonstrated that the theory's practice leads to positive organizational outcomes. This attribute alone makes LMX theory an important tool for effective public health leaders.

> ### Consider This
>
>
>
> "It is difficult to express anything at all with any degree of exactness, so that complete relationships are few and far between."
> —Gustave Flaubert[42(p328)]
>
> As you consider Flaubert's statement, how does it intersect with the concepts of the LMX theory?

Weaknesses of LMX Theory

Obviously, the most prevalent criticism of the LMX theory is that it appears to run counter to the basic idea of fairness. Followers are divided into two groups, and one group receives greater attention, opportunities, and rewards than the other. Certainly, discrimination may result, and the perception of privileged workplace groups can have a negative impact on interactions between followers.[24] No matter how hard the leader tries to bring out-group members into the in-group, the question remains: Does the theory produce inequalities?

Within the leader–follower dyadic relationship, the expectations of each member develop into a type of psychological contract.[43] Among the follower's key expectations are equity and organizational justice, as examined by Scandura.[44] The theory itself fails to address basic issues of distributive justice (relating to promotions, pay increases, and important job assignments), as well as procedural and interactional justice (relating to decision making, communication, and fairness). However, Harter and Evanecky[45] point out that, if all followers are free to become in-group members, LMX theory may not actively create inequalities. In addition, leadership efforts that engage with the theory to pursue partnership building may considerably reduce the concerns about inequity.

Another potential weakness for LMX theory involves determining how high-quality exchanges are created and, further, how partnership building occurs in the development of high-quality exchanges with all followers. Like many other leadership theories, LMX theory struggles with issues of concepts, definitions, and propositions. Questions also surround the limited research supporting the theory. No empirical studies have been conducted using dyadic measurements to analyze the process,[46] and some critics have questioned the validity of the scales used by investigators.

Despite these criticisms, LMX theory has been effective for many public health leaders, in part because it provides a single leadership theory that can be used with followers within the organization and with constituents and collaborators. It is one of the many tools available to help leaders better understand workplace dynamics and ultimately assist in maximizing public health service delivery.

Case Study: Oklahoma City Wellness Now

Launched in 2010, Oklahoma City's Wellness Now initiative is a grassroots community coalition of more than 100 agencies focused on improving the health and wellness of the residents of Oklahoma City and other parts of Oklahoma County.

The foundation for Wellness Now was laid more than 15 years ago through a series of economic development commitments collectively known as the Metropolitan Area Projects Plan. Among other activities, the plan vastly improved the built environment of Oklahoma City, and it began linking the city's economy with the holistic health and well-being of its citizens. In 2006, after Oklahoma City had been named one of the country's "fattest" cities, the city went on a diet—losing a collective 1 million pounds. The city also built hundreds of miles of walking paths and biking trails, as well as a 70-acre central park downtown. But the health improvement efforts did not stop there.

Wellness Now is housed within the Oklahoma City–County Health Department and led by an executive team that includes the Oklahoma

City mayor, the chair of the Oklahoma County Board of Commissioners, the director of the Health Department, the chair of the Board of Health, academic faculty from the Oklahoma University Health Sciences Center, and other prominent community leaders. Individual work groups led by Health Department staff focus on adolescent health, care coordination, health at work, maternal and child health, mental health, nutrition and physical activity, and tobacco use prevention.

Wellness Now conducts and reports on comprehensive and collaborative community health needs assessments and community health improvement plans. It hosts Open Streets events to encourage residents to get out and move. It reports annually on all of its work groups, priorities, resources, and even walkability studies. Importantly, the initiative began using a ZIP Code Wellness Score within the county to track outcomes and progress on critical measures of health and overall wellness. This score helps demonstrate the impact of social, physical, and environmental determinants on both individual and community health.

Like most major cities, Oklahoma City has more to do to improve the health of its community. However, with collaborative, community-owned, and community-developed initiatives such as Wellness Now, the potential for change is great.

Discussion and Application Questions

1. How might such a broad base of community partners be both a challenge and a benefit to effective public health leadership?
2. What is the importance of external partnerships to effective public health leadership?
3. What skills do public health leaders need to possess to effectively use LMX theory in leveraging partnerships, collaborations, and coalitions such as Wellness Now?

Summary

The leader–member exchange (LMX) theory of leadership, like the contingency theories, considers the interactional aspects of actors within organizations. Its unit of analysis is the dyadic pair, which consists of a leader and a follower within the work environment. In LMX theory, the leader practices individualized leadership, based on the individual needs of each follower in relation to the leader. Every follower is part of a unique dyadic relationship, which determines the behavior of the leader with the follower and the follower's response to the leader. The network of trust relationships that develop between leaders and followers is key to LMX theory.

The first stage in the development of individualized leadership is vertical dyad linkage, marked by an awareness that individual relationships exist between the leader and each follower. These relationships result in assignment of each follower to either an in-group or an out-group within the work setting. The in-group consists of followers who have higher degrees of exchange with the leader and who are willing to take on expanded roles, whereas the out-group consists of followers who are content to function solely based on the defined roles of their job description. Work-related activities that are not included as part of an employee's formal position description are considered extra-role behavior. The second stage in the development of individualized leadership focuses more explicitly on the exchange that occurs in a leader–follower relationship. The leadership-making model examines the way that the social/emotional exchange relationship progresses from being a relationship between two strangers, to a relationship between two acquaintances, to, eventually, a mature relationship. This progression occurs in three phases: (1) role finding, (2) role making, and (3) role implementation. A more advanced stage of individualized leadership is partnership building, in which leaders try to develop and maintain mature relationships with all of their followers, treating each person individually but positively.

A variety of elements can influence the exchange between a leader and follower, and measurement of LMX can therefore be a challenge. The scale known as the LMX-7, based on a seven-item questionnaire, measures the key dimensions of trust, respect, and obligation. Trust can be measured using a validated instrument called the Conditions of Trust Inventory, which considers 11 dimensions: availability, competence, consistency, discreetness, fairness, integrity, loyalty, openness, promise fulfillment, receptivity, and overall trust.

LMX theory is highly applicable to the field of public health. Measures such as the CTI are highly valuable both for public health organizations seeking to evaluate the effectiveness of initiatives to promote trust and for public health leaders practicing individualized leadership approaches. Workforce assessment tools can help leaders better understand the relationships within their organizations and make evidence-based decisions at the organizational level. Leaders, however, should be aware that the separation of followers into an in-group and out-group has a potential for unfairness, and they should not allow personal biases—whether based on race, ethnicity, age, gender, sexual orientation, or other attributes—to influence which followers are invited into the in-group.

Discussion Questions

1. Summarize the leader–member exchange theory of organizational leadership.

2. Discuss the concept of trust. How does it relate to public health practice?

3. Why are vertical dyadic pairs important in the practice of effective public health leadership?

4. How is trust measured in LMX theory?

5. Explain the Conditions of Trust Inventory. How is it used in LMX theory?

6. Compare and contrast in-groups and out-groups.

7. How does membership in an in-group or an out-group affect an individual follower?

8. What are Graen's stages in the development of LMX theory, and how are they related to one another?

9. What is organizational citizenship behavior? Explain its impact on the mission of a public health organization.

10. For deeper thought: Imagine you are the director of a local public health department. Describe job tension and explain how it affects your followers and your organization.

Web Resources

Lunenburg, F. C. 2010. "Leader–Member Exchange Theory: Another Perspective on the Leadership Process." *International Journal of Management, Business and Administration.* Accessed May 30, 2017. www.nationalforum.com/Electronic%20Journal% 20Volumes/Lunenburg,%20Fred%20C.%20Leader-Member%20Exchange%20 Theory%20IJMBA%20V13%202010.pdf.

Mind Tools. 2017. "Leader-Member Exchange Theory: Getting the Best from All Team Members." Accessed May 30. www.mindtools.com/pages/article/leader-member-exchange.htm.

Watson, M. L. 2004. "Can There Be Just One Trust? A Cross-Disciplinary Identification of Trust Definitions and Measurement." Institute for Public Relations. Accessed May 30, 2017. www.instituteforpr.org/wp-content/uploads/2004_Watson.pdf.

References

1. Dansereau, F., G. B. Graen, and W. G. Haga. 1975. "A Vertical Dyad Linkage Approach to Leadership Within Formal Organizations: A Longitudinal Investigation of the Role Making Process." *Organizational Behavior and Human Performance* 13 (1): 46–78.

2. Graen, G. B., and J. F. Cashman. 1975. "A Role Making Model of Leadership in Formal Organizations: A Developmental Approach." In *Leadership Frontiers*, edited by J. G. Hunt and L. L. Larson, 143–65. Kent, OH: Kent State University Press.

3. Changing Minds. 2017. "Leader-Member Exchange (LMX) Theory." Accessed February 6. http://changingminds.org/explanations/theories/leader_member_exchange.htm.

4. Berscheid, E. 1999. "The Greening of Relationship Science." *American Psychologist* 54 (4): 260–66.

5. Dansereau, F. 1995. "A Dyadic Approach to Leadership: Creating and Nurturing This Approach Under Fire." *Leadership Quarterly* 6 (4): 479–90.

6. Graen, G. B., and M. Uhl-Bien. 1995. "Relationship-Based Approach to Leadership: Development of Leader–Member Exchange (LMX) Theory of Leadership over 25 Years: Applying a Multi-level Multi-domain Perspective." *Leadership Quarterly* 6 (2): 219–47.

7. Daft, R. L. 2015. *The Leadership Experience*, 6th ed. Mason, OH: South-Western.

8. Hochwarter, W. 2005. "LMX and Job Tension: Linear and Non-linear Effects and Affectivity." *Journal of Business and Psychology* 19 (4): 505–20.

9. Ledlow, G. R., and M. N. Coppola. 2014. *Leadership for Health Professionals: Theory, Skills, and Applications*, 2nd ed. Sudbury, MA: Jones & Bartlett Learning.

10. Manzoni, J., and J. Barsoux. 1998. "The Set-Up-to-Fail Syndrome." *Harvard Business Review* 76 (2): 103–13.

11. Yukl, G. 2013. *Leadership in Organizations*, 8th ed. Upper Saddle River, NJ: Prentice Hall.

12. Graen, G. B. 1976. "Role-Making Processes Within Complex Organizations." In *Handbook of Industrial and Organizational Psychology*, edited by M. D. Dunnette, 1201–45. Chicago: Rand McNally.

13. Northouse, P. G. 2016. *Leadership: Theory and Practice*, 7th ed. Los Angeles: Sage.

14. Liden, R. C., S. J. Wayne, and D. Stilwell. 1993. "A Longitudinal Study on the Early Development of Leader–Member Exchange." *Journal of Applied Psychology* 78 (4): 662–74.

15. Atwater, L., and A. Carmeli. 2009. "Leader–Member Exchange, Feelings of Energy, and Involvement in Creative Work." *Leadership Quarterly* 20 (3): 264–75.

16. Harris, K. J., A. R. Wheeler, and K. M. Kacmar. 2009. "Leader–Member Exchange and Empowerment: Direct and Interactive Effects

on Job Satisfaction, Turnover Intentions, and Performance." *Leadership Quarterly* 20 (3): 371–82.

17. Graen, G. B., and M. Uhl-Bien. 1991. "The Transformation of Professionals into Self-Managing and Partially Self-Designing Contributors: Toward a Theory of Leadership-Making." *Journal of Management Systems* 3 (3): 25–39.

18. Graen, G. B., and T. Scandura. 1987. "Toward a Psychology of Dyadic Organizing." *Research in Organizational Behavior* 9 (1): 175–208.

19. Graen, G. B. 1989. *Unwritten Rules for Your Career: 15 Secrets for Fast-Track Success*. New York: John Wiley & Sons.

20. Zalesny, M. D., and G. B. Graen. 1986. "Exchange Theory in Leadership Research." In *Encyclopedia of Leadership*, edited by G. Reber, 714–27. Linz, Germany: Linz University Press.

21. Burns, J. M. 1978. *Leadership*. New York: Harper & Row.

22. Graen, G. B. 1990. "The Productive Leadership System." In *International Work Motivation*, edited by E. Fleishman, 200–33. Hillsdale, NJ: Lawrence Erlbaum Associates.

23. Uhl-Bien, M., and G. B. Graen. 1992. "Leadership-Making in Self-Managing Professional Work Teams: An Empirical Investigation." In *The Impact of Leadership*, edited by K. E. Clark, M. B. Clark, and D. P. Campbell, 379–87. West Orange, NJ: Leadership Library of America.

24. McClane, W. E. 1991. "Implications of Member Role Differentiation: Analysis of a Key Concept in the LMX Model of Leadership." *Group and Organization Management* 16 (1): 102–13.

25. Schriesheim, C. A., S. Castro, and C. C. Cogliser. 1999. "Leader–Member Exchange Research: A Comprehensive Review of Theory and Data-Analysis Procedures." *Leadership Quarterly* 10 (1): 63–113.

26. Deluga, R. J., and T. J. Perry. 1994. "The Role of Subordinate Performance and Ingratiation in Leader–Member Exchanges." *Group and Organization Management* 19 (1): 67–86.

27. Liden, R. C., S. J. Wayne, and D. Stilwell. 1993. "A Longitudinal Study on the Early Development of Leader–Member Exchanges." *Journal of Applied Psychology* 78 (4): 662–74.

28. Philips, A. S., and A. G. Bedeian. 1994. "Leader–Follower Exchange Quality: The Role of Personal and Interpersonal Attributes." *Academy of Management Journal* 37 (4): 990–1001.

29. Scandura, T. A., and C. A. Schriesheim. 1994. "Leader–Member Exchange and Supervisor Career Mentoring as Complementary Constructs in Leadership Research." *Academy of Management Journal* 37 (6): 1588–1602.

30. Gerstner, C. R., and D. V. Day. 1997. "Meta-analytic Review of Leader–Member Exchange Theory: Correlates and Construct Issues." *Journal of Applied Psychology* 82 (6): 827–44.

31. Deluga, R. 1994. "Supervisor Trust Building, Leader–Member Exchange and Organizational Citizenship Behaviour." *Journal of Occupational and Organizational Psychology* 67 (4): 315–26.

32. Butler, J. 1991. "Toward Understanding and Measuring Conditions of Trust: Evolution of a Conditions of Trust Inventory." *Journal of Management* 17 (3): 643–63.

33. Duarte, N. T., J. R. Goodson, and N. R. Klich. 1993. "How Do I Like Thee? Let Me Appraise the Ways." *Journal of Organizational Behavior* 14 (3): 239–49.

34. Liden, R. C., and G. Graen. 1980. "Generalizability of the Vertical Dyad Linkage Model of Leadership." *Academy of Management Journal* 23 (3): 451–65.

35. Tierney, P., and T. Bauer. 1996. "A Longitudinal Assessment of LMX on Extra-Role Behavior." In *Academy of Management Best Paper Proceedings*, 298–305. Briarcliff Manor, NY: Academy of Management.

36. Sparrowe, R. T., and R. C. Liden. 2005. "Two Routes to Influence: Integrating Leader–Member Exchange and Social Network Perspectives." *Administrative Science Quarterly* 50 (4): 505–35.

37. Stringer, L. 2006. "The Link Between the Quality of the Supervisor–Employee Relationship and the Level of the Employee's Job Satisfaction." *Public Organization Review* 6 (2): 125–42.

38. Harris, K., and M. Kacmar. 2006. "Too Much of a Good Thing? The Curvilinear Effect of Leader–Member Exchange on Stress." *Journal of Social Psychology* 146 (1): 65–84.

39. Mase, W. 2008. "Trust Relationships Among Public Health Workers: An Application of the Leader–Member Exchange Theory (LMX)." PhD dissertation, University of Kentucky.

40. National Association of County and City Health Officials (NACCHO). 2011. *2010 National Profile of Local Health Departments*. Washington, DC: National Association of County and City Health Officials.

41. Shortell, S., and A. D. Kaluzny. 2000. *Health Care Management: Organization Design and Behavior*, 4th ed. Clifton Park, NY: Delmar Cengage Learning.

42. Flaubert, G. (1869) 1964. *Sentimental Education*. London, UK: Penguin Books.

43. Hollander, E. P. 1978. *Leadership Dynamics: A Practical Guide to Effective Relationships*. New York: Free Press.

44. Scandura, T. A. 1999. "Rethinking Leader–Member Exchange: An Organizational Justice Perspective." *Leadership Quarterly* 10 (1): 25–40.

45. Harter, N., and D. Evanecky. 2002. "Fairness in Leader–Member Exchange Theory: Do We All Belong on the Inside?" *Leadership Review* 2 (2): 1–7.

46. Schriesheim, C. A., S. L. Castro, X. Zhou, and F. J. Yammarino. 2001. "The Folly of Theorizing 'A' but Testing 'B': A Selective Level-of-Analysis Review of the Field and a Detailed Leader–Member Exchange Illustration." *Leadership Quarterly* 12 (4): 515–51.

TRANSFORMATIONAL LEADERSHIP

Erik L. Carlton and James W. Holsinger Jr.

Learning Objectives

Upon completion of this chapter, you should be able to

- apply core aspects of transformational leadership;
- compare and contrast transformational and transactional leadership styles;
- use tools for measuring leadership style, especially transformational leadership;
- analyze the role of transformational leadership in public health settings;
- appraise principles of authenticity in transformational leadership;
- distinguish authentic transformational leadership from pseudotransformational leadership;
- analyze moderators of transformational leadership, especially followership; and
- assess the role of relationships in leadership, particularly transformational leadership.

Focus on Leadership Competencies

This chapter emphasizes the following Association of Schools and Programs of Public Health (ASPPH) leadership competencies:

- Describe the attributes of leadership in public health.
- Develop strategies to motivate others for collaborative problem solving, decision-making, and evaluation.
- Describe alternative strategies for collaboration and partnership among organizations, focused on public health goals.
- Create a shared vision.

(continued)

It also addresses the following Council on Linkages public health leadership competency:

- Analyzes internal and external facilitators and barriers that may affect the delivery of the 10 Essential Public Health Services.

Note: See the appendix at the end of the book for complete lists of competencies.

Introduction

Today more than ever before, developments in the public health landscape have created a need for leaders who not only are competent in the daily tasks of leading and managing in public health settings but also have a strong ethical focus and can get the most from themselves and their organizations.

Despite the many laws and regulations that govern leaders' actions, a variety of influences threaten to lure leaders into professional and ethical lapses. In every organization, economic and social forces drive large parts of the agenda. Whether in the private or public sector, leaders are constantly faced with pressures—both internal and external—to improve profitability, quality, safety, productivity, service, and satisfaction. The pace of organizational activities in the midst of such pressures can hypnotize even the best of leaders and drive them toward more rapid, but less carefully considered, decision making. Leaders can be lulled into a sense of temporal security, believing themselves to be supported by past assumptions when, in reality, new issues of the present and future loom before them. With budgetary uncertainties, organizations are called on to do more with less, and the temptation to cut corners, rather than cut organizational excess, is very real. Even in the best attempts to fulfill organizational missions in the face of these demands, leaders may default to their basic approaches and thereby fail ethically. Without a strong professional and ethical base, the capacity and integrity of leaders and the organizations they shepherd are at serious risk.

In public health in particular, leaders face increasingly complex challenges while being called on more and more to lead and collaborate with the communities where they live, work, and serve. Economic difficulties in many communities have left individuals unable to afford medical care, and funding shortfalls have limited the ability of public health agencies to provide basic care for the

 Consider This

"A rock pile ceases to be a rock pile the moment a single man contemplates it, bearing within him the image of a cathedral."

—Antoine de Saint-Exupéry[1(p129)]

Consider the transformation that occurs from a rock pile to a cathedral. How can this analogy apply to leadership of a public health organization?

indigent.[2,3] Since public health agencies perform more than just clinical roles, practitioners deal with additional challenges related to environmental health, sanitation, and other efforts to achieve and maintain population health. Essential human resources—the public health workforce—have been in the midst of major upheaval. The retirement of large numbers of highly experienced practitioners has resulted in a dearth of practical knowledge, as new staff members, when they can be hired, often lack the same level of public health education or experience.[4] The impact of national health reform on public health organizations and their employees, both in the short term and over the long term, is unknown.[5,6] At the same time, natural disasters and other crises can readily and without notice destroy the delicate balance of capacity and competence in public health practice.[7]

Today's public health challenges are at once fascinating, frustrating, and inspiring, and the need for creative, innovative, and effective leadership has never been greater.[8] Today's public health leaders must engage multiple stakeholders in activities that, by their very nature, are open to broad public scrutiny and debate.[9] Leaders therefore must be as skilled and astute politically as they are at managing the technical and systemic aspects of public health.[10,11]

These demands on today's public health leaders have attracted growing numbers of practitioners to **transformational leadership**, a leadership model that emphasizes efforts to produce positive change in individuals and social systems—particularly, enhancing followers' motivation, morale, and performance. Leaders who effectively use this approach are able to *transform* the raw material of human and organizational resources into people and systems prepared for today's challenges.

transformational leadership
A leadership model that emphasizes efforts to produce positive change in individuals and social systems—particularly, enhancing followers' motivation, morale, and performance.

Understanding Transformational Leadership

Leadership theories and their applications have evolved over time. Whereas leadership was once viewed as a set of characteristics and behaviors, today it is increasingly being approached as a relational process. This **dyadic framing of leadership**, which considers leadership through the lens of relationships, has encouraged leaders to be more inclusive, more empowering, and more considerate of the needs, motivations, and potential of the people they lead. As noted in chapter 1, the Association of Schools and Programs in Public Health[12,13] has outlined core leadership competencies for MPH and DrPH program graduates, and both sets of competencies define *leadership* in terms of creating a shared vision, motivating others, galvanizing organizational and community resources, and using the best strategies and practices to enhance services and solve problems. These are core aspects of transformational leadership.

dyadic framing of leadership
A way of viewing leadership with an emphasis on relational processes between leaders and followers.

In addition to possessing qualities well suited to today's public health challenges, transformational leaders have a certain personal appeal. They engage in a pattern of behaviors that "arouse inspirational motivation, provide intellectual stimulation, and treat followers with individualized consideration . . . [to] transform their followers' needs, values, preferences, and aspirations toward reaching their full potential and generate higher levels of performance."[14(pp328–29)] Transformational leaders have been described as inspirational, challenging, development oriented, and determined to maximize potential,[15] and they are known to challenge the status quo.[16,17,18]

charisma
The ability to connect with followers in a way that produces remarkable performance and attainment.

Transformational leadership relies on **charisma**—the ability to connect with followers in a manner that produces remarkable performance and attainment.[19] Leaders exhibit this charisma by articulating goals, taking risks, setting high expectations, and emphasizing a collective identity and vision.[20] They may also demonstrate charisma through self-sacrifice. Choi and Mai-Dalton[21] studied leadership sacrifice and its effect on follower behaviors, and they found not only that self-sacrificial leaders were more likely to be seen as charismatic and authentic but also that self-sacrificial behaviors increased followers' intention to reciprocate. Several authors have suggested that charisma is not something that leaders possess but rather the outcome of a relationship between leaders and followers.[16,22] Leadership is based on a symbiotic relationship between individuals who choose to lead and those who choose to follow.[23] Leadership and followership join at a relational nexus, and leaders are expected to be honest, forward-looking, competent, and inspiring—in short, credible.

Effective Public Health Leaders . . .

. . . embrace innovation and creativity.

leader attribution error
The tendency to overestimate the role of a single leader and underestimate, or altogether ignore, the roles of the many followers.

The transformational leadership model addresses several shortcomings of past leadership theories. Perhaps the greatest flaw in many leadership theories has been an *a priori* focus on leaders, their roles, and their behaviors. Many theorists have assumed that individuals have more power than they really do and therefore have emphasized the concept of being a "great leader" rather than understanding the dynamic and interpersonal nature of leader–follower dyads. This tendency to overestimate the role of a single leader and to underestimate (or altogether ignore) the roles of the many followers is known as **leader attribution error**.[24] Theories that make this error may be compelling and marketable, but they ultimately tend to be short-sighted and organizationally impotent. The vital aspect of leadership study and leadership development is not the identification of unique qualities that make individual leaders heroic; rather, it is the understanding of the ways leaders can function effectively in a variety of settings, with complex demands, and with multiple stakeholders. In other words, it is the way that leaders transact with, transform, and are transformed by their followers, organizations, and communities.

transactional leadership
Leadership that emphasizes setting clear objectives and goals for followers and using punishments and rewards to encourage compliance.

A number of more traditional leadership theories have approached the subject primarily in transactional terms—for instance, in leader–member exchanges where leaders provide support, direction, and reinforcement and followers provide an agreed-upon degree of performance.[14] This **transactional leadership** approach is typically associated with corrective, remedial, or reactive management styles, but it generally is not associated with risk taking, change, or motivation. Transformational leadership does not replace transactional leadership, and it does not exclude active transactional elements such as contingent rewards to encourage goal achievement or corrective action to address poor performance. Rather, it augments these elements with other aspects—specifically, idealized influence, intellectual stimulation, inspirational motivation, and individualized consideration, as discussed later in the chapter—to make the leadership transformational.[25,26]

In recent decades, numerous studies have examined transformational and transactional leadership, as well as **passive-avoidant leadership**, in which decision-making power is passed to followers. These three models collectively are known as **full-range leadership**. Of the three, only transformational leadership has been linked to improved quality, employee satisfaction, productivity, and perceived leadership efficacy.[28,29,30,31,32,33] The transactional and passive-avoidant styles, meanwhile, when used on their own, are seen as a prescription for mediocrity.[34,35]

> ### Spotlight
>
>
>
> Quotes from practitioners of transactional leadership[27]:
>
> "When placed in command, take charge."
> —Norman Schwarzkopf
>
> "The price of success is hard work, dedication to the job at hand, and the determination that whether we win or lose, we have applied the best of ourselves to the task at hand."
> —Vince Lombardi
>
> "The first rule of any technology used in a business is that automation applied to an efficient operation will magnify the efficiency. The second is that automation applied to an inefficient operation will magnify the inefficiency."
> —Bill Gates
>
> "Starbucks is not an advertiser; people think we are a great marketing company, but in fact we spend very little money on marketing and more money on training our people than advertising."
> —Howard Schultz

Transformational leadership does not neglect the basic expectations of employee performance, but it is essentially charismatic in nature, providing inspirational motivation, intellectual stimulation, and individualized consideration to followers.[36] Further, it is not an artifact of individual personality but rather an interpersonal construct, occurring only in relationships between a leader and a follower[37,38,39] and in the context of organizational work environments.[40] As such, transformational leadership may be less about personality traits and more about relationship traits and abilities, including emotional intelligence.[41] The potential that leaders have to transform organizations is based on their ability to tap into the values and motivations of the people they lead and then act accordingly.[42] In the process, leaders and followers engage one another in a manner that elevates the performance, motivations, and morality of all involved.[43] Among other findings, transformational leadership has been shown to increase employee satisfaction and retention and improve organizational financial, social, and ethical performance.

passive-avoidant leadership
A leadership style in which the followers are given the power to make decisions.

full-range leadership
A model that consists of the transformational, transactional, and passive-avoidant leadership styles.

In its truest sense, transformational leadership builds upon a base of effective transactional leadership. Some authors, in discussing subtle variations of transformational leadership theory, have failed to acknowledge this foundation, but without transactional elements, individual and organizational transformation will be limited or nonexistent. The core theorists are clear about the **augmentative effect** of transformational leadership—that transformational leadership augments transactional leadership.[26,44] This effect is illustrated in exhibit 7.1.

Transformational leadership can also be seen as a by-product of well-applied situational leadership. In situational leadership, as discussed in chapter 4, leaders use different types of support and direction depending on the followers' competency and motivation. In extending that approach, transformational leadership helps leaders harness the human potential in their organization by appropriately assisting the development of each follower.

One criticism that has been directed at transformational leadership is that it can, at times, be used to achieve immoral or unethical ends.[45] A common example is Adolf Hitler, who used the full range of transactional and transformational leadership components to take control of Germany and carry out a brutal campaign of violence. Recognizing this concern, Bass[46] distinguishes between **authentic transformational leadership** and **pseudotransformational leadership**. Authentic transformational leaders are motivated by altruism and integrity, whereas pseudotransformational leaders are driven by self-centeredness. True transformational leadership thus stands on a clear ethical foundation, raising the level of morality in the group or organization.[45] Given the situationally applied, morally based, authenticity-oriented nature of transformational leadership, it is not surprising that transformational leaders have been shown to use higher levels of moral reasoning than primarily transactional or passive-avoidant leaders.[46,47,48]

augmentative effect
The idea that transformational leadership augments, or enhances, transactional leadership.

authentic transformational leadership
Transformational leadership motivated by altruism and integrity.

pseudo-transformational leadership
Use of transformational leadership concepts for self-centered purposes.

EXHIBIT 7.1
The Augmentative Effect of Transformational Leadership

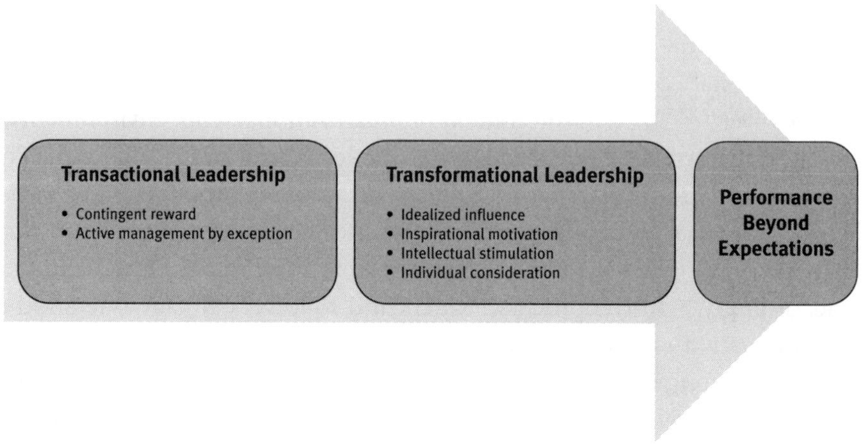

Ethics and Authentic Transformational Leadership

Authenticity in transformational leadership is closely related to leader integrity, which is discussed in greater detail in chapter 8. Grover and Moorman[47] and others[48] have outlined a basic model of leader integrity with four behavioral components: honesty, credibility, consistency, and ethics/morality. Each of these components is vital to leader integrity and, thus, essential for authenticity and transformational leadership. The lack of any or all of these components seriously undermines leadership and jeopardizes the leader's transformative potential. When leaders have integrity, they act in accordance with their thoughts and words.[49] To ensure integrity—and, thus, authenticity—in leadership, effective public health leaders must be both self-aware and self-sufficient.

Self-Awareness

Being aware of ethical frameworks and the ways they are acted out is perhaps the most central aspect in forming an ethical base to leadership. When the ethicist James Rest[50] identified four components of morality, moral sensitivity (or recognition) was the first one listed. Individuals who possess greater moral sensitivity are more tuned into ethical issues and better understand the ramifications of their actions, including how their words and actions influence others. Greater self-awareness can improve ethical judgments and decision-making, and it can heighten motivation to act ethically in accordance with one's ideal ethical self.

Self-Sufficiency

When individuals form a strong personal ethical framework and are aware of it, they are in a greater position to influence others. Leadership is influence, and influence occurs through both positional and personal power.[51] Personal power requires self-sufficiency—a certain degree of internal strength and completeness—which is only possible when leaders act with integrity from a strong and positive moral foundation. When individuals are not physically, emotionally, mentally, spiritually, ethically, and even fiscally self-sufficient, they risk sapping the strengths and motivations of others. If they are not careful, they risk being swayed by skewed perspectives and faltering in their ethical standards. Public health leaders must, therefore, be vigilant in understanding both the light and shadow sides of themselves and their leadership.

Authentic Leadership

Stated simply, authenticity in leadership amounts to being oneself and enabling others to be themselves as well. It comes from having a strong ethical foundation, being aware of it, and having the self-efficacy to encourage, if not inspire, others to be ethical. Such qualities can have a profound impact on followers and are therefore deeply empowering to leaders.[52] Authenticity both requires and provides a measure of intrapersonal and interpersonal resonance that allows leaders to understand, engage, and inspire followers.[53] Only leaders with strong ethical frameworks can be truly transformational.[43] The simplest framework for discerning authentic transformational leadership from pseudotransformational leadership involves three components: the ends sought, the means employed, and the consequences of the actions or approach. Exhibit 7.2 further distinguishes between the two approaches.

As Bass[46(p171)] points out, "Leaders are authentically transformational when they increase awareness of what is right, good, important, and beautiful, when they help to elevate followers' needs for achievement and self-actualization, when they foster in followers higher moral maturity, and when they move followers to go beyond their self-interests for the good of their group, organization, or society." Pseudotransformational leaders may be motivational and transformative, but they do so largely to pursue their own self-interests and not the interests of the collective.

Effective Public Health Leaders . . .

. . . are neither completely saints nor sinners; neither completely selfless nor selfish.[46]

Moderating Leader Effectiveness: Followership and the Transformational Leader

As noted earlier in the chapter, many past leadership theories have made the mistake of placing a myopic focus on leaders, their roles, and their behaviors. Such a focus tends to overlook the dynamic and interpersonal nature of the leader–follower dyad, which includes a number of factors that can have a

EXHIBIT 7.2
Authentic Transformational Leadership Versus Pseudotransformational Leadership

	Authentic Transformational Leadership	Pseudotransformational Leadership
Idealized influence	The leader displays selflessness, putting the organization first.	The leader may be subtly manipulative or display egoism.
Inspirational motivation	The leader empowers followers and inspires them to be better.	The leader uses coercion and may micromanage followers.
Intellectual stimulation	Innovation comes from the ranks; discourse is open and fluid.	Innovation follows the leader; groupthink may be present.
Individual consideration	Followers feel understood, appreciated, and developed.	Followers feel manipulated, underused, and/or trapped.

moderating effect on a leader's effectiveness. Leadership is relational in nature, and effective leaders must learn to value **followership**. Rousseau[54] stated, "Much trouble, we are told, is taken to teach young princes the art of reigning; but their education seems to do them no good. It would be better to begin by teaching them the art of obeying." Indeed, in most organizations, just as much potential—if not more—lies in developing the capacity of those who follow as in seeking to improve those who lead.

An evolution has occurred in what it means "to follow," and the days of passive subordination have given way to an era of dynamic, engaged followership. *Followership* can be defined as a follower's efforts to actively help an organization or a cause to succeed while independently exercising critical judgment in completing tasks and solving potential problems.[55] The way that followers respond to leaders, and the relationships they have, is as important as what leaders do or why they do it.[56] Today, fewer subordinates are content with or amenable to autocratic and directive superiors, and more want to be included in decisions that determine what they will do and how they will do it. Though most organizational structures maintain some form of managerial hierarchy, functionally and relationally these structures are becoming more horizontal. Indeed, as workforce education and specialization have increased, the idea of expertise—and thus leadership—has been redefined.[56] No longer are competence and skill the domain of superiors. Rather, those in leadership roles are surrounded by talented individuals in follower roles. The opportunity for followers to influence leaders and organizations has never been greater. Consequently, the concept of followership has taken on greater importance in research and practice.

Followership is related to the idea of **dynamic subordinancy** (sometimes spelled *subordinacy*), introduced by Zaleznik[57] in the 1960s. Individuals who show dynamic subordinancy assume responsibility for their own behavior and development, as well as for their contributions to the organization. Leaders, through training and supervision, can develop such an attitude, as well as an environment in which the attitude can be applied.[58] Plaintive obeisance is no longer appropriate for followers. Today's organizations thrive by seeking to fully engage all internal stakeholders.

Some researchers have begun examining the characteristics of followers that facilitate charismatic and/or transformational leadership. Ehrhart and Klein,[20] for

followership
A follower's efforts to actively help an organization or a cause to succeed while independently exercising critical judgment in completing tasks and solving potential problems.

Spotlight

Effective public health leaders must remember that leadership is relational in nature.

---

dynamic subordinancy
A condition in which individuals assume responsibility for their own behavior and development, as well as for their contributions to the organization, rather than simply relying on directional, autocratic leadership.

Consider This

"The people who are doing the work are the moving force.... My job is to create a space for them to clear out the rest of the organization and keep it at bay."
—Steve Jobs[59(p135)]

As an effective public health leader, what can you do to more fully empower your followers?

instance, found that followers' values and personality largely determined their preference for charismatic versus task-oriented leaders. Follower satisfaction and performance can be significantly influenced by how well the leader is able to meet or portray the style of leadership preferred by each follower. Leaders can therefore avoid losing followers if they understand and respond to the followers' motivations.[55] Dvir and Shamir[14] demonstrated that followers' development largely determined the extent to which transformational leadership is operationalized in the workplace.

The more leaders come to understand followers, the more they are able to tap into the human talent and potential within their organization, and the better they will be able to guide the organization toward positive outcomes. Likewise, the more followers engage their leaders in decision making, accountability, and performance, the greater influence they will have on their leaders and the organization. This symbiosis is not serendipitous. Rather, it is the function of a specific, value-driven, and behaviorally informed approach that can and should be practiced by leader and follower alike.

The topic of followership is discussed in greater detail in chapter 10.

Consider This

"The best of leadership is both transformational and transactional. Transformational leadership augments the effectiveness of transactional leadership; it does not replace transactional leadership."
—B. M. Bass and P. Steidlmeier[44(p191)]

As an effective public health leader, how do you utilize both transactional and transformational leadership?

Assessing Transformational Leadership

Multifactor Leadership Questionnaire (MLQ)
A 45-item questionnaire that can be implemented in both self-rated and other-rater formats to measure transformational, transactional, and passive-avoidant leadership.

The **Multifactor Leadership Questionnaire (MLQ)**, developed by Avolio and Bass,[15] is the most commonly used measure not only of transformational leadership but also of transactional and passive-avoidant leadership. It is a 45-item questionnaire that can be implemented in both self-rated and other-rater formats, or in multiple-rater options. The MLQ has been validated and extensively employed in a variety of research and consulting settings,[15,60,61,62,63,64,65,66] and it has been shown to be an effective tool in leadership development.[67,68]

The questions in the MLQ focus on four main areas: the three full-range leadership styles (i.e., transformational, transactional, and passive-avoidant) plus outcomes of leadership. Each of these areas includes a number of subscales or individual components.

Measuring Transformational Leadership

Transformational leaders move followers to have a greater vision of themselves and the opportunities and challenges of their environment. Such leaders are proactive. Instead of settling for expected performance, they strive to optimize individual, group, and organizational development and innovation. They influence associates, coworkers, and followers to strive for higher levels of performance and higher moral and ethical standards. The MLQ measures the following components of transformational leadership, sometimes known as the "four I's" (see exhibit 7.3):

1. **Idealized influence attributes and behaviors (IIA and IIB)** are what followers look for in leaders. Transformational leaders are admired, trusted, and respected, and followers identify with them and want to emulate them. Idealized attributes include the ability to instill pride in others, the tendency to put the good of the group above one's own self-interest, and a sense of power and confidence. Idealized behaviors include speaking about important values and beliefs, considering the moral and ethical consequences of decisions, and emphasizing a collective sense of mission.

   idealized influence attributes and behaviors (IIA and IIB) The collection of ideal qualities and actions that followers look for in leaders.

2. **Inspirational motivation (IM)** involves leaders' efforts to motivate others by providing meaning and challenge to the followers' work. Transformational leaders talk optimistically and enthusiastically about what needs to be accomplished, articulating a compelling vision of the future and expressing confidence that goals will be achieved. Ultimately, the followers come to envision that future for themselves.

   inspirational motivation (IM) The enthusiasm, encouragement, and optimism that a leader provides to inspire and motivate followers.

3. **Intellectual stimulation (IS)** is the way that leaders stimulate followers to be creative and innovative, and it typically involves questioning assumptions, reframing problems, and approaching old situations in new ways. Transformational leaders solicit new ideas and creative solutions from followers, and they do not ridicule or publicly criticize individuals' mistakes. They reexamine critical assumptions, seek differing perspectives when solving problems, and encourage others to approach issues from different angles.

   intellectual stimulation (IS) The degree to which a leader provides a stimulating environment through dialogue, innovation, creativity, and collaborative problem solving.

4. **Individual consideration (IC)**, as demonstrated by transformational leaders, involves acting as a coach or mentor to followers and paying attention to each individual's need for achievement and growth. Through individual consideration, leaders provide new learning opportunities and a supportive climate, and followers develop to successively higher levels of potential. Leaders who rank high in this component treat others as individuals rather than just as members of the group; consider each individual's unique needs, abilities, and aspirations; devote significant time to teaching and coaching; and help others develop their strengths.

   individual consideration (IC) The way in which a leader acts as a coach or mentor and pays attention to each individual's need for achievement and growth.

Measuring Transactional Leadership

Transactional leadership focuses on defining clear expectations for followers and promoting follower performance to achieve the expected levels. It includes

EXHIBIT 7.3
The "Four I's" of Transformational Leadership

Idealized Influence

The leader epitomizes ideal attitudes and behaviors, influencing followers through charismatic vision and action.

Inspirational Motivation

The leader motivates and inspires followers to work toward a common vision and/or shared goals.

The "Four I's" of Transformational Leadership

Intellectual Stimulation

The leader engenders innovation, creativity, and critical thinking in followers.

Individual Consideration

The leader individualizes efforts to understand followers and helps them realize their full potential.

contingent reward (CR)
A transactional leadership approach that sets expectations for followers and offers recognition or rewards when goals are achieved.

both constructive transactions, such as rewards for goal achievement, and corrective transactions, such as steps taken to address poor performance—both of which are among the core management functions in organizations. The two components of transactional leadership are as follows:

1. **Contingent reward (CR)** leadership clarifies expectations for followers and offers recognition or rewards when goals are achieved. Used effectively, it can encourage individuals and groups to achieve expected levels of performance. Leaders demonstrating this component provide others with assistance in exchange for their efforts, speak in specific terms about responsibility for achieving performance targets, make clear what one can expect to receive when performance goals are achieved, and express satisfaction when people meet expectations.

management by exception, active (MBEA)
A transactional leadership approach that involves setting clear standards for compliance, specifying what constitutes ineffective performance, closely monitoring for deviances and mistakes, and taking corrective action as quickly as possible when problems occur.

2. **Management by exception, active (MBEA)**, involves establishing clear standards for follower compliance and specifying what constitutes ineffective performance. It further implies actively monitoring follower performance and taking corrective action as quickly as possible when problems occur. Leaders who demonstrate this approach focus their attention on irregularities, mistakes, exceptions, and deviations from standards.

Measuring Passive-Avoidant Leadership

Passive-avoidant leadership, the last of the three full-range leadership styles, is apparent in leaders who do not specify agreements, clarify expectations, or provide goals and standards for followers. The passive-avoidant style includes two main types of behavior, both of which have a negative impact on followers and associates:

1. **Management by exception, passive (MBEP)**, is similar to MBEA except that the leaders take a more passive and reactive approach. They do not address situations and problems systematically; instead, they wait for things to go wrong before taking action. They show a firm belief in the "If it ain't broke, don't fix it" approach and, as a result, often fail to intervene until problems become serious.

2. **Laissez-faire (LF) leadership** can be seen in leaders who choose not to get involved when important issues arise, are often absent when needed, avoid making decisions, and are slow to respond to urgent questions. It is sometimes referred to as *nonleadership*.[62]

> **management by exception, passive (MBEP)**
> A passive-avoidant leadership approach in which the leader waits for things to go wrong before taking action.
>
> **laissez-faire (LF) leadership**
> A passive approach to leadership in which leaders are absent or uninvolved in important issues and decisions; sometimes referred to as *nonleadership*.

Measuring Leadership Outcomes

In addition to assessing transformational, transactional, and passive-avoidant leadership components, the MLQ also measures three specific leadership outcomes: extra effort (EE), effectiveness (EFF), and satisfaction with the leadership (SAT). Extra effort involves getting others to do more than is expected, heightening others' desire to succeed, and increasing others' willingness to try harder. Effectiveness is the degree to which leaders are successful in meeting others' job-related needs, in representing their group to higher authority, and in meeting organizational requirements. Satisfaction with the leadership reflects the leader's ability to work with others in a satisfying way.

Developing Transformational Leadership for Public Health

Effective public health leaders face a constant barrage of internal and external pressures to provide better services with greater accountability and higher ethical standards. Each day, they are called on to make difficult decisions in the face of funding cuts, staff turnover, increased patient loads during

---

Spotlight

The Multifactor Leadership Questionnaire can be used to develop a profile of attributes and behaviors related to styles of leadership, as well as general outcomes of leadership, and it can help leaders identify strengths and growth areas to enhance their work with others. However, it was not designed to link leaders to specific leadership styles. In assessing MLQ results, rather than labeling a leader as either transformational or transactional, a more appropriate approach might be to identify the leader as, for instance, more transformational than the norm or less transactional than the norm.

Leadership Application Case: Tears in the Office

The Leadership Application Case at the beginning of this book provides realistic scenarios for the application of key leadership concepts covered in the text. See the section marked "Chapter 7 Application" for the scenario and discussion questions that correspond with this chapter.

economic downturns, and uncertainties related to national healthcare reform. At the same time, they are tasked with leading others and ensuring that their followers' actions are effective and appropriate. Leader–follower interactions, small-group situations, organizational cultures, and interorganizational collaborations all present situations in which effective and ethical leadership is vital. In many scenarios, leaders may be tempted to avoid pressing decisions or to maintain the status quo to the best of their abilities. But if they instead choose transformational leadership, they can challenge the norm, take risks, and strive to transform themselves and their organizations to make a meaningful difference in the health of the public they serve.

A Framework of Competencies

Rowitz[69] distinguishes between the management and leadership skill sets for public health, and he arranges them along a continuum. He includes agency management skills (e.g., planning, organizing, controlling, budgeting) and organizational leadership skills (e.g., coaching, team building, problem solving) at one end of the continuum, and he places transactional leadership skills (e.g., relationship building, collaboration, communication) in the middle. At the other end of the continuum are strategic leadership skills (e.g., systems thinking, strategic planning, negotiation, policy analysis) and transformational leadership skills (e.g., innovation, change, systems transformation). Rowitz's model recognizes that a broad spectrum of management and leadership skills are vital to effective public health leadership, and, with the right competency framework and metrics, it can be highly useful in organizing and tracking leadership development efforts.

Drawing upon earlier public health leadership competency frameworks, a group of scholars and practitioners associated with the National Public Health Leadership Development Network (NLN) set out to develop a Leadership Competency Framework. The NLN group focused not only on identifying the major areas of leadership practice but also on considering future challenges that would require specific skills and abilities on the part of public health leaders. The framework developed over subsequent NLN conferences, ultimately consisting of 79 competencies across four areas[70]:

1. Core transformational competencies, including visionary leadership, sense of mission, and effectiveness as a change agent (see exhibit 7.4)
2. Political competencies, which relate to political processes, negotiation, ethics and power, and marketing and education
3. Transorganizational competencies, such as understanding organizational dynamics, interorganizational collaborating dynamics, and social forecasting and marketing
4. Team-building competencies, such as developing team-oriented structures and systems, facilitating development of teams and work groups, serving in facilitation and mediation roles, and being an effective team member

EXHIBIT 7.4
NLN Core
Transformational
Competencies

VISIONARY LEADERSHIP
1. Articulates vision and scenarios for change
2. Facilitates development of vision
3. Encourages others to share the vision
4. Applies innovative methods for strategic decision making

SENSE OF MISSION
1. Articulates and models professional values, beliefs, and ethics
2. Facilitates development of mission and purpose
3. Facilitates reassessment and adaptation of mission to vision
4. Facilitates development of strategies to achieve mission

EFFECTIVE CHANGE AGENT
1. Facilitates development of a learning organization
2. Creates systems and structures for transformational change
3. Creates evaluation systems for change strategies
4. Facilitates strategic and tactical assessment and planning
5. Facilitates identification of emerging and acute problems
6. Utilizes change theories and models in strategic development
7. Identifies emotional and rational elements in strategic planning
8. Creates critical dynamic tension within change strategies
9. Facilitates development of effective dialogue
10. Utilizes methods to empower others to take action
11. Models active learning and personal mastery
12. Models and facilitates cultural sensitivity and competence
13. Models utilization and application of systems thinking
14. Models critical thinking and analysis skills
15. Models appropriate risk-taking behavior
16. Models group process behaviors: listening, dialoging, negotiating, encouraging, and motivating
17. Models leadership traits: integrity, credibility, enthusiasm, commitment, honesty, caring, and trust

Source: Data from Wright, K., L. Rowitz, A. Merkle, W. M. Reid, G. Robinson, B. Herzog, D. Weber, D. Carmichael, T. R. Balderson, and E. Baker. 2000. "Competency Development in Public Health." *American Journal of Public Health* 90 (8): 1202–7.

The NLN framework is noteworthy in that it goes above and beyond the general practitioner competencies set forth elsewhere and outlines a vision for public health leadership, much of which focuses on transformational aspects. Like any skill, transformational leadership can be developed through a variety of means, and the effort might be most effective when these means are used in concerted combination with one another.

An initial measure of transformational leadership tendencies can be accomplished through an instrument such as the Multifactor Leadership Questionnaire, discussed earlier. The self-rating versions of these instruments can quickly provide initial insights about an individual leader, whereas a 360-degree review—in which the individual's leaders, followers, and peers all rate the individual's leadership behaviors and characteristics—can provide a greater breadth of perspective and less biased profiling. Such an assessment process informs the individuals being reviewed, helping them gain awareness of unknown tendencies in their leadership style.

Once the assessment has been completed and the leader's self-awareness has been heightened, targeted leader development efforts can be applied in areas where transformational skills were found to be less well developed. For example, an individual review and comprehensive 360-degree feedback might reveal that a leader provides intellectually stimulating environments and offers a high degree of individual consideration but is not highly inspirational or motivating. The leader might even come across as self-serving. Such feedback could help the leader focus personal and professional development efforts on being more visionary and demonstrating greater selflessness as a leader. Combining assessments and associated feedback with dedicated leadership development programs, such as mentoring programs, can be especially helpful (as discussed in chapter 13). External consultants can also play a meaningful role in development, and they can typically offer a more objective view of the organization and the leaders being measured.

Providing Opportunities

Finally, the importance of providing leaders with opportunities to practice transformational skills cannot be overlooked. Public health is a profession of many disciplines, but too often these disciplines remain isolated in functional silos. When such isolation occurs, individuals with great leadership potential can become locked into the routines of their job and have neither the opportunity nor the encouragement to lead in transformational ways.

A study by Carlton and colleagues[71,72] demonstrated that a breadth of transformational and transactional leadership styles were used in local public health departments, but it also suggested that transformational styles were more likely to be practiced in specific areas. For instance, the styles seemed more amenable to people working in administration or health education than to nurses in clinical practice or environmentalists conducting restaurant inspections. Such discrepancies can be addressed to some extent through cross-cutting teams or task forces dedicated to transformational organization or community change. Such groups can help provide individuals with opportunities to develop and apply transformational skills in addition to the standard transactional skills required in their areas of expertise.

 Consider This

"If you treat a man as he is, he will remain how he is; if you treat him as he ought to be and could be, he will become as he ought to be and could be."
—Johann Wolfgang von Goethe[73]

As an effective public health leader, could you use transformational leadership skills to implement Goethe's statement? If so, how would you do it? If not, what leadership model would you use instead, and why?

Case Study: The Smoking Ban in Lexington, Kentucky[74,75]

Lexington, Kentucky, for years had prided itself on being the center of the burley tobacco belt, and it was at one time part of the largest burley tobacco–producing county in the United States. However, on July 1, 2003, the Lexington–Fayette Urban County Government Council voted 11–3 to ban smoking in enclosed public spaces such as restaurants and bars. Suddenly, Lexington had become the first community in Kentucky to vote for such a ban to reduce the public health effects of smoking.

Two transformational leaders—Dr. Melinda Rowe, the Fayette County commissioner of health, and Dr. Ellen Hahn, a professor at the University of Kentucky College of Nursing and director of the Kentucky Center for Smoke-Free Policy—teamed up to lobby the Urban County Council to implement the policy. Local restaurant and bar owners, fearful that their clientele would abandon their businesses, fought the ban all the way to the Kentucky Supreme Court. But following a 6–1 ruling, the ban took effect on April 27, 2004.

The reasoning behind the ban was based on the potential health effects not only for people who smoke but also for nonsmokers who may be affected by second-hand smoke. Soon after implementation, health statistics began to show the ban's results. By 2005, asthma-related emergency room visits had gone down by 22 percent. In less than two years, the smoking rate in Fayette County decreased from 26 percent to 17.5 percent—meaning 16,500 fewer smokers—which resulted in healthcare savings of $21 million per year, according to the Kentucky Center for Smoke-Free Policy. Furthermore, an analysis of nicotine in public-space workers' hair quickly demonstrated a decrease of 56 percent. Dr. Hahn has estimated that a statewide smoking ban in Kentucky's public spaces would result in a smoking rate decrease of 32 percent.

The public health efforts in Kentucky to reduce the effects of smoking have continued since the original ordinance in Lexington. Jefferson County—the home of Louisville, the state's largest city—has joined the effort, as have an additional 10 counties and 24 other cities. One-third of the population of Kentucky is covered by smoking ordinances, although the rural areas of the state remain largely uncovered. A statewide ban has failed repeatedly in the Kentucky General Assembly.

(continued)

Discussion and Application Questions

1. Why have effective public health leaders had difficulty educating their communities about the need to stop smoking?
2. Is a city-by-city or county-by-county approach to banning smoking in public spaces the most effective approach? If not, how might a transformational leader implement a different approach?
3. What challenges does smoking present to effective public health leaders?
4. Imagine you are the new health department director of a county that does not have a ban on smoking in public spaces. How would you function as a transformational leader in such a situation?

Summary

Today's public health landscape demands leaders not only who are competent in their day-to-day work but also who have a strong ethical focus and can get the most from themselves and their organizations. The model of transformational leadership helps address this need by emphasizing ways that leaders can enhance followers' motivation, morale, and performance.

The transformational leadership model builds on past leadership theories and addresses some of their shortcomings. Rather than simply focusing on leaders and their attributes, the transformational model considers leadership in the context of dynamic interpersonal relationships with followers. It reflects an evolution in what it means "to follow," in which the days of passive subordination have given way to an era of active, engaged followership. Transformational leadership includes certain aspects of transactional leadership—such as contingent rewards to encourage goal achievement and corrective action to address poor performance—but it augments these elements with other aspects to make the leadership transformational.

Transformational leadership, transactional leadership, and passive-avoidant leadership may be examined together, with the three models collectively referred to as *full-range leadership*. The tool most commonly used in measuring these types of leadership is the Multifactor Leadership Questionnaire. The questionnaire systematically assesses transformational, transactional, and passive-avoidant leadership, as well as leadership outcomes. It considers four components of transformational leadership: (1) idealized influence attributes and behaviors, (2) inspirational motivation, (3) intellectual stimulation, and (4) individual consideration.

Ethics and morality are key to transformational leadership, and they help distinguish authentic transformational leadership from pseudotransformational leadership used for selfish purposes. Leaders must be both self-aware and self-sufficient to ensure integrity and authenticity in their leadership.

Scholars and practitioners associated with the National Public Health Leadership Development Network have created a Leadership Competency Framework that outlines a vision for public health leadership, much of which is based on a transformational leadership approach. Leaders who effectively use this approach are able to *transform* the raw material of human and organizational resources into people and systems prepared for today's challenges.

Discussion Questions

1. What are the "four I's" of transformational leadership?
2. How are transformational leadership and transactional leadership related?
3. Distinguish between authentic transformational leadership and pseudotransformational leadership. How is authenticity related to ethical leadership practice?
4. What is the role of followership in moderating transformational leadership?
5. Describe the importance of relationships in transformational leadership.
6. What are the core transformational competencies? How would you apply them to effective public health leadership?
7. Compare and contrast the transformational, transactional, and passive-avoidant leadership styles.
8. How does the Leadership Competency Framework affect the development of leaders in public health?
9. Describe the Multifactor Leadership Questionnaire, and explain its purpose. How might you use it in a public health organization?
10. For deeper thought: Imagine you are the director of environmental services for a county or city health department. How could you engage in transformational leadership in that role?

Web Resources

Johannsen, M. 2014. "The Transformational Leadership Style: What It Is and Isn't." Legacee. Published March 9. www.legacee.com/transformational-leadership/.

Mind Tools. 2017. "Transformational Leadership: Becoming an Inspirational Leader." Accessed June 19. www.mindtools.com/pages/article/transformational-leadership.htm.

Spahr, P. 2016. "What Is Transactional Leadership? How Structure Leads to Results." Updated October 19. http://online.stu.edu/transactional-leadership/.

References

1. de Saint-Exupéry, A. (1942) 1986. *Flight to Arras.* Translated by L. Galantiere. San Diego, CA: Harcourt Brace.

2. Brooks, R. G., L. M. Beitsch, P. Street, and A. Chukmaitov. 2009. "Aligning Public Health Financing with Essential Public Health Service Functions and National Public Health Performance Standards." *Journal of Public Health Management & Practice* 15 (4): 299–306.

3. Kinner, K., and C. Pellegrini. 2009. "Expenditures for Public Health: Assessing Historical and Prospective Trends." *American Journal of Public Health* 99 (10): 1780–91.

4. Gebbie, K. M., A. Raziano, and S. Elliott. 2009. "Public Health Workforce Enumeration." *American Journal of Public Health* 99 (5): 786–87.

5. Chernichovsky, D., and A. A. Leibowitz. 2010. "Integrating Public Health and Personal Care in a Reformed US Health Care System." *American Journal of Public Health* 100 (2): 205–11.

6. Milstein, B., J. Homer, and G. Hirsch. 2010. "Analyzing National Health Reform Strategies with a Dynamic Simulation Model." *American Journal of Public Health* 100 (5): 811–19.

7. Thomas, J. C., P. D. MacDonald, and E. M. Wenink. 2009. "Ethical Decision Making in a Crisis: A Case Study of Ethics in Public Health Emergencies." *Journal of Public Health Management & Practice* 15 (2): E16–E21.

8. Annett, H. 2009. "Leadership in Public Health: A View from a Large English PCT Co-terminous with a Local Authority." *Journal of Public Health* 31 (2): 205–7.

9. Koh, H. K., and M. Jacobson. 2009. "Fostering Public Health Leadership." *Journal of Public Health* 31 (2): 199–201.

10. Hunter, D. J. 2009. "Leading for Health and Wellbeing: The Need for a New Paradigm." *Journal of Public Health* 31 (2): 202–4.

11. Williams, J. C., J. Costich, W. D. Hacker, and J. S. Davis. 2010. "Lessons Learned in Systems Thinking Approach for Evaluation Planning." *Journal of Public Health Management & Practice* 16 (2): 151–55.

12. Association of Schools of Public Health Education Committee. 2009. *Doctor of Public Health (DrPH) Core Competency Model, Version 1.3.*

Published November. www.aspph.org/app/uploads/2014/04/ DrPHVersion1-3.pdf.

13. Association of Schools of Public Health Education Committee. 2006. *Master's Degree in Public Health Core Competency Model, Version 2.3.* Published August. www.aspph.org/app/uploads/2014/04/Version 2.31_FINAL.pdf.

14. Dvir, T., and B. Shamir. 2003. "Follower Developmental Characteristics as Predicting Transformational Leadership: A Longitudinal Field Study." *Leadership Quarterly* 14 (3): 327–44.

15. Avolio, B. J., and B. M. Bass. 2004. *Multifactor Leadership Questionnaire: Manual & Sample Set.* Menlo Park, CA: Mind Garden Inc.

16. Conger, J. A., and R. N. Kanungo. 1987. "Toward a Behavioral Theory of Charismatic Leadership in Organizational Settings." *Academy of Management Review* 12 (4): 637–47.

17. Conger, J. A., R. N. Kanungo, S. T. Menon, and P. Mathur. 1997. "Measuring Charisma: Dimensionality and Validity of the Conger-Kanungo Scale of Charismatic Leadership." *Canadian Journal of Administrative Sciences* 14 (3): 290–301.

18. Conger, J. A., R. N. Kanungo, and S. T. Menon. 2000. "Charismatic Leadership and Follower Effects." *Journal of Organizational Behavior* 21 (7): 747–67.

19. Yammarino, F. J., A. J. Dubinsky, L. B. Comer, and M. A. Jolson. 1997. "Women and Transformational and Contingent Reward Leadership: A Multiple-Levels-of-Analysis Perspective." *Academy of Management Journal* 40 (1): 205–22.

20. Ehrhart, M. G., and K. J. Klein. 2001. "Predicting Followers' Preferences for Charismatic Leadership: The Influence of Follower Values and Personality." *Leadership Quarterly* 12 (2): 153–79.

21. Choi, Y., and R. R. Mai-Dalton. 1999. "The Model of Followers' Responses to Self-Sacrificial Leadership: An Empirical Test." *Leadership Quarterly* 10 (3): 397–421.

22. Shamir, B., R. J. House, and M. B. Arthur. 1993. "The Motivational Effects of Charismatic Leadership: A Self-Concept Based Theory." *Organization Science* 4 (4): 577–94.

23. Kouzes, J. M., and B. Z. Posner. 2004. "Follower-Oriented Leadership." In *Encyclopedia of Leadership*, edited by G. R. Goethals, G. Sorenson, and J. M. Burns, 494–99. Oxford, UK: Sage Reference/ Berkshire.

24. Hackman, R. 2002. *Leading Teams: Setting the Stage for Great Performances.* Boston: Harvard Business School Press.

25. Bass, B. M., and B. J. Avolio. 1993. "Transformational Leadership: A Response to the Critiques." In *Leadership Theory and Research: Perspectives and Directions*, edited by M. M. Chemers and R. Ayman, 49–60. San Diego, CA: Academic Press.

26. Waldman, D. A., B. M. Bass, and F. J. Yammarino. 1990. "Adding to Contingent-Reward Behavior: The Augmenting Effect of Charismatic Leadership." *Group & Organizational Studies* 15 (4): 381–94.

27. Spahr, P. 2016. "What Is Transactional Leadership? How Structure Leads to Results." Updated October 19. http://online.stu.edu/transactional-leadership/.

28. Barbuto, J. E. 2005. "Motivation and Transactional, Charismatic, and Transformational Leadership: A Test of Antecedents." *Journal of Leadership & Organizational Studies* 11 (4): 26–40.

29. Bass, B. M., D. I. Jung, B. J. Avolio, and Y. Berson. 2003. "Predicting Unit Performance by Assessing Transformational and Transactional Leadership." *Journal of Applied Psychology* 88 (2): 207–18.

30. Boerner, S., S. A. Eisenbeiss, and D. Griesser. 2007. "Follower Behavior and Organizational Performance: The Impact of Transformational Leaders." *Journal of Leadership & Organizational Studies* 13 (3): 15–26.

31. Gellis, Z. D. 2001. "Social Work Perceptions of Transformational and Transactional Leadership in Health Care." *Social Work Research* 25 (1): 17–25.

32. Lowe, K. B., K. Galen Kroeck, and N. Sivasubramaniam. 1996. "Effectiveness Correlates of Transformational and Transactional Leadership: A Meta-analytic Review of the MLQ Literature." *Leadership Quarterly* 7 (3): 385–425.

33. Mary, N. L. 2005. "Transformational Leadership in Human Service Organizations." *Administration in Social Work* 29 (2): 105–18.

34. Bass, B. M. 1990. "From Transactional to Transformational Leadership: Learning to Share the Vision." *Organizational Dynamics* 18 (3): 19–31.

35. Friedman, A. A. 2004. "Beyond Mediocrity: Transformational Leadership Within a Transactional Framework." *International Journal of Leadership in Education* 7 (3): 203–24.

36. Bass, B. M., and B. J. Avolio. 1993. "Transformational Leadership and Organizational Culture." *Public Administration Quarterly* 17 (1): 112–21.

37. Howell, J. M., and B. Shamir. 2005. "The Role of Followers in the Charismatic Leadership Process: Relationships and Their Consequences." *Academy of Management Review* 30 (1): 96–112.

38. Jermier, J. M. 1993. "Introduction—Charismatic Leadership: Neo-Weberian Perspectives." *Leadership Quarterly* 4 (3–4): 217–34.

39. Klein, K. J., and R. J. House. 1995. "On Fire: Charismatic Leadership and Levels of Analysis." *Leadership Quarterly* 6 (2): 183–98.

40. De Hoogh, A. H. B., D. N. Den Hartog, and P. L. Koopman. 2005. "Linking the Big Five-Factors of Personality to Charismatic and Transactional Leadership; Perceived Dynamic Work Environment as a Moderator." *Journal of Organizational Behavior* 26 (7): 839–65.

41. Brown, F. W., and D. Moshavi. 2005. "Transformational Leadership and Emotional Intelligence: A Potential Pathway for an Increased Understanding of Interpersonal Influence." *Journal of Organizational Behavior* 26 (7): 867–71.

42. Haslam, S. A., and M. J. Platow. 2001. "The Link Between Leadership and Followership: How Affirming Social Identity Translates Vision into Action." *Personality and Social Psychology Bulletin* 27 (11): 1469–79.

43. Burns, J. M. 1978. *Leadership*. New York: Harper & Row.

44. Bass, B. M., and P. Steidlmeier. 1999. "Ethics, Character and Authentic Transformational Leadership Behavior." *Leadership Quarterly* 10 (2): 181–217.

45. Johnson, C. E. 2009. *Meeting the Ethical Challenges of Leadership: Casting Light or Shadow*. Los Angeles: Sage.

46. Bass, B. M. 1998. "The Ethics of Transformational Leadership." In *Ethics: The Heart of Leadership*, edited by J. Ciulla, 169–92. Westport, CT: Praeger.

47. Grover, S. L., and R. Moorman. 2009. "Challenges to Leader Integrity: How Leaders Deal with Dilemmas of Honesty." In *Ethical Dilemmas in Management*, edited by C. Gartsen and T. Hernes, 52–63. New York: Routledge.

48. Kouzes, J. M., and B. Z. Posner. 2007. *The Leadership Challenge*, 4th ed. San Francisco: Jossey-Bass.

49. Becker, T. E. 1998. "Integrity in Organizations: Beyond Honesty and Conscientiousness." *Academy of Management Review* 23 (1): 154–61.

50. Rest, J. 1994. "Background: Theory and Research." In *Moral Development in the Professions: Psychology and Applied Ethics*, edited by J. Rest and D. Narvaez, 1–25. Hillsdale, NJ: Lawrence Erlbaum Associates.

51. Fernandez, C. S. P. 2009. "The Power of Positive Personal Regard." In *Managing the Public Health Enterprise*, edited by E. L. Baker, A. J. Menkens, and J. E. Porter, 45–49. Sudbury, MA: Jones & Bartlett.

52. Palanski, M. E., and F. J. Yammarino. 2007. "Integrity and Leadership: Clearing the Conceptual Confusion." *European Management Journal* 25 (3): 171–84.

53. Goleman, D., R. Boyatzis, and A. McKee. 2002. *Primal Leadership: Realizing the Power of Emotional Intelligence.* Boston: Harvard Business School Press.

54. Rousseau, J. J. 1973. *The Social Contract and Discourses.* Markham, ON: Fitzhenry & Whiteside.

55. Kelley, R. E. 2004. "Followership." In *Encyclopedia of Leadership,* edited by G. R. Goethals, G. Sorenson, and J. M. Burns, 504–13. Oxford, UK: Sage Reference/Berkshire.

56. Kellerman, B. 2008. *Followership: How Followers Are Creating Change and Changing Leaders.* Boston: Harvard Business School Press.

57. Zaleznik, A. 1965. "The Dynamics of Subordinacy." *Harvard Business Review* 43 (3): 119–31.

58. Crockett, W. J. 1981. "Dynamic Subordinancy." *Training Development Journal* 35 (5): 155–64.

59. Fluegelman, A. (ed.). 1984. "The Making of the Macintosh." *Macworld* 1 (1): 126–35.

60. Avolio, B. J., and B. M. Bass. 1999. "Re-examining the Components of Transformational and Transactional Leadership Using the Multifactor Leadership Questionnaire." *Journal of Occupational & Organizational Psychology* 72 (4): 441–62.

61. Hartog, D. N. D., J. J. Van Muijen, and P. L. Koopman. 1997. "Transactional Versus Transformational Leadership: An Analysis of the MLQ." *Journal of Occupational & Organizational Psychology* 70 (1): 19–34.

62. Hinkin, T. R., and C. A. Schriesheim. 2008. "A Theoretical and Empirical Examination of the Transactional and Non-leadership Dimensions of the Multifactor Leadership Questionnaire (MLQ)." *Leadership Quarterly* 19 (5): 501–13.

63. Rowold, J., and K. Heinitz. 2007. "Transformational and Charismatic Leadership: Assessing the Convergent, Divergent and Criterion Validity of the MLQ and the CKS." *Leadership Quarterly* 18 (2): 121–33.

64. Rowold, J., and A. Rohmann. 2009. "Transformational and Transactional Leadership Styles, Followers' Positive and Negative Emotions, and Performance in German Nonprofit Orchestras." *Nonprofit Management & Leadership* 20 (1): 41–59.

65. Tejeda, M. J. 2001. "The MLQ Revisited: Psychometric Properties and Recommendations." *Leadership Quarterly* 12 (1): 31–52.

66. Tepper, B. J., and P. M. Percy. 1994. "Structural Validity of the Multifactor Leadership Questionnaire." *Educational & Psychological Measurement* 54 (3): 734–44.

67. Horwitz, I. B., S. K. Horwitz, P. Daram, M. L. Brandt, F. C. Brunicardi, and S. S. Awad. 2008. "Transformational, Transactional, and Passive-Avoidant Leadership Characteristics of a Surgical Resident Cohort: Analysis Using the Multifactor Leadership Questionnaire and Implications for Improving Surgical Education Curriculums." *Journal of Surgical Research* 148 (1): 49–59.

68. Spinelli, R. J. 2006. "The Applicability of Bass's Model of Transformational, Transactional, and Laissez-Faire Leadership in the Hospital Administrative Environment." *Hospital Topics* 84 (2): 11–18.

69. Rowitz, L. 2010. "Management and Leadership." *Journal of Public Health Management & Practice* 16 (2): 174–76.

70. Wright, K., L. Rowitz, A. Merkle, W. M. Reid, G. Robinson, B. Herzog, D. Weber, D. Carmichael, T. R. Balderson, and E. Baker. 2000. "Competency Development in Public Health." *American Journal of Public Health* 90 (8): 1202–7.

71. Carlton, E. L., J. W. Holsinger Jr., M. Riddell, and H. Bush. 2015. "Full-Range Public Health Leadership, Part 1: Quantitative Analysis." *Frontiers in Public Health*. Published April 30. http://journal. frontiersin.org/article/10.3389/fpubh.2015.00073/full.

72. Carlton, E. L., J. W. Holsinger Jr., M. Riddell, and H. Bush. 2015. "Full-Range Public Health Leadership, Part 2: Qualitative Analysis and Synthesis." *Frontiers in Public Health*. Published July 8. http://journal. frontiersin.org/article/10.3389/fpubh.2015.00174/full.

73. von Goethe, J. W. n.d. "Goethe Quotes." Accessed September 11, 2017. www.quotationspage.com/quote/27074.html.

74. *Lexington Herald Leader*. 2013. "Lexington Smoking Ban Also Snuffed Fears." Published June 30. www.kentucky.com/opinion/editorials/ article44431956.html.

75. Meehan, M. 2014. "10 Years After It Became Law, Fayette County's Smoking Law Is Gaining Acceptance." *Lexington Herald-Leader*. Published April 26. www.kentucky.com/living/family/ article44486688.html.

III

THE EFFECTIVE PRACTICE OF PUBLIC HEALTH LEADERSHIP

8

THE ETHICAL BASIS OF PUBLIC HEALTH LEADERSHIP

James R. Thobaben and James W. Holsinger Jr.

Learning Objectives

Upon completion of this chapter, you should be able to

- apply moral reasoning, using operating values or middle axioms, for public health;
- demonstrate how moral consideration should factor into public health decision making;
- illustrate how moral conflict might arise in public health leadership situations;
- explain how such conflict might be resolved (or at least addressed) to the extent necessary to make coherent decisions and address unavoidable disagreement; and
- differentiate basic types of moral reasoning.

Focus on Leadership Competencies

This chapter emphasizes the following Association of Schools and Programs of Public Health (ASPPH) leadership competencies:

- Demonstrate transparency, integrity, and honesty in all actions.
- Apply social justice and human rights principles when addressing community needs.

It also addresses the following Council on Linkages public health leadership competencies:

- Incorporates ethical standards of practice.
- Ensures use of professional development opportunities by individuals and teams.

Note: See the appendix at the end of the book for complete lists of competencies.

Introduction

Effective public health leaders must have a core understanding of moral reasoning and ethical decision making. They need to recognize that individuals and communities have values and that all people act in a moral manner, with greater or lesser consistency toward a desired end. Everyone—at least anyone capable of performing some minimal degree of analysis followed by intentional behavior—seeks some good. People, to varying degrees, consciously act on preferences. Even those individuals who are deemed immoral or whose values are considered repugnant make moral choices for the "good" that they choose to recognize. To use traditional language, the will follows the affections; to use psychosocial language, decisions follow attachments.

Public health leaders cannot allow themselves to be immobilized by an endless search for absolute, unassailable moral truths to guide every choice made, nor can they be amoral actors who refuse culpability or diffuse accountability with claims that the morally preferable option is not knowable or does not even exist. Rather, they must honor the values of the organization of which they are part and simultaneously acknowledge their own core values. These values, in turn, must be pragmatically expressed in light of the complexity of social structures, interpersonal relationships, plurality of worldviews, and limited predictability of epidemiological interventions.

The Starting Assumption: The Good of Public Health

In some sense, moral foundations exist prior to conscious moral calculations, at least assuming that any given moral choice or valuing of a virtue is something more than crass postevent self-justification. The basic core values by which right and wrong are defined are either selected by, socialized into, or culturally assumed by the one reasoning about moral decisions.

The good that is assumed in public health is the ongoing biological well-being of a population and the individuals who make up that population. This is the assumed mission, or reason for existing, for all public health organizations—an *a priori* foundational assertion. The vast majority of public health leaders share this assertion about the foundational good of their field. In pursuing the improvement (or at least maintenance) of the total health of a given human population, most public health organizations use some kind of utilitarian approach. In the tradition of Bentham and Mills, Rachels[1(p156)] defines this approach as doing "whatever will produce the greatest possible balance of happiness over unhappiness for everyone who will be affected by our action." Of course, people may have different interpretations of "biological well-being"— as well as different ideas about the boundaries of a "population"—and with those differences come variations in moral choices. The definitions of key terms must not be so vague as to be meaningless, or else endless debates or even the duplicitous serving of political agendas might result. A precise definition of the term health itself is therefore essential.

The World Health Organization Definition of Health

In 1946, the World Health Organization (WHO),[2] in its earliest days as a formal body, provided the following definition of *health*: "Health is a state of complete physical, mental, and social well-being and not merely the absence of disease or infirmity." This definition was written shortly after the end of World War II, and it reflects postwar hopes and fears, with genuine anxiety about the coming Cold War. It also reflects extraordinary belief in the power of science, along with great ambivalence about who might use that power. The WHO definition called civil society toward a positive goal, but critics today, with a comfortable perspective created by decades of reflection, have pointed out its flaws—for instance, that its focus on "complete" well-being might be considered "utopian, inflexible, and unrealistic."[3(p13)]

Reconsidering the Definition of Health

For public health purposes, a better approach to defining *health* is based on the idea of **plastic biological functionality**. Under this approach, the norm for human functioning is not anatomical or physiological normality but rather the biological capacity to operate given the social and ecological order. Plasticity represents the range defined by what is biologically possible given reasonably available assets, including technologies. In other words, a person with a functioning artificial limb is not less "normal" than one with all major appendages intact. Normality for this purpose is a statistical range of functional capacity, not a physical ideal.[4,5,6,7,8,9,10]

> **plastic biological functionality**
> A person's biological capacity to operate given the social and ecological order.

The legal power of public health is simply too great to allow expansive definitions of its mission. If *health* is defined as something more than physiological and anatomical functionality (or some equivalent), then the potential for abuse is significant. Such abuse may at first be intrusive, then onerous, and finally oppressive. For this reason, if for no other, *health* must be defined in a restricted way, based on plastic biological functionality.

Over the last several decades, WHO has done a better job in defining *health* in terms of functionality, as demonstrated in the International Classification of Impairment, Disability, and Handicap and its successor, the International Classification of Functioning, Disability, and Health. Still, the advantages of these newer categorizations make the mistakes of the original definition all the more glaring. The original WHO definition of health, if indiscriminately accepted, opens the possibility for what is arguably the most dangerous moral risk for public health leaders—that hubris might lead to the manipulative promotion of an internal institutional or a civic political agenda beyond the biological well-being of the public.

Mores, Morals, and Ethics

Although public health does tend to assume that certain outcomes should be sought using utilitarian reasoning, being a good moral leader is not a matter of simplistic ethical arithmetic. If it were, leaders faced with disagreements would simply unveil the purported truth of a decision to those who disagree, and the newly edified opponents would fall into line. The reality of public health, however, involves fundamental, strategic, and tactical disagreements that cannot be resolved by condescending or even well-considered instruction. Indeed, most moral disagreements arise not out of ignorance but out of the fact that, at the risk of sounding redundant, people disagree.

To understand how organizations and their leaders function morally, we must differentiate between **mores**, **morals**, and **ethics** as analytical concepts.[11] (In actual practice, people often conflate the terms *morality* and *ethics*, but some precision in use is helpful analytically.) The term *mores* describes social or organizational standards of good and bad and of right and wrong that are simply assumed by the group without formal expression. They generally involve unspoken social patterns that indicate what is met with approval or disapproval, which thereby creates a space for the allowable or tolerable. Although mores are informal and not specifically outlined, they still reflect very real value boundaries. Much can be learned about the actual operationalized values of an organization by examining its mores.

The term *morals* refers to standards that are formally expressed and recognized as motivations for choices and actions. If unexpressed mores are challenged—for instance, in the event of an internal or external threat, or perceived threat, to the group—then the values have to be evaluated, which can only occur through formal expression. As that expression of value is endorsed, the mores become morals. Morals often clarify relationships and boundaries, and they legitimize the social structures of the group. New organizations usually take shape around the intentional engagement of previous assumptions, with the new organizations seeking to effectively answer key moral questions.

Ethics refers to the critical analysis of morality. The analysis can be either descriptive (e.g., sociological, cultural, anthropological, psychological) or normative (e.g., philosophical, theological). The analysis of a moral choice may simply be an examination of how some value affects some choice,

mores
Standards of good and bad and of right and wrong that are simply assumed without formal expression.

morals
Standards and patterns of behavior that are formally expressed and legitimized.

ethics
The analysis of formally expressed and legitimized standards and patterns of behavior.

Consider This

"As we practice resolving dilemmas we find ethics to be less a goal than a pathway, less a destination than a trip, less an inoculation than a process."
—Rushworth Kidder[12(p174)]

How do you understand ethics? Do you agree or disagree with Kidder?

without a judgment on the value itself. Alternatively, moral decisions and behaviors can be analyzed in accordance with standards external to public health, such that the choice or action that the agent thought right/wrong, good/bad, or desirable/repulsive is itself evaluated as a proper or improper choice.

The Basic Models of Moral Authority

If an organization could function completely at the level of mores, then a leader might avoid any consideration of ethics and ignore any possibility of moral conflict. However, no such organizations exist. Even if a group is internally stable, the community around it changes. Public health in particular has many such changes, from rapidly developing biotechnologies to the globalization of both healthcare and disease. Effective public health leaders are therefore, by necessity, individuals who can successfully address moral concerns. They must be at least moderately skilled at ethical analysis, and they must have leadership characteristics that authenticate the moral direction of the organization. In other words, they must be people of **integrity**.

integrity
Consistency between claimed moral values and behavior.

A helpful tool for understanding ethical leadership is the categorization of moral authority developed by Max Weber.

> **Effective Public Health Leaders . . .**
>
> . . . practice doing what is legal, moral, and ethical.

Weber's Typology

An essay presenting Weber's typology was first published in 1922. In leadership theory terms, the typology is a blend of trait, behavioral, contingency, and transformational interpretations of authority.[13] Expressed in simplified form, Weber's[14] model includes three primary types of organizational authority, with some further subdivision:

1. The charismatic leader—sometimes called the *prophet*—whose effective leadership ability (charisma) is intrinsically held, or even supernaturally given
2. The role-holding leader—the *priest*—who uses traditional organizational power provided by sociocultural placement in the community
3. The management specialist leader—the *bureaucrat*—who has technical, rational-legal management skills (i.e., mastery of bureaucratic organizational skills)

The terms *prophet* and *priest*, though borrowed from religion, are not necessarily meant to have spiritual significance in this use. Likewise, the term *bureaucracy* is not meant pejoratively here, but rather as a descriptor of an organization with significant division of labor managed through formally described office and officer responsibilities. Weber's typology is illustrated in exhibit 8.1.

The prophet possesses charisma, which is understood as the capacity to morally lead based on the characteristics (or perceived characteristics) of that individual leader. In Weber's thought, charisma is the power to bring about organizational or social change by drawing others through the transformational process. In leadership theory, the prophetic leader might be called a visionary or a model example.[15,16] Weber[17(pp358–59)] explains:

> The term "charisma" will be applied to a certain quality of an individual personality by virtue of which he is considered extraordinary and treated as endowed with supernatural, superhuman, or at least specifically exceptional powers or qualities. These are such as are not accessible to the ordinary person, but are regarded as of divine origin or exemplary, and on the basis of them the individual concerned is treated as leader.

Prophetic leaders tend to emerge during periods when social structures or roles are radically threatened or changing.[18] Public health, as a field, took shape in the nineteenth century, during a time of great cultural and sociopolitical uncertainty concerning urbanization, industrialization, mass immigration, and developments in medical science. Similar confusion may arise today, particularly during major crises (e.g., a worldwide epidemic). In such events, traditional reasoning and structures often fail, or at least are deemed inadequate, creating an opportunity for prophetic leadership. To borrow a term from cultural anthropology, these times of upheaval and confusion may be

EXHIBIT 8.1
Models of Moral
Leadership

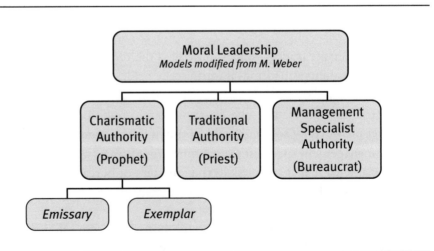

Source: Adapted from Weber, M. (1947) 1997. *The Theory of Social and Economic Organization*. New York: Free Press.

considered periods of **liminality**—that is, periods when clear cultural meaning is absent because of challenge or transformation. The typical outcome of a liminal period is a new or modified social structure, expressed in new roles or at least in new understandings of existing roles or the individuals filling them. In the most extreme situations, when liminality is not resolved, anomie and anarchy result, and organizations fall apart. Such extreme instances are inevitably disastrous from a public health perspective, as evident in the world's war zones and ungovernable regions.

liminality
The absence of clear cultural meaning during periods of challenge or transformation.

Leaders in the prophet category can be further distinguished by the type of charismatic inspiration they offer. Those who provide a vision based on an understanding of some transcendent good are deemed emissary prophets, whereas those who inspire through their own example are exemplary prophets. In public health, an emissary prophet is one who offers an image of improved health and a believable route to achieve it, inspiring public health practitioners and obtaining compliance, if not enthusiastic support, from the population served. Exemplar prophets use their own behavior to demonstrate practices that are recognized as repeatable, thus initiating systemic behavioral changes in public health practitioners or even the population. Exemplar behaviors are extremely important internally for public health organizations.

Among key figures in the history of public health, John Snow is regarded as a prophetic leader, both as an exemplar of correct public health behaviors and as an emissary of a new vision of health. He demonstrated, contrary to the scientific assertions of the time, how that vision of improved health might be achieved for an area of London facing a seemingly uncontrollable cholera outbreak. Similarly, Dorothea Dix can be considered a prophetic moral leader—both as an exemplar and an emissary—in transforming the public health of mental illness. Arguably, the World Health Organization, in advancing its definition of *health* following World War II, was trying (though not entirely successfully) to be prophetic in the emissary sense, offering a message of wellness and goodness to inspire individuals and nations to seek the goal of health.

Despite these examples, the dramatic authority figure is not typical in public health. Prophets, or leaders who can only function in a prophetic manner, are rarely useful over extended lengths of time. Charismatic prophets who lack traditional authority and bureaucratic mastery—no matter how profoundly they might speak in the moment—tend to eventually become either visionaries who ignore practical daily concerns or micromanagers who are unable to relinquish any organizational control. They often prove incapable of performing day-to-day functions, such as guiding the regular moral practice of public health, or, even worse, they become failed exemplars, ultimately dismissed as hypocrites.

In its purest form, charismatic authority has a distinctive nature unfamiliar to normal, routine structures, and it is based on social relationships and charismatic personal qualities.[18] Such leadership is not ideally suited to daily operations, but it may be necessary to ensure good moral choices when dramatic changes or conflicts arise, especially from the outside. For instance, if a genuinely dangerous epidemic looms or if the actions of a government or corporation are threatening the public's physical well-being, a prophet may be needed to lead the public health organization and the people at the periphery of the organization.

Traditional leaders of the priest category are often regarded as experts and have status granted through higher education in secular settings; they have authority based on their roles rather than their charisma. Whereas prophetic figures tend to rise during periods of upheaval or instability, traditional authority tends to dominate when times are normal or calm. Often, after a prophet leads dramatic change, a traditional leader attempts to establish and formalize those changes—a process of routinization. In a sense, charisma is shifted from the prophetic individual to the roles of traditional authority and eventually bureaucratic authority.

Over time, all organizations need regular practices that are predictable and moral in operation and outcome. In public health, this need supports the development of respectful authority based on traditional roles that mirror the roles found in other organizations in society. Many public health leaders of the early twentieth century spoke with cultural-priestly authority similar to that granted to physicians of that era. For instance, Charles-Edward A. Winslow, working from within the newly developing public health field, directed its growth and provided moral authority for the formation of its structures. This kind of traditional moral authority is efficient as long as the activities of the organization are fairly regular and the organization being directed is not too large. The leader sets a model of moral behaviors that governs internal and external interactions.

If the risk for prophetic leaders is that they might ignore or micromanage regular processes, the risk for traditional leaders is that they might not be able to adapt when changes are necessary—for instance, when a public health organization must respond to changes in the social ecology or dramatic epidemiological shifts. Roughly, a parallel can be drawn with Kuhn's[19] description of normal science, which resembles traditional moral authority, and revolutionary science, which corresponds with prophetic authority.

As an organization grows and eventually becomes more complex, routinization takes the form of bureaucratization. Large organizations, including large public health organizations, have very specific differentiated tasks, and these tasks require division into bureaus of responsibility. Such division can be useful in that it suggests that decisions are rational and impartial. Without it, overreliance on prophetic proclamations or traditional face-to-face authority can quickly look like favoritism, cronyism, or arbitrary use of power.

Of course, rational management, or bureaucracy itself, can also be problematic, particularly if the differentiation process disperses accountability to the point that no one in particular assumes moral responsibility for decisions. People with greater immediate interests, if they have the bureaucratic power to do so, may consume disproportionately more of what are supposed to be commonly held resources while distributing the cost to all. Public interests are often violated by bureaucratic interests and incentives that have perverse implications.[20] The budget of a government or large public organization is like a commons: It can be depleted, has nonexclusive ownership, and allows for use by self-maximizing moral actors who diffuse accountabililty.[20,21] As Weber suggested, such use is not simply a form of greed; rather, it is often based on the genuine belief that one's own organization must exist in a given form and "triumph" in the consumption of shared resources because it provides specific goods for society. Thus, focused self-preservation behaviors are often justifiable to the bureaucrats. Indeed, many bureaucratic organizations have so-called codes of conduct or codes of ethics that are little more than risk-management tools (or, less kindly, lawsuit-avoidance mechanisms).

Rational management and organizational authority, if they lack a morally good leader who expects moral behavior out of employees and others, can easily result in banal evil, where little ethical analysis takes place beyond a vaguely defined justification for organizational self-preservation.[22] One of the greatest moral responsibilities of an effective public health leader, then, is to actively prevent such abuse from occurring, while still encouraging specialization for expertise.

The Public Health Model of Moral Authority

In contemporary public health organizations, leadership legitimacy is variably based on all three of Weber's forms of authority. Traditional authority is provided through an "ordination" of leaders through academic degrees (e.g., DrPH, MD, PhD) from accredited institutions and certifications from professional organizations. Since managerial authority is attached to a place on an organizational chart, an individual assuming a position of leadership needs some competence in morally managing the intricacies (and occasionally the intrigues) of a public health bureaucracy. A leader must manage the bureaus of the organization consistently and with fairness. The effective public health leader must also have some level of prophetic charisma. This charisma is not simply charm but rather the authority of exemplary and visionary behaviors. Importantly, moral public health leaders need to legitimatize their claims in all three ways, varying in emphasis in accordance with organizational and epidemiological circumstances.

In addition to the three types of authority already discussed, Weber's typology also includes a fourth category—the laity, or the constituency being served (see exhibit 8.2). For the purposes of our discussion, the laity comprises the constituents and collaborators in public health. Often, the laity is juxtaposed with priestly, prophetic, and bureaucratic leaders. The laity may endorse traditional, ritualized authority figures such that the individuals in the moral community are strengthened and each has a place in it.[17] People need to know not only where they belong, but also how and for what purpose; if they do not, they might withdraw, resist, or rebel. Depending on the circumstances, the laity may strongly identify with charismatic leaders or completely reject their authority. Under bureaucratic authority, the laity is defined by common characteristics and pooled into categories, and both employees and served constituency members are "managed" with efficiency on the basis of their commonalities. As long as bureaucratic leaders recognize that each person is unique and distinct in ways pertinent to the broader community, this pooling can create valuable efficiencies for the organization; but if individual differences are ignored and people are simply assigned anonymously into categories, the pooling becomes immoral and will be counterproductive to the public's health. Ideally, public health procedures are developed such that the functioning of the bureaucracy serves the institutional end without turning the laity into discardable parts of a mindless machine. Specialization and even quantification are morally desirable if they efficiently serve good ends, but the hyperrationalization of some public health organizations risks reducing constituents to numbers on charts and employees to their Social Security numbers.

The best model for public health is not the exclusive use of one type of moral authority but rather a blending of the types. The effective public health leader must be able to function in generally predictable moral ways that are highly comparable for the sake of outcome analysis (bureaucratic), with legitimacy provided through traditional organizations that go beyond the specific

EXHIBIT 8.2
The Role of Constituents (Laity) in Moral Leadership

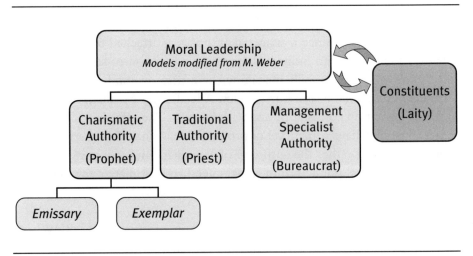

Source: Adapted from Weber, M. (1947) 1997. *The Theory of Social and Economic Organization*. New York: Free Press.

structure of public health (traditional/priestly), and with the ability, though only rarely needed, to lead through significant crises without sacrificing the core morality of the organization nor losing sight of the vision of public health (prophetic). Effective public health leaders need to know how to work for consensus within the organization and at least seek tacit agreement with people outside it. When making decisions, they must pay attention to the voices of

Leadership Application Case: A Breach of Trust

The Leadership Application Case at the beginning of this book provides realistic scenarios for the application of key leadership concepts covered in the text. See the section marked "Chapter 8 Application" for the scenario and discussion questions that correspond with this chapter.

constituents, collaborators, and fellow workers in the organization, as well as political leaders and scientists. Moral leaders seek not uniformity of thought but rather agreement on certain shared values and the functional rules that arise from those values. They then seek toleration (in the true sense) on matters not related to the organizational mission. Effective leaders also need to know how to morally coerce change when necessary.

Seeking Consensus and Using Middle Axioms

Moral public health leadership is not only a matter of understanding the social setting and adopting an effective style of authority; it is also a matter of how authority is used. The famous adage of Lord Acton[23]—"Power tends to corrupt, and absolute power corrupts absolutely"—has been cited so frequently that it has become a cliché, but it nonetheless rings true in public health administration. Given that public health leaders have considerable authority and may potentially use the state's police powers, they must lead with humility—both in understanding the good being sought (i.e., health in a population for the well-being of individuals) and in assessing the validity of the means for reaching that goal. Functionally, this humility is expressed in finding commonality and agreement whenever possible and acting in a restrained, prudent manner when use of force is necessary.

People may debate the reasoning behind the core public health values and, certainly, how those values can best be operationalized through the public health organization. After all, the foundations of morality are culturally or religiously based, and the individuals and groups involved in public health differ in their backgrounds and beliefs. Nonetheless, the central operating values of public health should be shared.

Middle axioms are basic moral principles that are generally shared even if individuals and groups do not agree on the principles' philosophical or theological foundations.[11] They reflect values that are structurally supported

middle axiom
A basic moral principle generally shared by individuals and groups even if they do not agree on the principle's philosophical or theological foundations.

EXHIBIT 8.3
Pyramid
for Moral
Cooperation
with People
Who Have
Different
Worldviews

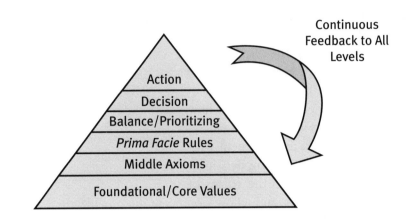

by society, even if people in the society do not agree on the reasons for why the values are accepted. Middle axioms, in turn, generate general applications or *prima facie* rules for given social sectors.

Among the truly essential middle axioms for public health are the following:

- People should not be harmed.
- People should be free (with freedoms expressed through negative rights, as discussed later in this chapter).
- People should be treated justly.
- The commonweal, including the natural world, should be protected to the extent possible.

Political thought in the United States assumes that human worth and freedom are expressed, in part, as natural rights. The value of the individual and the accompanying human rights exist prior to the social contract, and the social contract exists to protect that value and defend those rights. The endower of those rights is purposely left unspecified, and disagreement about that foundational belief is acceptable as long as the rights themselves are upheld. Exhibit 8.3 shows a pyramid, growing out of core values and middle axioms, that models moral cooperation among people who have different worldviews.

A list of operational rules with face validity for public health ethics can be found in the code of ethics advanced by the American Public Health Association,[24] as well as in an expanded discussion titled *Principles of the Ethical Practice of Public Health*,[25] which is discussed later in this chapter. The examples that follow show how society's middle axioms can generate rules for public health with face validity. In actual practice, such rules are often developed though a complicated history involving several middle axioms, so the following are only offered heuristically:

- Human life is a strong good and, therefore, generally, individuals should not be harmed (starting middle axiom).[26] Health (i.e., plastic biological functionality) is generally better for individuals than its absence (that absence being a condition caused by age-inappropriate decay or harm). Health is most accurately defined using the scientific study of the human organism (i.e., laboratory and clinical medical science) and the study of populations (i.e., epidemiology). Health is impacted both individually and corporately as it is conditioned by both internal (e.g., genetic) and corporate (e.g., cultural dietary patterns) factors, usually in an interactive manner. Therefore, the morality of human activities should, at least in part, be judged on the probable impact on individual and corporate human health. Further, public health as a means of promoting health is a legitimate entitlement.[27] The state should, consequently, fund public health services at a reasonable level, taking into account opportunity costs for society.

- Individuals are meant to be free (starting middle axiom). Part of freedom is the right to bodily integrity. The state should maximize the liberty (i.e., autonomy) of individuals. Even so, liberty is limited such that acts that will probably bring harm (not merely offense) to others should be restricted using state authority. Harm to another is caused not only by injurious behaviors directed at an individual but also by corporate activities that are significantly injurious. Public health interventions can be either helpful or harmful, or a combination of both. Given the requirement to maximize freedom, mechanisms for health protection and health improvement should be limited in proportion to other aspects of human thriving. The individual's life purpose (i.e., *telos*) should be respected. Individuals have quasi-self-ownership of their bodies. Legally, negative rights or rights of noninterference should be respected by effective public health leaders (e.g., rights to religious freedom, freedom of speech, freedom of assembly). Persons should be tolerated whenever possible. Similarly, persons should not be quarantined simply because an infectious agent may or may not be present and those individuals may or may not be vectors. A genuine risk, both in terms of infectiousness and severity, must be demonstrated. Likewise, privacy and confidentiality should be protected in cases of serious infections, unless the likely behavior of the infected person would very probably result in significant harm to another, who would otherwise not be vulnerable. Also, because of the shared liberty middle axioms, individuals should have the right to refuse treatments, unless to do so would pose a genuine threat to the public's health.

Check It Out

To review the code of ethics for public health as published in the *American Journal of Public Health*, visit www.ncbi.nlm.nih.gov/pmc/articles/PMC1447186/.

principlism
A system of
practical ethical
decision making
that concentrates
on the moral
principles of
autonomy,
beneficence,
nonmaleficence,
and justice.

Working lists of middle axioms and rules with face validity can be genuinely helpful, not because they provide easy answers but because they facilitate ethical discourse. **Principlism**, for instance, is an important list of middle axioms that (usually) includes autonomy, beneficence, nonmaleficence, and justice.[28,29] However, such lists can be problematic if they are assumed to have enough specificity to provide easy answers in particular circumstances. The reliance on these lists in such a manner can lead to the exclusion of other important values through carelessness or obliviousness. Effective use of the lists can also be threatened if the people in power define the axiomatic values in ways that serve their own beliefs or interests.

Public health authority is derived from the state's obligation to protect the common good for individual citizens (or residents). In the United States, the aim of the state is not to determine specific life goals for any individual but rather to protect life, liberty, and property (and/or the pursuit of happiness). The protection of these rights, further described in various constitutional amendments, assumes protection of the commons, the shared social and natural environments necessary for pursuit of the individual's purpose or life goals. The most basic purpose of public health under the authority of the state, then, is to protect the opportunity for individuals to pursue their life goals.

Operational rules for public health are generated from society's shared middle axioms in a process of prioritizing rules with face validity and negotiating how particular expressions of individual liberty and community well-being are best balanced. Ethical analysis often has layers of middle axioms and rules. Rules may at times be derived primarily from a single middle axiom, but they usually come from a combination of several.

Practically speaking, lists of axioms and sets of rules cannot eliminate the ethical gray area between moral certainty and moral uncertainty. They can shrink that area to the point that it is generally manageable, but the gray area cannot be eliminated. Many ethically complex circumstances cannot be resolved by drawing up a few rules. Consider laws about chewed tobacco products, for instance. Arguments about second-hand smoke do not apply to the chewing of tobacco in the same way that they apply to public smoking. The prohibition of chewing tobacco would depend on arguments about either cost to society or a paternalistic function of the state to protect its citizens, and the latter is problematic given the middle axioms dealing with freedom. Such a prohibition would also be problematic in that it would create inconsistency in the way that liberty and privacy arguments are applied for different behaviors. For instance, one might question why arguments about economic cost to society and the state's paternalistic function might be used to restrict chewing tobacco but not high-risk sexual behaviors on publicly run university campuses.

Still, this degree of complexity does not relieve leaders of their responsibility to make decisions with moral implications. Simply put, no moral argument for public health will be perfect, but the effective public health leader should make an effort to reach consistent, coherent, and generally acceptable positions—even if the effort requires teaching community members.

Justice and Rights

Public health organizations have typically focused on middle axioms and rules with face validity that can generally be subsumed under the category of **justice**. Justice, in short, involves giving each person his or her due. The language of justice has often been favored in public health because it suggests the empowerment of those who are otherwise vulnerable to adverse health conditions and because it implies a process (or, more formally, a procedure) by which competing interests can be balanced.

Such language can become clichéd or even manipulative, however. The use of justice language in public health is most often challenged when it is perceived to be validating the legality of unneeded intrusions into the lives of individuals and other organizations for reasons that go beyond a narrow definition of *health*. For instance, during debates over the Affordable Care Act of 2010, some religiously affiliated organizations objected to the inclusion of birth-control funding in the category of preventive care covered by the law. In spite of such disagreements, however, the very fact that the language of justice is being used means that a more or less coherent debate can occur in the public square.

Types of Justice

Justice can be retributive, commutative, or distributive. **Retributive justice** involves ensuring proportionate punishment for criminal behavior. A person who pollutes the commons without regard for public health and well-being may need to be punished. Retributive justice seeks not to inflict vengeance on the criminal but rather to rebalance society after a criminal act has put it out of kilter. Under retributive justice, like should be treated as like, and *equality* is the key watchword. **Distributive justice** is the dissemination of goods, both tangible and intangible, in an appropriate or equitable (though not necessarily equal) manner throughout society. The fair distribution of costs is also an important consideration in public health, especially in times of quarantine or other restrictions on the liberty of people who are not responsible for a health problem. **Commutative justice** is fairness in exchange and discourse, including such aspects as confidentiality and truth telling. Such justice may be violated if, for instance, a public health official intentionally deceives people to achieve some purported greater good.

Types of Rights

The expression of justice in the form of rights is extremely important in political discourse and in justifying the use of public health authority. As noted previously,

justice
The principle of being impartial and fair in resolving situations with competing claims or in assigning deserved rewards and punishments; giving each person his or her due.

retributive justice
The assignment of a proportionate punishment for criminal behavior.

distributive justice
The dissemination of goods and costs, both tangible and intangible, in an appropriate or equitable manner throughout society.

commutative justice
Fairness in exchange and discourse, including such aspects as confidentiality and truth telling.

negative right
A right of a person to be generally free from state interference with regard to speech, religion, assembly, or other matters; also called a *liberty right*.

positive right
A right or entitlement, often to a good or service, that arises out of a society's economic or structural capacity.

the natural rights of human beings are assumed to have existed prior to the formation of the state. The rights to freedom of speech, freedom of religion, and freedom of assembly, among others, are considered noninterference rights, because they suggest limits to state interference. Such rights are also called **negative rights**, or liberty rights. In most societies, people can also be said to have **positive rights**, or entitlements. Such rights arise out of the developing economic and structural capacity of society, and they may include rights to certain basic goods and services (e.g., education, adequate food). With regard to public health services, maintaining the environment as part of the commons would likely be considered protection of a negative right, whereas providing healthcare services for individuals would be considered a positive right. Unlike negative rights, positive rights depend on the resources available in a given society and, as a result, can vary widely. In the United States, questions about society's capacity—often discussed in terms of costs—are central to the debate over whether healthcare should be considered a right.

Some people also speak of "third-generation" rights, which usually involve rights of group self-determination. Such rights lack consistent legal support and have little effect on public health ethical analysis except in cases involving indigenous groups. Still, effective public health leaders should consider the impact of their decisions on cultural communities, even if third-generation rights are not clearly recognized.

Unsurprisingly, questions of justice can be extremely complex, and the various rights often come into conflict. In seeking to uphold justice, the public health leader should focus on the wellness of society overall while respecting to the greatest extent possible individual rights and group identities. The reasoning method of public health is primarily risk assessment—or *utility calculation*, in the ethics field—as conducted by a person of integrity and constrained by the rights of individuals. This general approach has had a dramatically positive impact on human health. Indeed, one can reasonably claim that decent food, basic inoculation, and the nonconsumption of sewage or otherwise contaminated water have had a greater impact than all postmorbid medical treatments combined. That very success, though, can lead to arrogance, which is dangerous when combined with civil authority. The effective public health leader, then, is not only one who acts to improve the biological well-being of the populace but also one who acts justly, acknowledging and protecting individuals' liberty.

Conflict and the Moral Public Health Leader

Conflict is less desirable than consensus, but consensus is not always possible—especially (or inevitably) when closely held values create opposite responses. Further, in some cases, people will disagree about how middle axioms and rules with face validity should be prioritized. In particular, concern for the best health outcome (as narrowly defined) may sometimes come into direct conflict with closely held social values, especially individual liberty. Such conflicts are common in such areas as mandated vaccination, quarantine, smoking restrictions, limitations on sugary beverage sales, trans-fat restaurant regulations, and some antipollution rules. Public health leaders should seek to minimize conflict, not only by acknowledging foundational values and clarifying shared middle axioms but also by considering how people and organizations morally reason. But sometimes, despite the leader's best efforts, compromise and cooperation are not achievable, and toleration of disagreement is not possible because of the potential consequences of inaction. The effective public health leader needs to know, therefore, how to enter into conflict in an ethically legitimate manner.

Although, in some cases, differing viewpoints can and should be accepted or at least tolerated, sometimes the leader must work against the intentions of another. Effective leaders do not approach every issue as yes/no or black/white, nor every person as either friend or foe. To the contrary, they use the moral authority they hold—drawing on prophetic charisma, traditional respect, or bureaucratic rationalized power, depending on the circumstances—to negotiate responses that serve their mission, which is to maximize the promotion of plastic biological functionality of the individuals who make up the public. Ideally, leaders do so through the recognition and application of shared middle axioms and agreed-upon rules. They should certainly be concerned with lowering factors that harm the public's health, but at the same time they must not deny other common values of the social order (e.g., liberty, property rights).

> ### Consider This
>
>
> "You can fool some of the people all of the time, and all of the people some of the time, but you cannot fool all of the people all of the time."
> —Abraham Lincoln[30]
>
> Is fooling people immoral? Unethical?

Unavoidable Conflict and Just Coercion Theory

Throughout history, leaders have developed analytical approaches to help them respond wisely to conflicts and social threats. Such approaches form the basis for **just coercion theory**, which refers, literally, to the morally proper compelling of other people. The theory—sometimes known as *just war theory*, though many find that name off-putting—uses generally accepted middle axioms of justice and various methods of moral reasoning (including utilitarianism, deontology, and virtue, discussed later in the chapter) to explain how authoritative power can and should be used. The theory has on occasion been applied to the field of public health,[31] where its balance of utility with other methods of moral reasoning presents advantages.

Public health administration, by its nature, involves at least the potential for restrictions on individual liberty for the public's good. Coercive action

just coercion theory
A theory that combines various moral reasoning methods— including utilitarianism, deontology, and virtue—to explain how governmental power can and should be used; also known as *just war theory*.

(e.g., quarantine), shame-inducing strategies (e.g., some antismoking advertisements), and at least some limits on individual freedom (e.g., crosswalks, jaywalking tickets) are common and arguably necessary. When applied properly, just coercion theory can be an extraordinarily useful tool both for establishing moral permission for certain coercive actions and for restraining or preventing other actions that might be immorally coercive. It can be used to make the best real-world choice when a leader has partial information, a probable but not assured outcome, and limited time for making a decision. When applied improperly, however, the theory can be used as a means for disguising self-interest or rationalizing self-righteousness.

Criteria for Just Coercion

Traditionally, just coercion theory has operated with two categories: the justice of entering into coercive action and the justice of how a coercive action is conducted. More recently, a third category has been suggested: justice, especially restorative justice, following a coercive action.[32] These categories are useful, but for the purposes of our discussion, we will combine the criteria for just coercion into a single list:

1. Just cause
2. Right intention
3. Legitimate authority
4. Last resort
5. Reasonable chance of success
6. Proportionality
7. Discrimination

Just Cause

The just cause criterion is based on whether the act of coercion is intended to correct an injustice or create a morally preferable condition. Applying the criterion to public health, Thobaben[11(p279)] writes: "In the case of public health, the *just cause* is always the health of the public. . . . The general assumption is that public health measures are intended to improve the physical well-being of individuals by improving the health of the population as a whole."

Right Intention

The second criterion, right intention, considers whether the motive of the moral actor coincides with just cause. Essentially, it is a virtue assertion about the character of the decision maker. Thobaben[11(p279)] explains: "*Right intention* can be defined as the matching of motive with just cause. In other words, does the moral agent's action coincide with what she or he says is the reason for coercing?" In matters of public health, the question occurs: Is the use of power occurring to serve the just cause, or is it really helping administrators to obtain promotions, politicians to procure more power, or practitioners to garner more status?

Legitimate Authority

The legitimate authority criterion typically centers on the sociopolitical status of the individual or group involved. Such status is usually, but not always, legally defined. Thobaben[11(p279–80)] explains that *legitimate authority* can be defined legally in the United States as "the agreed upon social authority" but notes that it does not always come from the federal government. He writes: "Following subsidiarity, it can mean that the family (as with fluoridated water consumption), the county or state (as with fluoridation of water supplies), or the federal government (as with funding of fluoridation research) is the locus of decision making."

Public health leaders generally know more than their broader constituencies do about matters of epidemiology, disease etiology, and so on, and this expertise affords them a degree of authority. However, it does not mean that those individuals are necessarily the best suited to determine what societal trade-offs should be made to achieve a specific public health outcome. Effective leaders strive to recognize what the societal costs are, and they work to educate others while at the same time being educated themselves. To not do so is, at best, disrespectful of the opinions and concerns of others; at worst, it is hubris. Expertise in public health should be honored, but public health leaders should not expect others to automatically defer to their opinions on the broader social morality. Under certain circumstances, however, leaders may have to resort to the use of police authority, albeit with great caution. As Thobaben[11(pp279–80)] points out, "Legitimate authority can extend to controlling persons who are not legally guilty, but legally threatening. For the public health a person's liberty can be restricted even if she or he does not deserve, on the basis of criminality, a limit on his or her freedom in the form of quarantine or compelled inoculation."

Last Resort

The last resort criterion suggests that a decision to use coercion should be reached only after prior efforts have proved futile, and it should be based on an evaluation of utility or efficaciousness of various steps. Coercion is a matter of degrees, and different levels of coercive authority may be appropriate depending on the severity of the consequences of inaction, weighed against the rights of individuals to not be coerced. Thobaben[11(p282)] explains: "Police power should be used for public health only as a *last resort*. For instance, instruction may be preferable, through public service announcements or through physicians.

Some argue that health education in schools is a last resort, arising because of the failure of parents to properly guide their own children. A better example is compelled quarantine after education and voluntary self-restriction have failed."

Reasonable Chance of Success

An action's reasonable chance of success is based on a utilitarian risk assessment and comparison with other potential actions and/or the status quo. The definition of *reasonable chance* here is comparative: The chance does not have to be more than 50 percent; it just has to be greater than the chances of success for the other options. A public health intervention meeting this criterion should lead to the lowest possible incidence of new cases, the best chance of lowering prevalence, and the diminishing of hazards related to incidence. Thobaben[11(p281)] writes that an action's reasonable chance of success reflects "a genuine probability of succeeding in comparison to the status quo and other alternatives" and that this probability, ideally, should be determined scientifically. In public health, the analysis required for this criterion inevitably lacks certainty, and moral choice is always constrained by the time available to decide and the authority to decide.[33] An important aspect of decision making is recognizing that choices are limited.

Proportionality

The proportionality criterion involves weighing the costs of any potential intervention against both the likely outcome and the status quo. Thobaben[11(p282)] writes: "The proportionality of a response to any risk is dependent on the availability of a range of responses. In public health, the evaluation of a hazard is properly yoked to a risk-benefit analysis of the possible responses, their efficacy and costs." Various public health models, including the US Preventive Services Task Force evaluation system, take into account both the benefits and harms of an intervention. Thobaben[11(p283)] explains that proportionality is "linked to the efficacy of the various possible interventions (including the status quo) as well as the comparability of the risk of the disease and the benefit of the treatment (to the individual or to the public)."

In weighing benefits and harms, public health leaders should be aware that some coercive interventions can threaten other social goods and damage leaders' moral position. Leaders should be conscious of two ethical concerns in particular—"dirty hands" and the "slippery slope." A "dirty hands" situation occurs when an effort to address a particular concern requires temporary moral compromises for which a correction will later be made. However, the danger is that the hands cannot be "washed clean" through subsequent compensatory action, or even that the compromise would set a corrupt precedent, leading to a habit of immorality and thereby "staining" the hands. The "slippery slope" danger is that conceding a morally debatable position will lead to increasingly immoral precedents, resulting in a morally reprehensible situation.

Discrimination

Discrimination, in this context, involves distinguishing between people who should be involved in the coercion and those who should not, and it can help protect bystanders or disempowered individuals. Thobaben[11(p283)] writes: "*Discrimination* is not a negative term under just coercion theory. To the contrary, it is a good thing to discriminate between combatants and noncombatants, those who must be coerced and those who need not be. So, if a person is not infected with a disease and another person is carelessly serving as the vector for that disease, then the state—assuming it is a debilitating or life-threatening illness—might intervene to protect the vulnerable and unwary." Nonetheless, sometimes innocent bystanders do get coerced. "For instance, the relative of a sick person may not have caused his or her illness in any way, nor have the disorder, but may still need to be quarantined for the sake of the population."

Effective Public Health Leaders . . .

. . . do the right thing, the right way, the first time.

Methods of Moral Reasoning

In considering the distinctive moral nature of public health leadership and the ethical use of the power intrinsic to such leadership, one should seek to understand the key reasoning methods and general moral reasoning tendencies as they relate to public health. With this understanding, the leadership virtues that promote the achievement of mission ends, as well as the vices that inhibit such achievement, can be effectively assessed. The morality of an organization and its leadership depends not only on foundational values but also on how those values are morally considered or ethically examined. This section of the chapter examines several key methods of moral reasoning (displayed in exhibit 8.4)—though, in actual practice, the distinctions can blur.

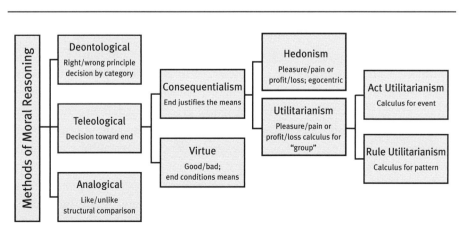

EXHIBIT 8.4
Methods of Moral Reasoning

deontological reasoning
Moral reasoning based on categories, which often yield sets of formal rules.

teleological reasoning
Moral thinking directed toward an end.

utilitarianism
A reasoning method based on comparing two or more options and choosing the one that does the most overall good for the most people.

hedonism
A reasoning method that prioritizes self-fulfillment and is contingent upon some significant degree of personal liberty; also known as *rational egoism*.

virtue reasoning
A reasoning method that emphasizes the development of the character of the individual or community as the moral end.

consequentialism
A type of teleological reasoning in which a desired end can justify the means; includes utilitarianism and hedonism.

Deontological Reasoning

Deontological reasoning is moral reasoning based on categories. Under this method, the construction of categories is the primary ethical task, and once categories are in place, moral choices should be relatively easy. Deontological reasoning often yields sets of formal rules, usually expressed in the language of *right/wrong*. The primary advantage of deontological reasoning is clarity; the primary disadvantage is its tendency toward casuistic legalism. In public health, sets of rules or codes (e.g., the public health code of ethics) are basically deontological sets of prescriptions. Importantly, the primary method of moral reasoning used in American law and in social contract theory is negative rights language, which is deontological.

Teleological Reasoning

Teleological reasoning is moral thinking directed toward an end (*telos*, in Greek). Traditionally, an end is a core valued good sought as an expression of the individual's nature or the organization's mission. The broad category of teleology includes the subsets of **utilitarianism**, **hedonism**, and **virtue reasoning**. Utilitarianism and hedonism together are known as **consequentialism**, and they share an emphasis on the consequences of reasoning, whether expressed in terms of interests, profit/loss, or pain/pleasure. Simplistically stated, consequentialist reasoning assumes that outcomes can be maximized and losses minimized such that, as the cliché says, "the end justifies the means." The distinction between *utilitarianism* and *hedonism* is that the former takes account of the group whereas the latter centers on the individual. (Note, however, that utilitarianism should not be equated with mechanistic organizational decision making and that hedonism is not the same as physical pleasure seeking.) Virtue reasoning focuses on the development of the character of the individual or community as the moral end.

Utilitarian Reasoning

Utilitarian reasoning is the process of comparing two or more options and choosing the one that does the most overall good for the most people. It comes in two forms: **act utilitarianism** and **rule utilitarianism**. The former is utilitarianism in its purest form, with every moral decision made on the basis of a comparative analysis of the particular situation with the aim of maximizing the group good. Of course, in real-world practice, leaders may not be able to pause and fully analyze each specific situation, and so rule utilitarianism is common. Under rule utilitarianism, general practices are established that have strong tendencies toward maximizing utility. In public health, rule utilitarianism can be seen in vaccination requirements intended to protect the public's well-being or, even more strongly, in environmental laws that regulate externalities associated with significant and probable public health risks.

In public health, utilitarianism can be used to include moral concerns in calculations of disease incidence, prevalence, and severity, and of cost of prevention and care. The primary advantages of utilitarian reasoning are that it simplifies moral complexity and allows the possibility of quantifying decisions. However, it also has disadvantages. First, the values being measured, which must be determined prior to determining utility, can be completely arbitrary. Second, the values, especially those having to do with abstract public health concepts such as whole health or human thriving, are notoriously difficult to measure. And third, outliers are almost inevitably further marginalized, since the addressing of their needs tends to be more costly.

act utilitarianism
A reasoning approach in which every moral decision is made on the basis of a comparative analysis of the particular situation with the aim of maximizing the group good.

rule utilitarianism
A reasoning approach in which general practices are followed that have strong tendencies toward maximizing the group good.

Hedonism

Hedonism, also known as *rational egoism*, is the process of prioritizing self-fulfillment, and it is contingent upon a significant degree of personal liberty. In popular usage, the term *hedonism* may imply crass, sensate living, but, philosophically, the pleasure sought can be something beyond mere physical experience. Although the US government, with its emphasis on social contract theory and negative rights, is strongly rooted in deontological moral reasoning, the Declaration of Independence includes a hedonistic assertion of the right to "the pursuit of happiness." This assertion refers not to an individual's right to frivolity but rather to one's right to work toward an individual ultimate end; thus, it is actually a mixture of hedonistic, deontological, and virtue reasoning. With regard to public health, a legitimate appeal to hedonism might be the assertion that, for instance, smoking can be directly linked to physical suffering and loss of income. The primary advantages of hedonistic reasoning are that it emphasizes the liberty of the individual and that it values industriousness and talent, which will actually strengthen the community over time. One disadvantage is its tendency to disregard the necessity of at least some communal activity and accountability.

Virtue Reasoning

Virtue reasoning differs from the two forms of consequentialism in that, rather than the end *justifying* the means, the end *conditions* the means. In other words, the end, or goal, shapes the behavior or character of the moral actor. Usually when an individual or organization is described as morally good or bad, an evaluation is being made on the basis of expressed character or displayed virtue. A good physician is one whose character is virtuous (at least in terms of professional behaviors) and whose skill set is developed and well applied. A good public health organization is one that acts in a manner consistent with its purpose. Similarly, a good public health leader is one who uses proper authority to serve the organization, leading in a manner consistent with that organization's mission.[33,34]

Analogical Moral Reasoning

analogical reasoning
Moral reasoning based on structural comparisons between situations.

In addition to deontological and teleological reasoning, public health leaders may also employ **analogical reasoning**, particularly in times of significant uncertainty. Analogical reasoning involves structural comparisons between situations, and it is usually expressed in the language of *like/unlike*. Typically, this form of reasoning is used either to initiate ethical consideration of a new problem or to explain a moral choice heuristically to someone else. In public health, analogical reasoning is often used when new crises arise. For instance, when the first cases of AIDS were recognized, public health organizations initially used methods drawn from past responses to epidemics and mathematical modeling that relied on assumptions of common structure in disease expansion.

A key strength of analogies is that they allow for simple explanations. A key disadvantage is that they can be erroneously constructed, especially when something is said to be similar to another concern but actually is not, thus generating a sort of analogical false positive.

Reasoning Methods and the Moral Decision-Making Process

The reasoning method employed does not necessarily drive a conclusion one way or another, but it does shape the moral decision-making process. Metaphorically, the various methods are the personality styles of the moral decision. Individuals and organizations tend to emphasize one method but frequently use two or three methods simultaneously (even if they do not acknowledge doing so). Most public health organizations tend toward utilitarian reasoning in defining their function and evaluating their level of success.

Each of the reasoning methods has its own moral vulnerabilities, and public health's tendency toward utilitarianism can too readily be used to overrule the deontological reasoning of human rights. Consider the numerous occasions throughout history when public health arguments have been used to justify suppression of nonmajority political, religious, sexual, or cultural behaviors. The Soviet Union was well known to have used concerns about mental illness and public health as instruments of social control. At various points in US history, the decisions of individuals and groups with social power—lawyers, judges, physicians, scientists, and public health leaders—have led to such injustices as eugenics policies, the Tuskegee epidemiological studies, and the US-led syphilis experiments in Guatemala.[35] When outliers are not protected as rights holders, or when some vague understanding of health is used in utility calculations to justify state coercion, the vulnerable inevitably suffer.

In addition to its use in public health, utilitarian reasoning is dominant in economics and arguably the primary moral reasoning method found in politics. However, it does not similarly dominate in the spheres of science, religion, or family. Moral conflicts frequently arise over which type of reasoning should be used in a given sphere or, even more so, in a given institution.[36] Individuals and organizational authorities often will talk past one another or be dismissive of others' preferred styles of reasoning. A moral public health leader, however, must work around such disputes and recognize that all methods are used in all spheres and organizations, just to different degrees.

Public health leaders who use only utilitarianism are the same leaders who are likely to rely almost exclusively on bureaucratic authority, and in doing so, they will almost inevitably fail both themselves and their organizations. They will find that the constituents of the organization simply cannot or do not follow their leadership, and they will either ignore the problem or legalistically follow the rules and excessively compartmentalize responsibility. Any outliers or awkward or complex circumstances will create situations that are unmanageable until additional rules are created, finally leading to a tangle of casuistic public health regulations or even intentional abuse.

Especially during genuine upheaval or systemic uncertainty, exemplar or perhaps emissary charismatic moral leadership is required. Simplistic bureaucratic adherence and the calculation of utility will not work. Outcomes matter, but an organization is not simply a "black box" into which inputs are placed and from which outputs are drawn. An organization is made up of individuals. It is as much a community of face-to-face relationships as it is a set of formal social structures, as much organic as it is mechanical, and as much a guildlike expert association as it is a businesslike corporate entity.[37]

> ### Effective Public Health Leaders . . .
>
> . . . know that everything accomplished should be legal, moral, and ethical.

Ethical Public Health Leadership for the Twenty-First Century

Utilitarianism carries significant risks if practiced in an absolute sense, but it nonetheless should remain the primary moral reasoning method for public health. In a sense, the appropriate form is a restricted utilitarianism, not pure utilitarianism. Organizations that were designed to serve the public's health should place a primary emphasis on meeting public health ends to the extent possible within limits created by the rights of individuals, the economic constraints of society, and the prevailing cultural and political realities. In other words, public health organizations should operate using utilitarian reasoning that is bounded and controlled by deontologically defined rights and the **prudence** of virtuous leaders. The "good" leader in public health, then, is personally virtuous and recognizes societal boundaries and individual rights, while at the same time maximizing the improvement of plastic biological functionality in the population.

prudence
Applied wisdom.

Considering "Good" and "Right"

By the beginning of the 21st century, phrases such as "good leader" and "morally right choice," for some people, had taken on just the slightest authoritarian tone. The idea of good or morally right choices implies that other choices are bad or morally wrong, a label that some may consider offensive (which is ironic, given that offense assumes a common value and expectations that the value is recognized). Indeed, in the United States in the early decades of the 2000s, many discussions about morality were being reduced to personal reflections on taste. In public health practice, however, refusal to recognize what is good or right will result in organizational drift or even purposelessness. Anyone who has held a leadership role in public health knows that choices about cigarette smoking, behaviors contributing to morbid obesity, lack of childhood inoculations, unprotected sexual behaviors, careless disposal of pollutants in drinking water, and so on are not morally neutral.

No society, and no organizations within a society, can operate without functional assertions about what is right or good. All human interactions, to varying degrees and in varying ways, are shaped by moral claims. To use a public health example, drivers may stop at a stop sign for any number of reasons. They might stop because they do not want to get a ticket (aversion to social consequences against the self, a hedonistic response). Or perhaps they stop because they do not want to be harmed or cause harm to others and they consider the "cost" of stopping to be minimal (utilitarianism). They might find that the stop sign reflects a reasonable moral rule for a civil society (deontology), or they may simply want to be law-abiding individuals (virtue). Underneath the law itself is a shared moral claim that human life, at least some human life, is a moral good and that its protection is a morally right action that should be enforced with morally just policing authority directed by a morally good (at least in some sense) leader.

People may be immoral, but they cannot be amoral—at least not if they live in a society. In the broad sense, morality is the basis for law, and law is the ordering of society. Society and social institutions are always based on prior mores and moral claims. In turn, specific laws, regulations, and rules—and the institutions that generate and enforce them—can be judged as more or less right, good, or desired based on the socially shared moral ideals (which, in the United States, is largely based on middle axioms).

The Ethical Analysis of Moral Outcomes

How, then, can public health leaders know that they are acting in a moral way? How can their moral choices be evaluated? The answer is by considering the outcomes—that is, by examining how their decisions, in comparison with other possible options (including inaction), result in movement toward the society's shared good.

Leaders should develop specific measurements of moral success at three levels of analysis:

1. *Success in achieving the institutional mission of improved public health.* Leadership decisions should be effective in serving the institutional mission such that specific outcomes are achieved (improved public health is a morally desirable end). Leaders should be prudent in their decision making (utility and virtue) such that conflicts are minimized and effective use of funds is maximized so that lost opportunity costs are lowered relative to public health outcomes.

2. *Morally appropriate internal functioning of the organization.* Such functioning occurs when leaders accept accountability for the institutional systems, and it can often be assessed through content analysis of internal memos and external public communication. Leaders should treat other people both as functionaries in the organization (a utilitarian evaluation) and as ends in themselves, or their own moral persons (deontological reasoning). Appropriate internal functioning stems from leaders who hold employees accountable in a consistent, encouraging manner; maintain confidentialities of clients and employees; are honest and transparent to the extent allowable by law and regulation; and are tolerant of differences that do not directly bear on performance toward the institutional mission. Effective leaders make clear to the people being supervised that the leaders themselves—as well as others in the organization—will be held morally responsible for their behaviors and decisions.

3. *Moral evidence in the public health activities of the leader.* Leaders should be public health exemplars, temperately practicing what they preach (virtue reasoning). They can do so, for instance, by not smoking, by being reasonable in food consumption, by not participating in high-risk sexual behaviors, and by driving their automobile safely. They should strive to be organizationally courageous— neither impetuous nor cowardly.

> ### Spotlight
>
> The four classical virtues of prudence, courage, temperance, and justice are traditionally viewed as good habits, or patterns of behavior that can be developed through moral practice. Prudence is wisdom applied in decision making. Courage is the willingness to prudentially act for the moral good. Temperance is the influence of personal habits that allow the best moral choice to be implemented. Justice is rendering to each person his or her due, prudentially, such that the social order is strengthened for the well-being of each and all.

Defining Ethical Standards for Public Health

In 2002, the Public Health Leadership Society (PHLS)[25] listed a series of beliefs and values that would form the key assumptions underlying its *Principles of the*

Ethical Practice of Public Health. The first of these key assumptions, *Health,* affirms Article 25 of the Universal Declaration of Human Rights, stating that humans have a right to be provided the resources necessary to maintain their health. The second key assumption, *Community,* is based on six component beliefs: (1) that humans are interdependent and social in nature; (2) that institutions must have public trust to be effective; (3) that public health is based on collaboration; (4) that humans depend on their physical environment; (5) that all community members should have the opportunity to engage in the public discourse; and (6) that public health has a primary concern to identify and promote the requirements for health in the community. Similarly, the third key assumption, *Bases for Action,* is based on four beliefs: (1) that knowledge is both powerful and important; (2) that public health knowledge is primarily based on science; (3) that people take actions based on what they know; and (4) that the information on which people would like to base their actions is not always available. From these assumptions, the PHLS developed a set of principles that clearly spell out the need for public health to prevent adverse health outcomes in the community; to respect the rights of individuals; to receive input from community members; to empower the disenfranchised; to implement effective policies and programs; to provide the community with all relevant information; and to respect the community's diverse beliefs, values, and cultures. Public health institutions should have professionally competent employees who engage other community organizations collaboratively and build the trust of the community.

The National Board of Public Health Examiners (NBPHE)[38] sets forth a similar collection of principles in the code of ethics for its Certified in Public Health (CPH) credential. The code begins by stating that "All CPH professionals are entrusted with the duty of protecting, promoting and progressing the health of the public," and it lists a series of provisions that reflect this "responsibility of the highest order." Professionals are to place the health and safety of community members above their own interests; demonstrate integrity, honesty, and fairness; protect confidential information as needed; carry out actions in a timely fashion; remain free from bias; maintain competency through recertification; and appropriately reflect their academic and professional qualifications at all times.

The standards as expressed by the PHLS and the NBPHE underscore the attributes of professionalism, as discussed in chapter 2, while at the same time establishing core ethical principles.

 Check It Out

To read the Public Health Leadership Society's *Principles of the Ethical Practice of Public Health*, go to www.apha.org/~/media/files/pdf/membergroups/ethics_brochure.ashx.

To see the Certified in Public Health code of ethics of the National Board of Public Health Examiners, go to www.nbphe.org/code-of-ethics/.

Maintaining an Ethical Compass

Batra[39] states: "Integrity is a lot like being pregnant. Either you're pregnant, or you aren't. There's no middle ground. It's the same with integrity. Either you're behaving with integrity, or you're not."

One of the simplest ways for leaders to apply moral reasoning to day-to-day decision making is through the so-called headline test. As they make a decision, they consider how that decision might appear as a headline in a newspaper or blog the next day. Giving some thought to a decision's potential headlines can serve as a powerful reminder of the importance of ethics, and it can help leaders avoid ethical blunders. Few can forget the Enron scandal that dominated news coverage in the early 2000s, in which ethical failings produced such headlines as "Is There Anything Enron Didn't Do?"[40] and "How Enron Alienated Just About Everyone."[41] Public health leaders should recognize that all of their actions have the potential of being newsworthy, so passing the headline test should be a specific objective in their decision making. Concern about headlines, however, should not be used as an excuse for cowardice or bureaucratic avoidance of responsibility.

Leaders in public health should use ethical rubrics, or *prima facie* rules of conduct, to ensure that their ethical compasses point to true north. One rubric, for instance, might emphasize that simply doing what is legal does not necessarily result in ethical conduct. The law regulates relationships between individuals and organizations, but some lawful actions can result in damage to individuals, communities, and populations in ways that would not be considered ethical. Another ethical rubric might stress the importance of doing the right thing the right way the first time. Obviously, doing the wrong thing the right way the first time results in disaster, as does doing the right thing the wrong way the first time, and doing the right thing the right way the second time is far more costly than doing it right the first time. The effective public health leader ideally recognizes that the quality practice of public health is always less expensive than doing slipshod work that leaves wrecked lives and communities in its wake. The ethical practice of public health leadership based on simple, effective, and applicable rubrics will almost always pass the headline test.

Case Study: Mandating Human Papillomavirus Vaccination for Young Men[42,43,44]

At a media briefing on October 25, 2011, the Centers for Disease Control and Prevention (CDC) announced that its Advisory Committee on Immunization Practices (ACIP) now recommends routine vaccination of males aged 11 to 12 years to prevent human papillomavirus (HPV) infection and

(continued)

HPV-related disease. The committee stated that the HPV4 vaccine can be administered to boys as young as 9 years of age and that males aged 13 to 21 who were not previously vaccinated should be.

Related to the briefing, the CDC reported that approximately 18,000 HPV-associated cancers affect American women annually, with cervical cancer being the most common. At the same time, about 7,000 HPV-associated cancers affect American men each year, with head and neck cancers being the most common. More than 80 percent of anal cancers are caused in whole or in part by HPV. The prevalence rate for genital warts is approximately 1 out of every 100 sexually active adults in the United States. The CDC also noted that risk for HPV-related disease is highest among men who have sex with men and among individuals infected with HIV.

The ACIP recommendation of HPV vaccination for young men raises several ethical questions. A deontological question centers on young men's right of noninterference, as well as the rights of parents to make decisions concerning their children. A utilitarianism question also arises, because HPV vaccination is a low-cost intervention that not only saves lives but also reduces healthcare expenditures. Could not young men be compelled to receive the vaccine both because they are "participants" in society and because, deontologically, they have a duty to young women they might otherwise infect? Should the public health agency use coercive authority in a way that targets the entire high-risk pool of young men, even if some individuals assert they only participate in "safe" behaviors?

From a perspective of hedonism, the effort to vaccinate young men may be found to benefit the public health organization and its leaders professionally. The effort could also appeal to the personal pleasure and avoidance of pain for potential vaccination recipients. A virtue perspective might consider whether the vaccination campaign is compatible with the mission of the public health organization and improves the ongoing well-being of population members. From an analogical perspective, leaders might consider how an aggressive HPV vaccination campaign might compare with John Snow's removal of the Broad Street pump handle to combat an outbreak of cholera in London in 1854.

Discussion and Application Questions

1. In this situation, how might a leader demonstrate effective public health leadership?
2. Do you think an understanding of the ethical principles behind the situation will help or hinder the public health leader in making a decision about initiating the vaccination campaign?
3. What personal and professional issues might an effective public health leader face in making a decision about initiating this campaign?

Summary

This chapter seeks to provide a core understanding of moral reasoning and ethical decision making relevant to public health leadership. The assumed mission for all public health organizations is to promote the ongoing biological well-being of the population and the individuals who make up that population. This mission, accepted by the vast majority of public health leaders, reflects a basic assertion about the foundational good of the field.

In examining the moral functioning of public health, we distinguish between mores, morals, and ethics. Mores are social or organizational standards of good and bad and of right and wrong that are assumed by the group without formal expression. Morals are standards that are formally expressed and recognized as motivations for choices and actions. Ethics is the critical analysis of morality.

Max Weber's typology of organizational authority identifies three main types: (1) the charismatic leader, or prophet; (2) the role-holding leader, or priest; and (3) the management specialist leader, or the bureaucrat. Prophetic leaders rely on charisma, and they tend to emerge during periods when social structures are threatened or changing. Priestly leaders possess traditional authority based on their roles, and they tend to dominate when times are normal or calm. As organizations grow and become more complex and specialized, leadership authority takes an increasingly bureaucratic form. Today's public health leaders must be able to function in generally predictable ways within the organization (bureaucratic), with legitimacy provided through traditional roles and expertise (traditional/priestly), and with the ability to lead through crises without sacrificing the organization's core morality (prophetic).

Significant debate may surround the reasoning behind core public health values and the ways that those values can best be operationalized. After all, individuals' morality is largely based on culture and religion, and people differ in their backgrounds and beliefs. Nonetheless, the central operating values of public health should be agreed upon. Middle axioms are basic moral principles that are generally shared by individuals and groups even if they do not necessarily agree on the principles' philosophical or theological foundations. Working lists of middle axioms—such as principlism, which includes autonomy, beneficence, nonmaleficence, and justice—can help facilitate ethical discourse.

Justice and rights are key concepts in the moral practice of public health. Justice may be retributive (ensuring proportionate punishment for criminal behavior), distributive (involving the appropriate or equitable dissemination of goods), or commutative (emphasizing fairness in exchange and discourse). The rights to freedom of speech, freedom of religion, and freedom of assembly are examples of noninterference rights, or negative rights. In most societies, people also have positive rights, or entitlements, that arise out of the society's economic and structural capacity.

Public health leaders should seek to minimize conflict by acknowledging foundational values, clarifying shared middle axioms, and considering how people and organizations morally reason. Nonetheless, disagreement sometimes is inevitable, particularly in instances where the pursuit of a public health outcome requires the sacrifice of an individual's liberty or other values (e.g., mandated vaccination, quarantine, smoking restrictions). Public health leaders, therefore, need to be able to address these matters in an ethically legitimate manner. Just coercion theory provides some guidance in this area, as it uses generally accepted middle axioms of justice and various methods of moral reasoning to explain how governmental power can and should be used.

The effective public health leader needs to understand the key moral reasoning methods as they relate to public health. Deontological reasoning is moral reasoning based on categories, which often yield sets of formal rules. Teleological reasoning is moral thinking directed toward an end, and it includes utilitarianism, hedonism, and virtue reasoning. Analogical reasoning is moral reasoning based on structural comparisons between situations. Utilitarianism—which involves comparing two or more options and choosing the one that does the most overall good for the most people—is the most commonly used method in public health, but it should not be practiced in an absolute sense. Rather, public health organizations should operate using utilitarian reasoning that is controlled by deontologically defined rights and the prudence of virtuous leaders.

Discussion Questions

1. Discuss the good that is assumed in public health. What is its impact on the practice of public health leadership?
2. Describe the World Health Organization's definition of health. What are its ethical implications?
3. Define *mores*, *morals*, and *ethics*. What is their importance to public health practice?
4. What are the three forms of leadership legitimacy exhibited by contemporary public health organizations? Explain how each is exemplified.
5. Identify and describe the essential middle axioms of public health.
6. Define *justice* and its three basic subtypes. Provide public health examples of each.
7. Apply the concept of unavoidable conflict to the practice of public health, and provide examples of the application of just coercion theory.

8. Apply the concept of proportionality to the practice of public health leadership. What are the "dirty hands" and "slippery slope" ethical concerns?

9. Describe the main methods of moral reasoning. How do they apply to the practice of public health?

10. For deeper thought: As the director of your county's health department, you have taken the lead in passing a countywide smoking ban in restaurants and bars. You, personally, have quit smoking tobacco products, but you still use e-cigarettes. Discuss which ethical principles your use of nicotine supports and which it violates.

Web Resources

Public Health Leadership Society. 2002. *Principles of the Ethical Practice of Public Health.* Accessed June 30, 2017. www.apha.org/~/media/files/pdf/membergroups/ethics_brochure.ashx.

Thomas, J. C., M. Sage, J. Dillenberg, and V. J. Guillory. 2002. "A Code of Ethics for Public Health." *American Journal of Public Health.* Published July. www.ncbi.nlm.nih.gov/pmc/articles/PMC1447186/.

References

1. Rachels, J. 2007. *The Legacy of Socrates: Essays in Moral Philosophy.* New York: Columbia University Press.

2. World Health Organization. 1946. *Preamble to the Constitution of the World Health Organization.* Accessed February 6, 2017. www.ncbi.nlm.nih.gov/pmc/articles/PMC2567708/.

3. Krabbe, P. F. M. 2017. *The Measurement of Health and Health Status: Concepts, Methods and Applications from a Multidisciplinary Perspective.* London, UK: Elsevier.

4. Amundson, R. 2000. "Against Normal Function." *Studies in the History and Philosophy of the Biological and Biomedical Sciences* 31 (1): 33–53.

5. Bauman, Z. 2000. "The Consumer's Body." In *Liquid Modernity,* 76–82. Cambridge, UK: Polity Press.

6. Katz, S., and B. L. Marshall. 2004. "Is the Functional 'Normal'? Aging, Sexuality and the Bio-marking of Successful Living." *History of the Human Sciences* 17 (1): 53–75.

7. Thagard, P. 1999. *How Scientists Explain Disease.* Princeton, NJ: Princeton University Press.

8. Wachbroit, R. 1994. "Normality as a Biological Concept." *Philosophy of Science* 61 (4): 579–91.

9. Gould, S. J. 1981. *The Mismeasure of Man.* New York: Norton.

10. Foucault, M. 1973. *The Birth of the Clinic: An Archaeology of Medical Perception.* New York: Pantheon Books.

11. Thobaben, J. R. 2009. *Health-Care Ethics: A Comprehensive Christian Resource.* Downers Grove, IL: IVP Academic.

12. Kidder, R. M. 2009. *How Good People Make Tough Choices: Resolving the Dilemmas of Ethical Living.* New York: Harper.

13. Doyle, M. E., and M. K. Smith. 2001. "Classical Models of Managerial Leadership: Trait, Behavioural, Contingency and Transformational Theory." *Infed.* Accessed February 6, 2017. http://infed.org/mobi/classical-models-of-managerial-leadership-trait-behavioural-contingency-and-transformational-theory/.

14. Weber, M. 1947. *The Theory of Social and Economic Organization.* New York: Free Press.

15. Thomas, J. 2009. "Public Health Ethics." In *Principles of Public Health Practice*, 3rd ed., edited by F. D. Scutchfield and C. W. Keck, 133–48. Clifton Park, NY: Delmar Cengage Learning.

16. Manz, C. C., K. S. Cameron, K. P. Manz, R. D. Marx, and J. Neal (eds.). 2008. *The Virtuous Organization: Insights from Some of the World's Leading Management Thinkers.* Singapore: World Scientific Publishing Company.

17. Weber, M. (1947) 1997. "The Principal Characteristics of Charismatic Authority and Its Relations to Forms of Communal Organization." In *The Theory of Social and Economic Organization*, 358–62. New York: Free Press.

18. Turner, V. W. 1977. *The Ritual Process: Structure and Anti-structure.* Ithaca, NY: Cornell University Press.

19. Kuhn, T. S. 1996. *The Structure of Scientific Revolutions.* Chicago: University of Chicago Press.

20. Baden, J., and D. S. Noonan. 1998. *Managing the Commons.* Bloomington, IN: Indiana University Press.

21. Hardin, G. 1968. "The Tragedy of the Commons." *Science* 162 (3859): 1243–48.

22. Arendt, H. 1963. *Eichmann in Jerusalem: A Report on the Banality of Evil.* New York: Viking.

23. Online Library of Liberty. 2017. "Acton on Moral Judgements in History." Accessed February 6. http://oll.libertyfund.org/pages/acton-on-moral-judgements-in-history.

24. Thomas, J. C., M. Sage, J. Dillenberg, and V. J. Guillory. 2002. "A Code of Ethics for Public Health." *American Journal of Public Health.* Published July. www.ncbi.nlm.nih.gov/pmc/articles/PMC1447186/.

25. Public Health Leadership Society. 2002. *Principles of the Ethical Practice of Public Health.* Accessed February 6, 2017. www.apha. org/~/media/files/pdf/membergroups/ethics_brochure.ashx.

26. National Library of Medicine. 2017. "The Hippocratic Oath." Accessed February 6. www.nlm.nih.gov/hmd/greek/greek_oath.html.

27. Harvard T. H. Chan School of Public Health. 2017. "Harvard Chan Core Values." Accessed February 6. www.hsph.harvard.edu/ orientation/harvard-chan-core-values/.

28. National Commission for the Protection of Human Subjects of Biomedical and Behavioral Research. 1979. *The Belmont Report.* US Department of Health and Human Services. Accessed February 6, 2017. www.hhs.gov/ohrp/regulations-and-policy/belmont-report/ index.html.

29. Beauchamp, T. L., and J. F. Childress. 1994. *Principles of Biomedical Ethics.* New York: Oxford University Press.

30. Quotations Page. 2017. "Quotation Details: Quotation #27074." Accessed February 6. www.quotationspage.com/quote/27074.html.

31. World Health Organization. 2008. *Addressing Ethical Issues in Pandemic Influenza Planning: Discussion Papers.* Accessed February 6, 2017. www.who.int/csr/resources/publications/cds_flu_ethics_5web. pdf.

32. Orend, B. 2002. "Justice After War." *Ethics and International Affairs* 16 (1): 43–56.

33. Pellegrino, E. D., and D. C. Thomasma. 1993. *Virtues in Medical Practice.* New York: Oxford University Press.

34. Kass, L. R. 1988. *Toward a More Natural Science: Biology and Human Affairs.* New York: Free Press.

35. Presidential Commission for the Study of Bioethical Issues. 2012. "President's Bioethics Commission Posts Additional Documents Related to Its Historical Investigation of the 1940s U.S. Public Health Service STD Studies in Guatemala." Published February 23. https:// bioethicsarchive.georgetown.edu/pcsbi/node/665.html.

36. Walzer, M. 1984. *Spheres of Justice: A Defense of Pluralism and Equality.* New York: Basic Books.

37. Tönnies, F. (1935) 1957. *Community and Society.* Lansing, MI: Michigan State University Press.

38. National Board of Public Health Examiners. 2017. "Code of Ethics." Accessed June 30. www.nbphe.org/code-of-ethics/.

39. Batra, V. 2011. "*Integrity* Is Defined as Walking the Talk." ThinkLink. Published March 3. http://thinklink.in/integrity-defined-walking-talk/.

40. Elkind, P., and B. McLean. 2002. "Is There Anything Enron Didn't Do?" *Fortune* April 29, 23–24.

41. Carney, D. 2002. "How Enron Alienated Just About Everyone." *Bloomberg*. Published January 15. www.bloomberg.com/news/articles/2002-01-15/how-enron-alienated-just-about-everyone.

42. Advisory Committee on Immunization Practices. 2011. "Recommendations on the Use of Quadrivalent Human Papillomavirus Vaccine in Males." *Morbidity and Mortality Weekly Report* 60 (50): 1705–9.

43. Markowitz, L. E., E. F. Dunne, M. Saraiya, H. W. Chesson, C. R. Curtis, J. Gee, J. A. Bocchini Jr., and E. R. Unger. 2014. "Human Papillomavirus Vaccination: Recommendations of the Advisory Community on Immunization Practices (ACIP)." *Morbidity and Mortality Weekly Report* 63 (5): 1–29.

44. Petrosky, E., J. A. Bocchini Jr., S. Hariri, H. Chesson, C. R. Curtis, M. Saraiya, E. R. Unger, and L. E. Markowitz. 2015. "Use of 9-Valent Human Papillomavirus (HPV) Vaccine: Updated HPV Vaccination Recommendations of the Advisory Committee on Immunization Practices." *Morbidity and Mortality Weekly Report* 64 (11): 300–4.

THE CULTURAL BASIS OF PUBLIC HEALTH LEADERSHIP

James W. Holsinger Jr.

Learning Objectives

Upon completion of this chapter, you should be able to

- compare and contrast the terms *culture* and *organizational culture*;
- discuss diversity, prejudice, multiculturalism, and ethnocentrism;
- distinguish between the various categories of cultural phenomena;
- analyze socialization and explain the difference between internal integration and external adaptation;
- explain cultural cohesion and its importance to the development of a culture;
- discuss adaptive and high-performing cultures;
- compare positive and negative leader attributes, based on the GLOBE study findings;
- analyze three different approaches to diversity in organizations;
- describe the glass ceiling and the labyrinth; and
- compare and contrast the preferred leadership styles of women and men.

Focus on Leadership Competencies

This chapter emphasizes the following Association of Schools and Programs of Public Health (ASPPH) leadership competencies:

- Describe alternative strategies for collaboration and partnership.
- Communicate an organization's mission, shared vision, and values to stakeholders.
- Guide organizational decision-making and planning based on internal and external environmental research.

(continued)

It also addresses the following Council on Linkages public health leadership competencies:

- Explains the ways public health care and other organizations can work together or individually to impact the health of a community.
- Ensures use of professional development opportunities by individuals and teams.

Note: See the appendix at the end of the book for complete lists of competencies.

Introduction

culture
The shared learning of a group or organization, including such elements as values, beliefs, customs, behavior, emotions, and cognition.

organizational culture
Traditional or customary ways of thinking and acting that are shared by members of an organization and that individuals must acquire, to some extent, to be accepted into the organization.

diversity
The presence of people from a variety of cultures, backgrounds, or ethnicities.

multiculturalism
The presence of multiple cultures, or subcultures, within a larger system.

Leadership in public health, or in any organizational setting, involves a wide variety of cultural processes. **Culture** is a complex concept, defined by Schein[1(p111)] as "(a) a pattern of basic assumptions, (b) invented, discovered, or developed by a given group, (c) as it learns to cope with its problems of external adaptation and internal integration, (d) that has worked well enough to be considered valid and, therefore (e) is to be taught to new members as the (f) correct way to perceive, think, and feel in relation to those problems." Alternatively, the term can be thought of as the climate and practices of a group of people, indicating the values or beliefs that guide them,[2] or simply as a group's customs and way of life.[3] Within any larger culture, smaller subcultures exist. Public health practitioners, for instance, function within a set of cultures including that greater culture of their nation; the culture of their state, province, or territory; the culture of the field of public health; and the culture of their own organization.

An **organizational culture** consists of the traditional or customary ways of thinking and acting that are shared, to some extent, by members of an organization and that individuals must acquire, to some extent, to be accepted into the organization.[4] Every organization shares certain key values, norms, assumptions, and understandings,[5] and such elements are constantly being learned, shared, and transmitted to new members.[6] Leaders—through their visions and values, reactions to crises, role-modeling, and attention to followers—play a powerful role in shaping organizational culture. They develop systems, programs, structures, and even cultural forms such as rituals, symbols, and ceremonies,[7] all of which help set the tone for the organization.

A discussion about public health leadership and organizational culture requires an understanding of **diversity** and **multiculturalism**. Diversity is the presence of people from a variety of cultures, backgrounds, or ethnicities, and multiculturalism is the presence of multiple cultures, or subcultures, within a larger system. A culture will often include subcultures defined by such characteristics as gender, race, age, ethnicity, country of origin, or sexual orientation.

In a diverse workplace, **prejudice** and **ethnocentrism** are common concerns. Prejudice is a preconceived opinion, attitude, or belief that is based not on actual experience or reason but rather on generalized ideas about certain groups. Prejudice is rarely a positive construct; in fact, it is almost universally negative. It typically leads people to make faulty assumptions about individuals based on their race, ethnicity, age, or other characteristics, and such assumptions can be difficult to change and resistant to evidence to the contrary.[9] Ethnocentrism, a related concept, occurs when individuals hold their own culture or subculture at the center of their worldview, thereby placing their own values and beliefs above those of other cultures or subcultures. Individuals with an ethnocentric worldview often perceive their own culture to be "better" than the other cultures, making them intolerant toward the opinions, practices, and traditions of others.

Because prejudice and ethnocentrism limit people's ability to relate with others, both concepts impede effective public health leadership. Public health leaders, therefore, must find a balance between their own ways of doing things and others' ways of doing things, striving to overcome ethnocentrism while still maintaining their own values.[9] An appreciation for multiculturalism and diversity can help leaders better understand why people are so different, what followers' behaviors mean, and why modifying their behaviors can be so difficult.

> ### Spotlight
>
>
> "The people of each society store in their memories a particular complex set of symbols which they all learn. This is the content of their culture, and it determines their characteristic modes of information which appear in their speech, actions, and rituals; their artifacts of all sorts; and their social structure."
> —James G. Miller[8(p749)]

prejudice
A preconceived opinion, attitude, or belief that is based not on actual experience or reason but rather on generalized ideas about certain groups.

ethnocentrism
A tendency for individuals to place their own cultural group at the center of their worldview.

Aspects of Culture

Organizational culture functions at three levels with differing degrees of visibility. The first level consists of surface-level elements such as dress, office layout, ceremonies, symbols, and slogans—all things that can be seen and heard while watching and listening to the members of the group. The second level is less visible, and it consists of deeper values and understandings that are held in common by the group's members. Values at this level are expressed but not easily observed, and they can be said to represent "the way we do things around here." The third level consists of underlying assumptions and core beliefs that are so deeply embedded in the culture that the group members might not even be consciously aware of them. Often, assumptions originate as expressed values but eventually turn into such deeply held beliefs that they become taken for granted. As core

> ### Consider This
>
>
> "Son, I'm sorry, I made a mistake."
> —General George S. Patton Jr.[10(p257)]
>
> Do you find it difficult to apologize for your mistakes? If so, why? If not, why not?

values become more deeply engrained, members of the organization develop a sense of identity and a commitment to the organization's core values and way of doing things.

Schein[2] identifies ten major categories of cultural phenomena, as shown in exhibit 9.1. The observed behavioral regularities that occur when people interact include such aspects as the type of language people use and the customs, traditions, and rituals that people consider important. Group norms are the values and standards that evolve within the group, whereas espoused values are clearly announced principles about what the group intends to achieve. A formal philosophy, such as the ten essential public health services, may be enunciated by the group. Implicit "rules of the game" outline the way things get done in the group and must be taught to new members to ensure that they get along with leaders and coworkers. The organizational climate is determined by the way members of the group interact with one another and with constituents and collaborators. Embedded skills are special competencies that are deeply ingrained in the organization (even if they do not appear in writing) and must be passed on to new members. Closely related to embedded skills are the shared habits of thinking that guide members' thoughts, language, and perceptions, as well as the shared meanings and understandings that develop as members interact. These too must be taught to new members as they assimilate. Group members also characterize themselves through shared symbols, or "root metaphors," which, even if they are not consciously appreciated, reflect the emotions that members feel for being a part of the group.[2] Collectively, these aspects of culture contribute to a deep sense of attachment among group members, producing structural stability.

EXHIBIT 9.1

Major Categories of Cultural Phenomena

1. Observed behavioral regularities when people interact
2. Group norms
3. Espoused values
4. Formal philosophy
5. Rules of the game
6. Climate
7. Embedded skills
8. Habits of thinking, mental models, and/or linguistic paradigms
9. Shared meanings
10. "Root metaphors" or integrating symbols

Source: Data from Schein, E. H. 1992. *Organizational Culture and Leadership,* 2nd ed. San Francisco: Jossey-Bass.

Ideally, the various facets of the organizational culture bind together in integrative patterns that produce a paradigm of wholeness. Unfortunately, however, not all organizations develop this type of culture, and many are troubled by ambiguity and conflict. When a group becomes dysfunctional, the leader bears the responsibility of determining the dysfunctional attributes and managing the cultural change necessary to help the group survive in the external environment. The culture of a public health organization is deeply embedded in the wider culture, and it must be appropriate for meeting the greater needs of the communities and populations the organization serves. A key focus for public health leadership, then, is developing a subculture that will provide for the greater good.

> **Consider This**
>
> "Corporate culture at its most basic level is the sum of an organization's behavior and practices."
> —Jeff Rosenthal and Mary Ann Masarech[11(p4)]
>
> Why is an organization's culture important?

Socialization

Socialization is the process by which a person learns the deeply held assumptions that make up the heart of a culture. Often, when we consider the introduction of newcomers to the group, we focus on the ways they learn the basic rules, rituals, and behaviors that are outwardly apparent. Such instruction, however, covers only the surface aspects of the culture.[2] The true heart of the culture must be learned once the newcomer has been accepted as a permanent member of the group and admitted to its inner sanctums. Newcomers should be encouraged to actively engage in the socialization effort, through which they come to understand how group members perceive, feel, and think about important aspects of the group's life together. These patterns of perceptions, feelings, and thoughts, when placed in the situational context of the external environment, determine outward behavior. By studying the socialization process through which newcomers learn, we can better understand the deeper assumptions that underlie the group's culture.

socialization
The process by which a person learns the deeply held assumptions that make up the heart of a culture.

Internal Integration

Internal integration—the process by which culture establishes unity and collective identity within the group—depends on how the group establishes standards for membership, assigns power and status, and administers rewards and discipline. Organizations must develop principles for dealing with unpredictable and uncontrollable events, as well as mechanisms for dealing with workplace aggression and intimacy. Consensus must also be built around the symbols used within the organization.[12] By doing so, the organization develops a collective identity based on its culture, which enables group members to effectively work together. Unwritten rules strongly influence employee behavior

internal integration
The process by which culture establishes unity and collective identity within the group.

and play a major role in determining organizational performance. Therefore, for an organization to be highly effective, its leaders must ensure that these rules conform to the organization's objectives.[13] A strongly integrated culture—one that encourages trust, collaboration, and teamwork—makes employees more likely to effectively work together and share information, knowledge, and ideas.

External Adaptation

external adaptation
The cultural function through which members of an organization understand and adjust to the external environment.

Another major function of an organization's culture is to develop an understanding of the external environment and an ability to adapt to that environment. In public health organizations, such **external adaptation** involves understanding advocacy groups, constituents, and collaborators and being able to respond quickly to their needs and the needs of the population being served. Clearly, the culture of a public health organization should emphasize commitment to the core values of public health practice, including the ten essential public health services, and it should make clear the expectations for organizational success.[5] Such a culture will improve the organization's ability to respond rapidly to environmental threats and to natural and human-made disasters, which in turn reduces the level of anxiety, confusion, and uncertainty both for members of the organization and for the communities they serve. As public health organizations engage with the external environment, they gain valuable experience and develop effective solutions that can be passed on to future generations. Such experiences contribute to the shared assumptions of the organizational culture, thereby providing internal integration for the members, while also helping the organization adapt to its external environment.

Developing an Effective Organizational Culture

cultural cohesion
The extent of consensus for specific values among an organization's employees and their agreement with the way things are done.

An effective organizational culture is strong and cohesive, shows an ability to adapt, and is driven toward high performance. Effective public health leaders can work to develop and influence such a culture in a variety of ways.

Cultural Cohesion

Cultural cohesion is the extent of agreement about the way things are done and consensus about specific values among members of an organization. A strong and cohesive organizational culture occurs when there is widespread consensus on values; when consensus is lacking, the culture is weak. With regard to organizational culture, strength and cohesion are closely related. However, Arogyaswamy and Byles[14] prefer the term *cohesion*, in part because the word *strength* may introduce bias or suggest that a strong culture always performs well.

ideology
A coherent set of beliefs that holds individuals together, based on cause-and-effect relationships.

Arogyaswamy and Byles[14] used two descriptors to understand an organization's culture: (1) values, or people's principles and standards of behavior based on a judgment of what is important in life; and (2) **ideology**, which is a coherent set of beliefs that holds individuals together, based on cause-and-effect relationships.[15] With these descriptors, they examined the **internal fit** and **external fit** of the culture as it relates to organizational success. Internal fit is determined by the culture's cohesion and consistency, whereas external fit is determined by the development and implementation of strategies that are aligned with the outside environment. In a culture with a tight internal fit, members have strong agreement and consistency with regard to their values and ideologies, which results in a constant set of shared assumptions and beliefs. When the internal fit is looser, inconsistency in values and ideologies can lead to conflict and dysfunction, even if generally compatible values are present. Arogyaswamy and Byles[14] state that the formulation of an organization's strategy is influenced by organizational conditions (including resources and capabilities) and environmental properties, with the organization's culture being an important part of the process. For instance, when public health organizations are faced with changes related to national healthcare reform or changes in their state Medicaid program, they should consider not only the changing external conditions but also the organization's culture. Thus, the external fit reflects how strongly the organization's culture and its strategy relate to each other.

Tight cultural fits, both internal and external, are not necessarily a formula for success. Effective leaders should seek to understand and encourage cultural cohesion within their organizations, but they also must consider a variety of other variables (e.g., size of the organization or units, degree of interdependence, characterization of competitive advantage) as they deal with the changing landscape of public health practice.

Adaptation Versus Nonadaptation

Organizational cultures can be either adaptive or nonadaptive in nature, and the two styles display significantly different behaviors. In public health organizations with an adaptive culture, leaders pay close attention to collaborators, constituents, and advocacy groups; value the members of their communities and populations; and have relationships based on trust. They are willing to initiate change processes as necessary to assist their employees in meeting the needs of the people they serve, even if the changes involve risk. In organizations with a nonadaptive culture, leaders are more insular; act in a bureaucratic and political manner; and care mostly about themselves, their immediate team, and the services they have provided in the past. Such leaders are risk averse and prefer to maintain the status quo. They tend not to change their strategies to take advantage of the changes in the external environment.

When a public health organization fails to adapt and its culture fails to align with the needs of the external environment, a **culture gap** occurs. A culture gap reflects the difference between the values and behaviors that an organization actually has and those that are appropriate for the context in which the organization functions. In today's public health landscape, a culture gap can be debilitating.

internal fit
The degree to which an organization's culture has consensus and consistency in its values and ideologies.

external fit
Alignment of an organization's culture and strategies with the outside environment.

culture gap
The difference between the values and behaviors that an organization actually has and those that are appropriate for the context in which the organization functions.

If an organization has a nonadaptive posture, its leaders need to recognize that it is not functioning based on positive and important values, or that those values are not strongly held by the group members, and they need to change direction.

High Performance

Leaders in public health must understand the role of the organization's culture in meeting current challenges and creating new opportunities for the future. A culture thrives when it cultivates adaptation and strengthens organizational performance through change that energizes and motivates employees. Such efforts unify employees by establishing shared goals and a sense of higher mission, and they shape employees' behaviors in alignment with the organization's strategic prioritites.[5] Effective leaders use the organizational culture to exercise strategic objectives and engage people in innovative functions.[16]

Adaptive, high-performing cultures can be summarized in three basic rules[5]:

Consider This

"Relying on formal rules, policies, and procedures will not result in outstanding anything, be it customer service, innovation, or quality."
— Jennifer A. Chatman and Sandra Eunyoung Cha[16(pp22–23)]

If rules, policies, and procedures do not improve quality or enhance customer service or innovation, why should you follow them?

1. The whole is greater than the sum of its parts, and the boundaries between parts are reduced.
2. Trust and equality are core values.
3. Change, risk taking, and improvement are encouraged.

Several key processes can help public health leaders sustain a high-performance culture. These processes do not have to be carried out sequentially, since none is ever fully completed. The first process involves clarifying the mission and values of the organization. Leaders should examine the organization's core values and ensure that they have been fully integrated into the culture, the way the organization does its work, and the way it carries out its mission. The next process is relentless communication, which involves the ongoing use of two-way dialogue to instill the values and shape the culture. Beyond communicating, leaders also must model the espoused values in their actions; without the support of the leader's actions, the values will be seen as meaningless. Consistency is essential. Modeling of values should occur not only at the very top of the organization but also across the senior leadership team and at the middle management level. (Middle managers often are the weakest link in modeling values.) The alignment of the organization's practices with its espoused values can be a struggle, but all members of the organization should be held accountable. Leaders should manage performance by holding employees accountable not only for results but also for the behaviors used to achieve those results.

The final key process is engaging the employees. Although individual accountability and the alignment of practices are important, engagement occurs by capturing employees' hearts and minds, not by mandating their compliance. Public health leaders need to personally connect with their organization's values, demonstrate integrity in their actions, and clearly lead from personal conviction. They need to stay in tune with constituents, collaborators, and stakeholders and make every effort to develop messages that have meaning and empathy.[11] In short, they need to inspire followers to own their organization's culture and goals.

Effective Public Health Leaders . . .

. . . "unite [their] followers with a 'corporate mission.'"

—Donald T. Phillips[17(p113)]

Ways to Influence Culture

Effective public health leaders can influence the culture of their organizations in a variety of ways, whether through their own behavior or through structures, systems, programs, and cultural forms. They can act directly to shape culture by communicating their own values when they express the organization's vision and by confirming the importance of values and ideals in their day-to-day work. These cultural leadership behaviors will be discussed in greater detail later in the chapter. Leaders can also influence the culture through the design of management programs and systems, including formal processes such as budgeting, planning, reporting, performance evaluation, and employee training and mentoring. Managers can shape the socialization process for new employees by designing appropriate orientation and training programs that enhance awareness and understanding of the organizational culture. In addition, mentoring efforts (discussed in chapter 13) with both new and old employees can be an effective tool for inculcating the espoused values and visions.

Leaders can demonstrate the importance of the organization's values through their approach to rewards, recognition, and personnel decisions. What is rewarded is what is valued, and priorities are demonstrated through recognition and praise. Failing to recognize employee contributions or rewarding individuals regardless of their acceptance of the espoused values will send a false message and be counterproductive. The criteria for success and thereby rewards should be clearly enunciated, and decisions concerning them should be consistent.

Similarly, leaders can influence the culture through the way the organization is structured. Centralized and decentralized organizational structures send clear messages in and of themselves. If the organization speaks about employee initiative and shared responsibility but is structured in a hierarchical fashion, the messages it sends are inherently inconsistent. If egalitarianism is an espoused value, it should be reflected in the organization's office sizes, accoutrements, and other aspects. Cultural forms such as formal rituals, ceremonies, symbols, and stories play an important role in sending a consistent message and strengthening employee identification with the organization.

Global Study of Leadership

The practice of public health in the twenty-first century is global in nature, and numerous individuals immigrate to the United States from other countries each year. Therefore, today's public health leaders must possess a basic understanding of cultural differences if they are to lead their organizations effectively and engage with the diverse constituencies within the population.

The GLOBE Study's Dimensions of Culture

Culture consists of a variety of dimensions, and the effective public health leader must be able to understand these dimensions and the relationships that exist between them. Scholarly theories about culture can provide valuable guidance, but leaders should recognize that theories and concepts developed in one part of the world may not be applicable to other parts.[18] Hall[19] divided culture into two primary categories, individualistic and collectivist, based on whether the focus of the culture is placed with the individual or the group. Later investigators[20] classified culture into two dimensions, egalitarian/hierarchical, based on the level of shared power, and person/task, based on whether the emphasis is primarily placed on people or tasks. Hofstede[21,22] conducted a study of more than 100,000 individuals in more than 50 nations and identified five major cultural dimensions: (1) power distance, (2) uncertainty avoidance, (3) individualism/collectivism, (4) masculinity/femininity, and (5) long-term/short-term orientation.

In 2004, building on the earlier work of other investigators, House and colleagues[23] published the results of their Global Leadership and Organizational Behavior Effectiveness (GLOBE) research program. The authors presented nine cultural dimensions, each of which may be applied to a society, an organization, or a group; thus, the word *culture* is used broadly to include all of these levels. The GLOBE study's dimensions are as follows:

1. **Uncertainty avoidance** is the extent to which the culture uses established social norms, including laws, rules, and societal structures, to minimize uncertainty and increase predictability.
2. **Power distance** is the degree to which stratification within the culture results in the unequal sharing of power. Attributes that might contribute to stratification include power and authority, status and prestige, and wealth and material possessions.
3. **Institutional collectivism** is the degree to which the culture encourages collective activity, either institutionally or societally, and

---

uncertainty avoidance
The extent to which a culture uses established social norms to minimize uncertainty and increase predictability.

power distance
The degree to which stratification within a culture results in the unequal sharing of power.

institutional collectivism
The degree to which a culture encourages collective activity and is identified with the broader interests of society.

is identified with the broader interests of society instead of individual accomplishments.

4. **In-group collectivism** is the degree to which the culture is based on family cohesiveness, devotion, and loyalty.

5. **Gender egalitarianism** is the degree to which the culture minimizes gender differences in societal roles and encourages gender equality.

6. **Assertiveness** is the extent to which individuals in the culture are aggressive, assertive, or confrontational in relationships. This quality depends to some extent on societal encouragement.

7. **Future orientation** is the extent to which members of the culture engage in such activities as planning, investing in the future, and delaying gratification for the purpose of preparing for the future. A culture that ranks low in future orientation tends to engage in spontaneous activity while enjoying the present.

8. **Performance orientation** is the degree to which the culture encourages and rewards performance excellence and the attainment of challenging goals.

9. **Humane orientation** is the degree to which the culture encourages and rewards members' support for community values, sensitivity and caring for others, altruism, and generosity.

Incorporating responses from more than 17,000 managers across 62 countries, the GLOBE investigators matched the nine dimensions to ten regional clusters—Anglo, Germanic Europe, Latin Europe, Sub-Saharan Africa, Eastern Europe, the Middle East, Confucian Asia, Southern Asia, Latin America, and Nordic Europe—to determine the key cultural dimensions for leadership in various parts of the world. For the purposes of our discussion, we will focus on four clusters—Anglo, Confucian Asia, Latin America, and the Middle East—that vary in the way the dimensions are emphasized.

The Anglo cluster, which includes the United States, showed a high level of performance orientation and a lower level of in-group collectivism. Leaders in this cluster tended to emphasize competitiveness and a results orientation and focused less on family attachment. The Confucian Asia cluster, which includes China, South Korea, and Japan, had high scores in performance orientation, institutional collectivism, and in-group collectivism. Leaders in that cluster were found to be results driven, but they also tended to work together in groups and were devoted to their families. The Latin America cluster showed a high level of in-group collectivism but scored low on performance orientation, future orientation, institutional collectivism, and uncertainty avoidance. Leaders in these societies tended to be devoted to their families but not strongly engaged with societal and institutional groups. The Middle East cluster received a high score for in-group collectivism and low scores for future orientation, gender

in-group collectivism
The degree to which a culture is based on family cohesiveness, devotion, and loyalty.

gender egalitarianism
The degree to which a culture minimizes gender differences in societal roles and encourages gender equality.

assertiveness
The extent to which individuals are aggressive, assertive, or confrontational in relationships.

future orientation
The extent to which a culture engages in advance planning and other forward-looking activities.

performance orientation
The degree to which a culture encourages and rewards performance excellence and the attainment of goals.

humane orientation
The degree to which a culture encourages and rewards members' support for community values, sensitivity and caring, altruism, and generosity.

Leadership Application Case: John Marshall's Three Rubrics

The Leadership Application Case at the beginning of this book provides realistic scenarios for the application of key leadership concepts covered in the text. See the section marked "Chapter 9 Application" for the scenario and discussion questions that correspond with this chapter.

egalitarianism, and uncertainty avoidance. Leaders in that cluster were found to be devoted to their families and their own people, though they tended to treat people differently based on gender. They did not place heavy emphasis on policies and procedures, orderliness, or consistency. They tended to focus on current issues rather than attempt to control the future.

The GLOBE Study's Cultural Leadership Profiles

One of the key strengths of the GLOBE leadership study is its broad international scope, which distinguishes it from other leadership studies that have had a strong North American bias. As noted previously, leadership theories developed in one part of the world often do not apply in others.[24] The GLOBE researchers sought to link leadership behaviors with the culture clusters while incorporating **implicit leadership theory**[25]—the idea that individuals have certain beliefs and convictions about the traits and behaviors that distinguish leaders from nonleaders and effective leaders from ineffective leaders.[9] In this theory, leadership is like beauty—it is in the eye of the beholder.[26]

implicit leadership theory
The idea that individuals have certain beliefs and convictions about the traits and behaviors that distinguish leaders from nonleaders and effective leaders from ineffective leaders.

To assess the ways that different cultures practiced leadership, the GLOBE researchers focused on six leadership behaviors:

1. Charismatic/value-based leadership involves leaders' efforts to inspire and motivate followers, while also expecting a high level of performance, based on strongly espoused values. Leaders who use these behaviors are considered trustworthy, inspirational, and visionary, while at the same time being decision and performance oriented.

2. Team-oriented leadership focuses on building teams around a common purpose. Leaders using this behavior are seen as collaborative and diplomatic, as well as administratively competent.

3. Participative leadership occurs when leaders involve followers in the decision-making process and use followers' expertise to implement decisions. Such leaders encourage active participation and are nonautocratic in their approach.

4. Humane-oriented leadership emphasizes leaders' efforts to be considerate, generous, modest, sensitive, and compassionate in their interactions with followers.

5. Autonomous leadership is independent and individualistic in its nature. Leaders using this behavior are autonomous and unique in their approach.

6. Self-protective leadership is marked by leaders' tendencies to protect themselves and to think only of the security and safety of themselves and their group.

The GLOBE investigators used assessments of these behaviors to develop leadership profiles for each regional cluster. The Anglo leadership profile was strongly charismatic and values based, favoring leaders who were participative and sensitive to followers and others. People in the Anglo cluster valued autonomy and team orientation, and they preferred leaders who were motivational, visionary, and considerate. The study found that the least effective form of leadership in the Anglo cluster was a self-protective style prone to saving face. The leadership profile for Confucian Asia, on the other hand, described a self-protective leader who was also team- and humane-oriented. Leaders in that cluster normally did not invite followers to engage in goal setting or decision making. Instead, they tended to make independent decisions, though at the same time they worked well with others and cared about them. The Latin America leadership profile placed great importance on charismatic/value-based, team-oriented, and self-protective leadership behaviors, and it placed the least importance on autonomous leadership. Leaders tended to be inspiring and collaborative but also self-serving at times, with only a moderate interest in including people in decision making. Finally, the leadership profile of the Middle East cluster, in contrast to the three other clusters discussed here, emphasized status and saving face. Charismatic/value-based, team-oriented, and participative leadership behaviors were not found to be essential for effective leadership. Leaders in the Middle East cluster were also found to be family oriented and independent.

Although the GLOBE study identified significant leadership differences across the various clusters, it also identified a number of universally positive and negative leadership attributes, shown in exhibit 9.2. On a global basis, the exceptional leader is one who demonstrates a high level of integrity, is charismatic/value driven, and has superb interpersonal skills.[26] The ineffective leader is characterized as asocial, malevolent, and self-focused.

> ### Check It Out
>
> For more information on the GLOBE study, go to http://globeproject.com.

Strengths and Weaknesses of the GLOBE Study

Like any research project, the GLOBE study has both strengths and weaknesses. A clear strength is the sheer magnitude of the study, with the participation of 17,000 managers from 62 countries. The study also had a well-thought-out quantitative research design that used standardized instruments to assess leadership and its cultural aspects. Notably, it expanded the Hofstede[21,22] template

EXHIBIT 9.2
Global Leader
Attributes

Positive Leader Attributes		Negative Leader Attributes
Trustworthy	Motivated	Loner
Has foresight	Decisive	Irritable
Positive	Communicative	Ruthless
Confidence builder	Coordinative	Asocial
Intelligent	Honest	Nonexplicit
Win–win problem solver	Encouraging	Dictatorial
Administratively skilled	Motive arouser	Noncooperative
Excellence oriented	Dependable	Egocentric
Just	Effective bargainer	
Plans ahead	Informed	
Dynamic	Team builder	

Source: Data from House, J. R., P. J. Hanges, M. Javidan, P. W. Dorfman, and V. Gupta (eds.). 2004. *Culture, Leadership, and Organizations: The GLOBE Study of 62 Societies*. Thousand Oaks, CA: Sage.

of five cultural dimensions to nine, providing a broader and more elaborate methodology for the study of leadership. The GLOBE study provided a clear demonstration of the complexity of the leadership process and the way culture influences it, while at the same time identifying a number of universally accepted attributes of positive and negative leadership—a contribution of significant interest to public health leaders. Unfortunately, the GLOBE study did not produce a unitary theory of the means by which culture impacts leadership. In addition, the study's basis on the implicit leadership theory may be considered a limitation in that it assumes leadership is based on how one is perceived as a leader by others.[9] Furthermore, the GLOBE approach is in some ways akin to the trait approach (discussed in chapter 3), and in a like manner it fails to consider the effects of the situation or context on leadership practice. Nonetheless, insights from the GLOBE study can help leaders to understand their own cultural biases and preferences, to work effectively with people from different backgrounds, and to meet the needs of followers and constituents in an increasingly diverse population.

Diversity in Organizations

Diversity is a culturally determined construct that can take into account a wide range of variables, including age, race, ethnicity, education, gender, sexual orientation, and socioeconomic level. The word *diversity* has meant different things to different people at different times, and researchers have shown little consensus on how the concept affects organizational processes and outcomes.[27] Stevens, Plaut, and Sanchez-Burks[28(p412)] have defined *diversity* as "the degree to which a workgroup or organization is heterogeneous with respect to personal and functional attributes." Clearly, as older Americans have begun working longer, as women and minorities have assumed jobs previously unavailable to them, and as the demographic composition of the United States has shifted, diversity within US organizations has been increasing.[29]

Diversity encompasses all the ways in which people differ, including those ways that affect how people work, interact with each other, and define who they are.[30] Organizations can welcome and engage their diverse workforce by promoting a culture of **inclusion**. An inclusive culture considers a broad spectrum of personal traits and attributes, going beyond traditional notions of diversity to incorporate such elements as personality, function, competency, income, parenthood, language, work styles, and military experience, among others (see exhibit 9.3). It considers qualities that were present at birth as well as those that were acquired during the course of people's lives. All the dimensions of both the traditional and inclusive models of diversity have the potential to influence the ways individuals define themselves and the ways they are viewed by their coworkers. Effective leaders, therefore, must maintain an inclusive environment and recognize the unique strengths that each person brings.

inclusion
The practice of welcoming diversity and encouraging participation from people representing a wide variety of backgrounds and characteristics.

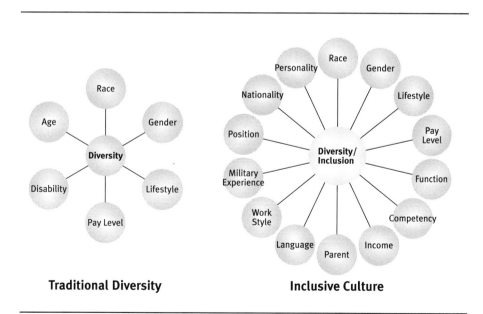

EXHIBIT 9.3
Model of an Inclusive Culture

Traditional Diversity

Inclusive Culture

Source: Oshiotse, A., and R. O'Leary. 2007. "Corning Creates an Inclusive Culture to Drive Technology Innovation and Performance." *Global Business and Organizational Excellence* 26 (3): 7–21. Reprinted with permission of John Wiley & Sons.

The Value of Diversity

A growing body of research confirms the value that diversity brings to organizations. Richard,[31] for instance, finds that workforce diversity aids in the development of human capital as a strategic asset and produces a valuable cultural mix in the human resource base. In 2013, *New York Times Magazine*[32] reported that 91 percent of jobseekers—and nearly all minority jobseekers—preferred organizations with diversity programs. In public health, in particular, organizations that recruit and value a diverse workforce have tended to attract and retain the best human talent.[7] Public health organizations with a diverse workforce tend to have practitioners who can relate culturally to the constituents, and therefore they are better suited to meet the needs of the diverse population. Diversity contributes through learning, flexibility, and increased morale, both for the workforce and the population it serves. An additional benefit is diversity of thought—a breadth and depth of opinions, ideas, and experiences that improve innovation, problem solving, and creativity.[5]

Consider This

"If everybody in the room is the same, you'll get a lot fewer arguments and a lot worse answers."
—Ivan Seidenberg[33(p54)]

How does hiring a diverse group of people improve the performance of a public health organization?

Despite the known benefits of organizational diversity, creating and maintaining an inclusive organizational culture—one in which each individual feels respected—can be difficult. Ethnocentrism and prejudice, as discussed earlier in the chapter, are common obstacles. **Stereotyping** leads many people to hold exaggerated or irrational negative beliefs about minority employees. Essentially, stereotypes are shortcuts in thinking, in which people assign characteristics to group members without regard for individuals' distinctive differences.[9] **Discrimination**—the acting out of prejudice—has generally become less blatant than it once was, but it still occurs. Often, discrimination is passive or unconscious in nature, to the point that people make discriminatory decisions without even realizing they are doing so. Such unconscious bias can affect hiring and promotion decisions, the assignment of work, performance reviews, and the treatment of employees on a day-to-day basis, thereby negating the benefits of a diverse culture.

stereotyping
Having exaggerated or irrational negative images or beliefs about members of certain groups.

discrimination
Actions that are based on prejudice.

Given the importance of diversity, effective public health leaders must work to create a culture of inclusion, to challenge the status quo when needed, and to establish conditions that will eliminate bias even in its unconscious forms. Ensuring that all employees are treated equally requires an active effort on the part of the leader.

Approaches to Diversity

Public health organizations can approach diversity in a variety of ways. Three of the most common ways are through the colorblind approach, the multicultural approach, and the all-inclusive workforce.

With roots in the American cultural ideals of equality, individualism, assimilation, and meritocracy,[34] the **colorblind approach** looks to create a common affiliation for all individuals within the broader organization, developing an overarching identity while ignoring cultural group identities.[35] It seeks to increase individuals' identification with the organization while decreasing the importance of individual differences.[36] The colorblind approach emphasizes unity and cohesion, and it stresses individual accomplishments and qualifications that override diversity and other factors. Thomas and Ely[37] have found that the colorblind approach is the most commonly used method for dealing with diversity in American culture and organizations. When a public health organization adopts a colorblind approach, the individuals most likely to identify with it are those who feel a need to belong or who believe strongly in individual merit.[28] Once individuals accept this approach, they tend to remain with the organization because they have become personally identified with it. Minority and majority group members, however, tend to view colorblindness from different perspectives. Although, in theory, the approach is based on merit and equal treatment of all employees, some minorities find it allows for the majority group to be culturally dominant and therefore is not truly colorblind in practice.[38] Minorities often consider the colorblind approach exclusionary, whereas majority group members find it more inclusive. The colorblind approach may magnify problems within organizations that lack diversity or even contribute to higher levels of racial bias. As a result, it may risk alienating or disenfranchising minority group members or even lead to the development of a racist culture.[39]

A second approach, the **multicultural approach**, specifically identifies employee differences as a benefit of a diverse workforce and as a source of organizational strength.[40] Organizations that adopt a multicultural ideology recognize and preserve group identities based on race, ethnicity, religious affiliation, and other characteristics.[28] As a result, they are typically attractive places for minority group members to work. To implement such an approach, organizations may emphasize the use of mentoring and networking, as well as diversity training for all employees. By raising cultural awareness, they hope to reduce bias among nonminority employees. If multicultural efforts are not actively maintained, they may fade over time, and they may encounter resistance from nonminority employees. Often, nonminority employees will support general equal employment opportunity programs but will oppose affirmative action efforts that focus on specific minority groups.

Given that some minority members feel excluded under the colorblind approach and that some nonminority members feel excluded under the multicultural approach, the **all-inclusive workforce**, a third approach, makes it a point to emphasize that diversity includes all employees—both minority and majority. The all-inclusive model recognizes the importance of all groups and fosters the continuation of subgroup identity within an overarching organizational identity.

colorblind approach
An approach to organizational diversity that seeks to develop an overarching identity for all individuals within the organization while ignoring cultural group identities

multicultural approach
An approach to organizational diversity that considers employees' cultural differences as a benefit and a source of organizational strength.

all-inclusive workforce
An approach to organizational diversity that fosters the continuation of subgroup identity within an overarching organizational identity.

By making both minorities and nonminorities feel respected and included, it aims to strengthen diversity while decreasing conflict and resistance. Stevens, Plaut, and Sanchez-Burks[28] propose that the all-inclusive model allows organizations to realize the benefits of diversity by facilitating relationships between differing groups. The approach fosters trust and commitment, as well as internal commitment and satisfaction, which are important for both minorities and nonminorities.[41] When all employees feel included, all are able to strive to reach their maximum potential. No demographic group is marginalized, so positive intergroup interaction and relations can occur.

All three of the approaches to diversity can be applied in the public health workplace, and leaders should thoughtfully consider which approach is best suited for their particular context. To effectively implement any diversity approach, leaders must understand the process of change and learning necessary for creating an inclusive culture. The process, as modeled in exhibit 9.4, has three main aspects: awareness, skills, and managing self.[30] It requires individuals to be aware of themselves, others, and their environment; to learn the skills needed to engage others in a different way; and to manage themselves and show a personal commitment to continued learning and application of skills. The key inclusion skills include inviting others into a relationship, inquiring into differences, and intervening when necessary to prevent exclusion. Of central importance to the model are the four principles of courage, awareness, respect, and empathy (CARE). Courage is necessary if individuals are to honestly evaluate themselves and commit to lasting behavioral change. Awareness in an all-inclusive culture goes beyond simply being aware of differences; it involves a deeper awareness of how differences affect the work environment and the organization, in addition to an awareness of individuals' own need to apply new skills in the workplace. Respect in this model involves both self-respect and respect for the diversity of coworkers. Individuals can often discover meaningful similarities once they truly respect one another's differences. Finally, empathy represents a greater understanding of how others feel, as well as a greater understanding of oneself, and it can help build trust in and respect for others.

The creation of a diverse workplace enables the organization to take full advantage of the benefits of diversity. It should minimize or eliminate biases, inequities, and opportunity gaps for people within the organization, while also making a positive difference in the lives of the diverse communities and populations being served.

Women in Leadership

The inclusion of women in leadership positions, a key aspect of workplace diversity, has changed significantly over time. For many years, sex-based discrimination greatly limited the opportunities for women, based on the outdated

EXHIBIT 9.4
Creating an
Inclusive
Culture

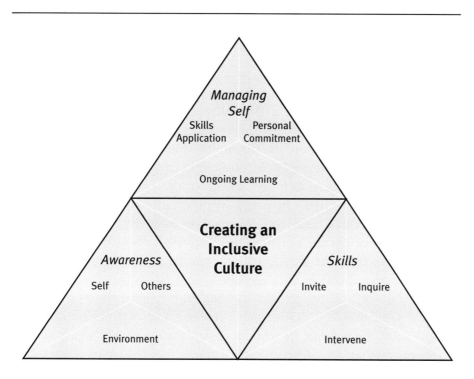

Source: Oshiotse, A., and R. O'Leary. 2007. "Corning Creates an Inclusive Culture to Drive Technology Innovation and Performance." *Global Business and Organizational Excellence* 26 (3): 7–21. Reprinted with permission of John Wiley & Sons.

and unsupported notion that men alone possessed the skills necessary for leadership. Through the continued advancement of women leaders, traditional notions of gender roles in the workplace have evolved, and gender egalitarianism today is regarded as an important cultural value. This trend is especially apparent in the field of public health: In 2010, more than 50 percent of top public health agency officials were women.[42] Still, even with this progress, gender stereotypes and role expectations have been slow to change, and sex-based discrimination—often in more subtle forms than in the past—continues to affect women in the workplace.[43]

Understanding the Labyrinth

When speaking about the biases and other obstacles that limit women's advancement in the workplace, people often speak of a metaphorical "glass ceiling." First coined in 1986, the term suggests that women rising through the ranks of an organization may be able to see up to the executive suite but are unable to break through the invisible barrier that keeps them from occupying it. More recently, however, some writers have proposed that a "labyrinth" might serve as a more appropriate metaphor for today's organizations.[44] Negotiating a labyrinth is neither simple nor easy, and it requires persistence, awareness of one's progress, and the ability to analyze what lies ahead. However, whereas a glass ceiling is impenetrable, a labyrinth does have a possible route to its center. Thus, rather than being trapped beneath a ceiling, women seeking leadership positions must negotiate the many walls that surround them as they pursue their goal. In attempting to explain the reasons for the labyrinth, people have typically attributed the obstacles women face to either human capital, gender differences, or prejudice.

In seeking to attribute the labyrinth to human capital, observers have suggested that women have less investment in education, less training, and less work experience than men do.[45] However, these arguments are not consistently supported by data—particularly with regard to education, given that women today receive a majority of bachelor's degrees and nearly a majority of advanced degrees. Research suggests that women are roughly equal to men in the degree to which they identify with their work and are committed to their work roles.[46] Evidence does not suggest that women leave jobs more often than men do; however, women have been shown to sustain greater losses after changing jobs, particularly if the job change occurs because of family obligations.[47] A more subtle form of the human capital explanation is the "female choice" argument, which postulates that women choose not to engage in leadership positions because they are concerned that such positions will interfere with family obligations.[45] However, the notion that the "mommy track" and domestic responsibilities preclude women from desiring leadership positions has been disabused.[48] Ultimately, outside of the possibility that women have less job experience and consistency of employment than men, the human capital argument fails to explain the conditions of the labyrinth. Some evidence does suggest that women receive less formal training and fewer developmental opportunities than men do; however, these differences are likely reflections of prejudice against women leaders.[49]

 Check It Out

To read a *Harvard Business Review* article about women and the labyrinth, go to https://hbr.org/2007/09/women-and-the-labyrinth-of-leadership.

The second proposed explanation for the labyrinth focuses on gender differences in such areas as commitment, motivation, self-promotion, negotiation, traits, style, and effectiveness. Research on leadership differences between women and men has suggested that women tend to use more democratic and participative styles.[50] Women who lead in an autocratic style are often devalued, particularly when they are evaluated by men. Burns[51] first considered the use of transformational leadership by women, and research has suggested that women's leadership styles tend to be slightly more transformational than men's and that women use contingent-reward behavior more effectively than men do.[52] Evidence also suggests that women tend not to be self-promoting in leadership positions.[53] In terms of leadership traits, research indicates that women and men are roughly equal in terms of intelligence, initiative, social skills, and the ability to persuade and that women rank more highly in integrity, assertiveness, and risk taking.[44] Thus, the gender differences that are supported by research are minor and tend to favor women, which weakens the idea that those differences are the reason for the labyrinth.

The third explanation is that the labyrinth and the leadership gap stem from prejudice and stereotyping.[55] Empirical evidence abounds that gender stereotypes significantly affect the perception and evaluation of women leaders and have a direct impact on their aspirations to become leaders. Such stereotypes, despite their well-documented inaccuracies, remain pervasive in American culture and appear highly resistant to change. Stereotypes often leave women leaders with conflicting expectations: For instance, as leaders, they are expected to be tough, but as women, they are expected to not be masculine. In today's organizations, the degree of prejudice at each individual level, or at each rung of the ladder, might not be enough to stop a female leader's advancement; however, the sum of all the discrimination that occurs at every level represents a significant barrier.

> ### Consider This
>
>
> "In government, in business, and in the professions there may be a day when women will be looked upon as persons. We are, however, far from that day as yet."
>
> —Eleanor Roosevelt[54]
>
> Does Mrs. Roosevelt's statement, from 1940, hold true today? If so, why? If not, why not?

Women's Leadership Styles

A variety of researchers have examined the ways that women differ from men in terms of leadership style and manner of communication. In comparing the conversational styles of women and men, Tannen[56] distinguishes between "rapport talk," which emphasizes emotional connections and a sense of community, and "report talk," which focuses more on providing information. Traditionally, rapport talk has been associated with women and report talk with men, and some have argued that rapport talk by women has no place in the workplace. Such notions have become outdated, however, and women have long demonstrated their ability to engage in report talk. In today's organizations, both rapport and report talk are necessary for engaging the workforce, and leaders, whether male or female, must be able to use both styles effectively.

Women's use of transformational leadership has been shown to be highly effective in today's culturally diverse workplace. Indeed, as the needs of society evolve, some have suggested that a new type of gender gap may be developing, with women being better able to pay attention, comply with the rules, communicate competently, and deal with interpersonal relationships.[57] A study by Bass and Avolio[58] found that women leaders ranked higher than male leaders in the transformational measures of idealized influence, inspirational motivation, individualized consideration, and intellectual stimulation. Such findings suggest that female leaders tend to earn the trust and respect of their followers, appeal to followers emotionally and symbolically, treat followers equitably based on each one's needs, and engage followers to think in new ways and question current ways of doing things. The study found women leaders to be both more effective than male leaders and more satisfying to work for. Compared to male leaders, women are less likely to emphasize competition, aggression, vertical hierarchies, and the formal authority of their positions. Instead, their style tends to be more interactive, caring, participatory, and inclusive.[52,59] Interactive leadership is a collaborative and consensual approach in which the leader's influence is based on relationships rather than position power and authority.[60] This relationship orientation allows for effective leadership with less emphasis on the top-down exercise of power.

The interactive approach to leadership represents values at the forefront of today's culturally diverse and globally connected public health landscape. Thus, gender differences in leadership style should not be considered a performance hindrance but rather a way to enhance the organization's effectiveness. As evident by the women who occupy more than 50 percent of the top leadership positions in US city and county health departments, women have clearly demonstrated their ability to lead. Perhaps in public health, Eleanor Roosevelt's hope has come true.

Case Study: Tuskegee Syphilis Study

The Tuskegee Study of Untreated Syphilis in the Negro Male—described as "arguably the most infamous biomedical research study in US history"[61]—was carried out by the US Public Health Service from 1932 to 1972. It took place on the campus of the Tuskegee Institute (now University), a historically black institution in Alabama, in collaboration with the institute. The study set out to observe the natural progression of syphilis and its effects on various organ systems, and it did so using a group of 600 African American men as research subjects.

Of the 600 participants, 399 men who were infected with syphilis made up the experimental group, and 201 men who did not have the disease made up the control group. The participants were "enticed and enrolled in the study with incentives including: medical exams, rides to and from the clinics, meals on examination days, free treatment for minor ailments and guarantees that provisions would be made after their deaths in terms of burial stipends paid to their survivors."[62(p42)] Originally, the study was supposed to consist of an observation phase followed by a treatment phase; however, when funding for the treatment phase was lost, the study continued, without informing the infected participants of its nature. During the course of the study, treatment was withheld from infected participants even after penicillin became widely available for treatment of syphilis in 1947. The study was established with the intent that the infected participants would never be informed of their health status.

On July 25, 1972, Jean Heller, a journalist from the Associated Press, reported details about the study, and the story captured national media attention. Responding to the controversy, the assistant secretary of health and scientific affairs of the US Department of Health, Education, and Welfare (now the Department of Health and Human Services) established an ad hoc advisory panel to review the study. The panel determined that, although the men participated freely, the research protocol for the study failed to ensure the safety of the participants. The study did not obtain informed consent from the participants, who were never informed of the purpose of the study or of the consequences of not being treated for the disease. In addition, the participants were not offered an opportunity to leave the study once penicillin became the drug of choice for treating syphilis. The panel therefore determined that the study was ethically unjustified and recommended that it be stopped.

By the time the study ended in November 1972, a number of participants had died, approximately 40 of their wives had contracted syphilis, and approximately 19 of their children had been born with congenital syphilis. Eventually, outcry over the study led to federal laws and regulations requiring institutional review boards for the protection of human subjects.

Discussion and Application Questions

1. In your opinion, what has been the cultural legacy of the Tuskegee study within the African American community in the United States?
2. What actions could effective public health leaders have taken to avert the devastating effects of the Tuskegee study?
3. In your opinion, why did US Public Health Service leaders fail to intervene and end the study?

Summary

Leadership in public health, or in any organizational setting, involves a wide variety of cultural processes. Culture is a complex concept that encompasses the values, beliefs, customs, behavior, emotions, and way of life for a group of people. Within any larger culture, smaller subcultures exist. An organizational culture consists of the traditional or customary ways of thinking and acting that are shared by members of an organization and that individuals must acquire in order to be accepted. Leaders—through their visions, values, and behavior—play a powerful role in shaping organizational culture.

Organizational culture includes a variety of aspects that, ideally, bind people together with a sense of unity and wholeness. The extent to which members agree about specific values and the way things are done is called cultural cohesion. Newcomers to a group learn the core elements of the culture through the process of socialization. Internal integration is the process by which a culture establishes unity and collective identity, and external adaptation is the process through which members understand and adjust to the external environment. Successful organizational cultures are adaptive in nature. They can initiate change, take risks, and keep up with the needs of a changing environment. A culture is most effective when it cultivates adaptation and strengthens organizational performance through change that energizes and motivates employees. Leaders can influence organizational culture in a variety of ways, whether through their own behavior or through structures, systems, programs, and cultural forms. The Global Leadership and Organizational Behavior Effectiveness (GLOBE) research program provides valuable information about leadership approaches from cultures throughout the world.

Diversity—the presence of a variety of cultures, ethnicities, backgrounds, and abilities within a group of people—can be highly beneficial for organizations, and organizations can engage a diverse workforce by promoting a culture of inclusion. However, maintaining such a culture can be difficult, especially if members of certain groups are targeted by stereotyping or prejudice. Leaders should strive to eliminate any such bias, even when it occurs in subtle or unconscious forms. The colorblind approach, the multicultural approach, and the all-inclusive workforce represent ways that leaders can promote diversity in their organizations.

A key aspect of workplace diversity involves the inclusion of women in leadership positions. Aspiring women in the workplace have traditionally faced significant barriers to advancement (whether a "glass ceiling" or a "labyrinth"), and these barriers have been largely linked to gender prejudice. However, outdated notions about gender roles have evolved over time, and women are increasingly taking on top leadership positions, particularly in public health.

Discussion Questions

1. Explain the concept of culture, and describe its impact on a public health organization.
2. Why is the socialization of new public health employees important?
3. Compare and contrast a public health organization's need to develop internal integration with its need to adapt to the external environment.

4. Define *culture cohesion*. What are its component parts?

5. What are adaptive and high-performing cultures? Explain their usefulness in public health organizations.

6. List and describe the dimensions of an organizational culture.

7. What are the global positive and negative leadership attributes? How have they been determined?

8. Why is diversity important in public health?

9. What are the diversity approaches for public health organizations?

10. For deeper thought: You, as the leader of a public health organization, are considering the key issues facing your female employees. Describe what you can do to help them move past the glass ceiling and/or beyond the labyrinth.

Web Resources

Eagly, A., and L. L. Carli. 2007. "Women and the Labyrinth of Leadership." *Harvard Business Review.* Published September. https://hbr.org/2007/09/women-and-the-labyrinth-of-leadership.

The Economist. 2009. "The Glass Ceiling." Published May 5. www.economist.com/node/13604240.

Global Leadership and Organizational Behavior Effectiveness. 2017. "About the Studies." Accessed July 5. http://globeproject.com/studies.

References

1. Schein, E. H. 1990. "Organizational Culture." *American Psychologist* 45 (2): 109–19.

2. Schein, E. H. 1992. *Organizational Culture and Leadership*, 2nd ed. San Francisco: Jossey-Bass.

3. Gudykunst, W. B., and S. Ting-Toomey. 1988. *Culture and Interpersonal Communication.* Newbury Park, CA: Sage.

4. Jacques, E. 1951. *The Changing Culture of a Factory.* London, UK: Tavistock Institute.

5. Daft, R. L. 2015. *The Leadership Experience*, 6th ed. Mason, OH: South-Western.

6. Bate, P. 1964. "The Impact of Organizational Culture on Approaches to Organizational Problem-Solving." *Organizational Studies* 5 (1): 43–66.

7. Hickman, G. R. 2010. *Leading Organizations: Perspectives for a New Era*, 2nd ed. Thousand Oaks, CA: Sage.

8. Miller, J. G. 1978. *Living Systems*. New York: McGraw-Hill.

9. Northouse, P. G. 2016. *Leadership: Theory and Practice*, 7th ed. Los Angeles: Sage.

10. Sewell, P. W. (ed.). 2001. *Healers in World War II*. Jefferson, NC: McFarland.

11. Rosenthal, J., and M. A. Masarech. 2003. "High-Performance Cultures: How Values Can Drive Business Results." *Journal of Organizational Excellence* 22 (2): 3–18.

12. Yukl, G. 2013. *Leadership in Organizations*, 8th ed. Upper Saddle River, NJ: Prentice Hall.

13. Scott-Morgan, P. B. 1993. "Barriers to a High-Performance Business." *Management Review* 82 (7): 37–41.

14. Arogyaswamy, B., and C. M. Byles. 1987. "Organizational Culture: Internal and External Fits." *Journal of Management* 13 (4): 647–59.

15. Beyer, J. M. 1981. "Ideologies, Values, and Decision-Making in Organizations." In *Handbook of Organizational Design*, vol. 2, *Remodeling Organizations and Their Environments*, edited by P. C. Nystrom and W. H. Starbuck, 166–202. New York: Oxford University Press.

16. Chatman, J. A., and S. E. Cha. 2003. "Leading by Leveraging Culture." *California Management Review* 45 (4): 20–24.

17. Phillips, D. 1992. *Lincoln on Leadership*. New York: Warner Books.

18. Den Hartog, D. N., and M. W. Dickson. 2004. "Leadership and Culture." In *The Nature of Leadership*, edited by J. Antonakis, A. T. Cianciolo, and R. J. Sternberg, 249–78. Thousand Oaks, CA: Sage.

19. Hall, E. T. 1976. *Beyond Culture*. New York: Doubleday.

20. Trompenaars, F. 1994. *Riding the Waves of Culture*. New York: Irwin.

21. Hofstede, G. 1980. *Culture's Consequences: International Differences in Work-Related Values*. Beverly Hills, CA: Sage.

22. Hofstede, G. 2001. *Culture's Consequences: Comparing Values, Behaviors, Institutions, and Organizations Across Nations*. Thousand Oaks, CA: Sage.

23. House, J. R., P. J. Hanges, M. Javidan, P. W. Dorfman, and V. Gupta (eds.). 2004. *Culture, Leadership, and Organizations: The GLOBE Study of 62 Societies*. Thousand Oaks, CA: Sage.

24. Hofstede, G. 1993. "Cultural Constraints in Management Theories." *Academy of Management Executive* 7 (1): 81–94.

25. Lord, R., and K. J. Maher. 1991. *Leadership and Information Processing: Linking Perceptions and Performance*. Boston: Unwin-Everyman.

26. Dorfman, P. W., P. J. Hanges, and F. C. Brodbeck. 2004. "Leadership and Cultural Variation: The Identification of Culturally Endorsed

Leadership Profiles." In *Culture, Leadership, and Organizations: The GLOBE Study of 62 Societies*, edited by J. R. House, P. J. Hanges, M. Javidan, P. W. Dorfman, and V. Gupta, 669–719. Thousand Oaks, CA: Sage.

27. Williams, K. Y., and C. A. O'Reilly. "Demography and Diversity in Organizations: A Review of 40 Years of Research." In *Research in Organizational Behavior*, edited by B. M. Staw and L. L. Cummings, 77–140. Greenwich, CT: JAI Press.

28. Stevens, F. G., V. C. Plaut, and J. Sanchez-Burks. 2010. "Unlocking the Benefits of Diversity: All-Inclusive Multiculturalism and Positive Organizational Change." In *Leading Organizations: Perspectives for a New Era*, 2nd ed., edited by G. R. Hickman, 411–24. Thousand Oaks, CA: Sage.

29. Milliken, F. J., and L. L. Martins. 1996. "Searching for Common Threads: Understanding the Multiple Effects of Diversity in Organizational Groups." *Academy of Management Review* 21 (2): 402–33.

30. Oshiotse, A., and R. O'Leary. 2007. "Corning Creates an Inclusive Culture to Drive Technology Innovation and Performance." *Global Business and Organizational Excellence* 26 (3): 7–21.

31. Richard, O. C. 2000. "Racial Diversity, Business Strategy, and Firm Performance: A Resource-Based View." *Academy of Management Journal* 43 (2): 164–77.

32. *New York Times Magazine*. 2013. "Diversity Initiatives Shown to be Critical to Job Seekers." September 14, 100.

33. Colvin, G. 1999. "The 50 Best Companies for Asians, Blacks, and Hispanics." *Fortune*, July 19, 53–58.

34. Plaut, V. C. 2002. "Cultural Models of Diversity: The Psychology of Difference and Inclusion." In *Engaging Cultural Differences: The Multicultural Challenge in a Liberal Democracy*, edited by R. Shweder, M. Minow, and H. R. Markus, 365–95. New York: Russell Sage.

35. Hogg, M. A., and D. A. Terry. 2000. "Social Identity and Self-Categorization Processes in Organizational Contexts." *Academy of Management Review* 25 (1): 121–40.

36. Chatman, J. A., and F. J. Flynn. 2001. "The Influence of Demographic Heterogeneity on the Emergence and Consequences of Cooperative Norms in Work Teams." *Academy of Management Journal* 44 (5): 956–74.

37. Thomas, D. A., and R. J. Ely. 1996. "Making Difference Matter: A New Paradigm for Managing Diversity." *Harvard Business Review* 74 (5): 79–90.

38. Markus, H. R., C. M. Steele, and D. M. Steele. 2000. "Colorblindness as a Barrier to Inclusion: Assimilation and Nonimmigrant Minorities." *Daedalus* 129 (4): 233–59.

39. Bonilla-Silva, E. 2003. *Racism Without Racists: Color-Blind Racism and the Persistence of Racial Inequality in the United States.* Lanham, MD: Rowman and Littlefield.

40. Cox, T. 1993. *The Multicultural Organization.* San Francisco: Barrett-Koehler.

41. Morrison, E. W., and E. J. Milliken. 2000. "Organizational Silence: A Barrier to Change and Development in a Pluralistic World." *Academy of Management Review* 25 (4): 706–25.

42. National Association of County and City Health Officials (NACCHO). 2011. *2010 National Profile of Local Health Departments.* Washington, DC: National Association of County and City Health Officials.

43. Heilman, M. E. 2001. "Description and Prescription: How Gender Stereotypes Prevent Women's Ascent Up the Organizational Ladder." *Journal of Social Issues* 57 (4): 657–74.

44. Eagly, A. H., and L. L. Carli. 2007. "Women and the Labyrinth of Leadership." *Harvard Business Review* 85 (9): 63–71.

45. Eagly, A. H., and L. L. Carli. 2004. "Women and Men as Leaders." In *The Nature of Leadership*, edited by J. Antonakis, A. T. Ciancolo, and R. J. Sternberg, 279–301. Thousand Oaks, CA: Sage.

46. Bielby, W. T., and D. D. Bielby. 1989. "Family Ties: Balancing Commitments to Work and Family in Dual Earner Households." *American Sociological Review* 54 (5): 776–89.

47. Keith, K., and A. McWilliams. 1999. "The Returns to Mobility and Job Search by Gender." *Industrial and Labor Relations Review* 52 (3): 460–77.

48. Smith, P. B. 2002. "Culture's Consequences: Something Old and Something New." *Human Relations* 55 (1): 119–35.

49. Baroff, M. B. 2015. "My Leadership Engine." *Frontiers in Public Health* 3 (137): 1–3.

50. van Engen, M. L., and T. M. Williamsen. 2004. "Sex and Leadership Styles: A Meta-analysis of Research Published in the 1990s." *Psychological Reports* 94 (1): 3–18.

51. Burns, J. M. 1978. *Leadership.* New York: Harper & Row.

52. Eagly, A. H., M. C. Johannesen-Schmidt, and M. L. van Engen. 2003. "Transformational, Transactional, and Laissez-Faire Leadership Styles: A Meta-analysis Comparing Women and Men." *Psychological Bulletin* 129 (4): 569–91.

53. Bowles, H. R., and K. L. McGinn. 2005. "Claiming Authority: Negotiating Challenges for Women Leaders." In *The Psychology of Leadership: New Perspectives and Research*, edited by D. M. Messick and R. M. Kramer, 191–208. Mahwah, NJ: Lawrence Erlbaum Associates.

54. Roosevelt, E. (1940) 2017. "Women in Politics." *Selected Writings of Eleanor Roosevelt*. Accessed July 5, 2017. http://newdeal.feri.org/er/er13.htm.

55. Hoyt, C. L., and M. M. Chemers. 2008. "Social Stigma and Leadership: A Long Climb Up a Slippery Ladder." In *Leadership at the Crossroads: Leadership and Psychology*, vol. 1, edited by C. L. Hoyt, G. R. Goethals, and D. R. Forsyth, 165–80. Westport, CT: Praeger.

56. Tannen, D. 1990. *You Just Don't Understand: Women and Men in Conversation*. New York: Ballantine.

57. Conlin, M. 2003. "The New Gender Gap." *Business Week*, May 26, 74–82.

58. Bass, M., and B. J. Avolio. 1994. "Shatter the Glass Ceiling: Women May Make Better Managers." *Human Resource Management* 33 (4): 549–60.

59. Stelter, N. Z. 2002. "Gender Differences in Leadership: Current Social Issues and Future Organizational Implications." *Journal of Leadership Studies* 8 (4): 88–99.

60. Rosener, J. B. 1995. *America's Competitive Secret: Women Managers.* New York: Oxford University Press.

61. Katz, R. V., S. S. Kegeles, N. R. Kressin, B. L. Green, M. Q. Wang, S. A. James, S. L. Russell, and C. Claudio. 2007. "The Tuskegee Legacy Project: Willingness of Minorities to Participate in Biomedical Research." *Journal of Healthcare for the Poor and Underserved* 17 (4): 698–715.

62. Satcher, D. 2011. "Tuskegee Legacy: The Role of the Social Determinants of Health." In *The Search for the Legacy of the USPHS Syphilis Study at Tuskegee*, edited by R. V. Katz and R. C. Warren, 41–48. Lanham, MD: Lexington Books.

FOLLOWERSHIP

Jennifer Redmond Knight and James W. Holsinger Jr.

Learning Objectives

Upon completion of this chapter, you should be able to

- compare and contrast the major followership styles,
- appraise the levels of followership engagement and understand how they relate to the major followership styles,
- discuss the seven paths of followership,
- describe the attributes of leaders and followers,
- understand the seven factors that affect leader–follower interactions,
- explain the Followership Continuum,
- compare the key leadership theories that focus on followers, and
- describe the relationship between leadership and followership.

Focus on Leadership Competencies

This chapter emphasizes the following Association of Schools and Programs of Public Health (ASPPH) leadership competencies:

- Describe alternative strategies for collaboration and partnership among organizations, focused on public health goals.
- Collaborate with diverse groups.
- Develop capacity-building strategies at the individual, organizational, and community level.

It also addresses the following Council on Linkages public health leadership competencies:

- Collaborates with individuals and organizations in developing a vision for a healthy community.

(continued)

- Provides opportunities for professional development for individuals and teams.
- Ensures use of professional development opportunities by individuals and teams.

Note: See the appendix at the end of the book for complete lists of competencies.

Introduction

Leadership has been the focus of extensive research and theorizing for many years, but the concept of followership has received considerably less attention. As noted in chapter 7, followership emphasizes the active efforts by followers to help the organization to succeed while independently exercising critical judgment. Followership has long been considered "secondary" to leadership, but those views are shifting. Researchers today are increasingly recognizing that followers have a powerful influence in their organizations and an impact on organizational outcomes that extends well beyond the formal recognition they receive.[1] Effective followers share a common purpose with the leader, believe in what the organization is trying to accomplish, want both the leader and the organization to succeed, and work energetically to those ends.[2] Without followers, there can be no leaders.

Public health organizations often have had a tendency to try to reach every person with the same health message in the same way, and they become frustrated when the desired health improvements do not occur.[3] The problem with such an approach is that it fails to take into account followers' distinct characteristics and their active role in the leader–follower relationship. Consider the way that advertising and marketing companies critically evaluate followers to determine what motivates them to action. Advertisers recognize that not all followers are the same and that different messages and approaches may be more effective for certain products and audiences. Public health has implemented some of these strategies in "social marketing" efforts, and a shift toward followership can now be seen in certain grassroots advocacy and public policy efforts. The identification of key followers who strategically work together has been critical to influencing smoke-free policies in public places, increasing tobacco taxes, improving access to clinical preventive services, and stimulating environmental changes aimed at reducing obesity.

 Consider This

"True leadership only exists if people follow when they have the freedom not to."

—Jim Collins[4(p13)]

As a public health practitioner, are there any reasons why you may choose not to follow a particular leader?

Many leadership theories and concepts—including transactional leadership, authentic leadership, servant leadership, transformational leadership, situational leadership, and emotional intelligence traits and competencies—focus on both the leader and the follower.[5,6,7,8,9,10,11,12] Leaders differ from one another in the characteristics they possess and in the styles they use, and they typically lead differently depending on the situation and the followers involved. Similarly, followers vary in their characteristics and styles, and they do not follow in the same way in every situation. Their behavior may depend on the leader's characteristics, their relationship with the leader, and past interactions and consequences between leaders and followers.[1] Good leaders and good followers both are important for accomplishing the organization's goals.

Effective public health leaders must be able to understand, appreciate, and apply the concepts of both leadership and followership, and they must recognize the significant crossover that exists between the two. Everyone is a follower. Not everyone follows all of the time, but everyone is a follower some of the time. Most individuals in leadership positions simultaneously act as followers.[13] Covey's[14] seven habits for highly effective people—discussed later in this chapter—are not simply guidelines for leaders; they apply to people who are leaders, followers, or, like most of us, a combination of both.

Effective Public Health Leaders . . .

. . . recognize that both good leaders and good followers are important for accomplishing the public health organization's goals.

Attributes of Followership

As the study of followership has advanced, a variety of follower styles and attributes have been identified. When people speak negatively of "being a follower," they often do so based on a stereotype of a certain type of follower (i.e., a passive, sheepish one); however, followership takes many forms, each with strengths and weaknesses, and certain forms are called for in specific situations. An essential aspect of followership is self-awareness. Just as leaders have leadership preferences, followers have followership preferences, and followers need to be aware of the type of follower they are in a given situation. Another essential aspect is social awareness. Followers must understand their leader's working style and agenda, and they must know how to react accordingly.[15] Social awareness is especially important during times of major change or potential turnover in leaders.

Basic Follower Types

One approach to categorizing follower styles, advanced by Kelley,[16] focuses on the level of independent, critical thinking that the follower displays and the degree to which the follower is active and positive or passive and negative. Another approach,

star or exemplary follower
A follower who thinks critically with positive energy and active engagement.

partner
A follower who both supports and is willing to challenge the leader.

sheep or passive follower
A follower who is dependent, does not think critically, and has negative energy or passive engagement.

resource
A follower who neither supports nor challenges the leader.

alienated follower
A follower who thinks independently but has negative energy or passive engagement.

individualist
A follower who is not fully supportive but is willing to challenge the leader.

yes-person/ conformist follower
A follower who has positive energy and engagement but is dependent and does not think critically.

implementer
A follower who is supportive but unwilling to challenge the leader.

offered by Chaleff,[2] focuses on the follower's level of support and willingness to challenge leaders. Between the two approaches, several basic follower types emerge. **Star or exemplary followers** are those who think independently and critically while maintaining positive energy and active engagement.[16] Such followers may also be considered **partners**—people who both support the leader and are willing to challenge the leader.[2] **Sheep or passive followers** are dependent and do not think critically; they tend to have negative energy and are passive in their engagement.[16] Sheep are similar to the follower type known as **resources**—those followers who neither support nor challenge the leader.[2] **Alienated followers** are those who think independently and critically but who exude a negative energy or are passively engaged.[16] They are similar to **individualists**, who are not fully supportive of their leaders but are willing to challenge them.[2] **Yes-person/conformist followers** have positive energy and engagement but are also highly dependent and do not think critically.[16] They are closely related to **implementers**, who are highly supportive of their leaders but unwilling to challenge them.[2]

Kellerman[1] categorizes followers based on level of engagement, which can vary depending on the situation, the attributes of the followers and leaders, and the cause they are following. The followers occupy five main levels: isolates, bystanders, participants, activists, and diehards (see exhibit 10.1). **Isolates** are completely detached and silent, and therefore often ignored. **Bystanders** observe the group or organization but choose not to participate. **Participants** engage with leaders, other followers, and the group or organization. They may support or oppose the leader. Regardless of how they participate, they try to make an impact through following. **Activists** also engage with the leader, other followers, and the group, but they act with an increased amount of passion and energy to support or oppose the leader or the organization. **Diehards**, the final type of follower, go a step farther than the activists. If they are loyal to their leaders, they may feel so strongly that they are willing to risk injury or even death to support them. Conversely, if they oppose their leaders, they may be willing to risk injury or death to remove them from power.

Consideration of the basic follower levels and types is particularly relevant to the field of public health, where an understanding of the population is essential. Some followers lack engagement and interest in implementing change that improves the health of communities. Positive health changes should not be expected if an organization pours most of its resources into efforts to reach isolates, bystanders, sheep, or diehards. Even if these followers desire improved public health, they are probably not going to participate or become engaged, or they may simply never change; thus, the considerable time and money spent trying to reach them may not be a wise investment. Instead, organizations should primarily focus on any and all of the other follower types, with specific understanding of the needs, desires, triggers, and support associated with each type. By adopting this more tailored approach, organizations move closer to implementing positive population-level health changes.

This categorization of followers is in many ways consistent with the **stages of change theory** and the **diffusion of innovation theory** with regard

EXHIBIT 10.1
Followership
Levels of
Engagement

Level of Engagement	Description	Relationship to Followership Style
Isolate	Detached, silent, uninterested, uninformed Does not care about leaders and does not respond Does the minimum necessary to get by	N/A
Bystander	Observes but does not participate Deliberate decision to stand aside; disengage from their leaders	Sheep or passive follower Resource
Participant	Engaged Favors or opposes leaders, groups, and organizations	Yes-person/conformist follower Implementer Alienated follower Individualist
Activist	Eager, energetic, engaged Feels strongly about leaders; works hard to support or oppose leaders	Star follower Partner
Diehard	Deeply devoted to leaders or deeply focused on removing leaders All-consuming passion; prepared to die if necessary	Star follower Partner

Sources: Data from Kellerman, B. 2008. *Followership: How Followers Are Creating Change and Changing Leaders*. Boston: Harvard Business School Press; Kelley, R. E. 2004. "Followership." In *Encyclopedia of Leadership*, vol. 2, edited by G. R. Goethals, G. J. Sorenson, and J. M. Burns, 504–13. Thousand Oaks, CA: Sage; and Chaleff, I. 2009. *The Courageous Follower: Standing Up to & for Our Leaders*, 3rd ed. San Francisco: Berrett-Koehler.

to health behavior. Under the stages of change theory, people are said to be either in a stage of precontemplation (not thinking about the change at all), contemplation (thinking about the change but not doing anything about it), preparation (making plans for action), action (making the change initially), or maintenance (having implemented the change for more than six months). Under the diffusion of innovation theory, people are categorized as innovators, early adopters, early majority, late majority, or laggards.[17] By recognizing followers' stages of change or receptivity to an innovation, public health organizations can target their interventions in the most efficient and effective manner possible.

Another important aspect of followership is the path or goal that motivates the follower. Followers differ in the degree to which they desire self-expression or self-transformation and whether they focus on relationship building or personal goals. Kelley[16] describes seven common follower paths:

isolate
A follower who is detached and silent, thus often ignored.

bystander
A follower who observes the group but chooses not to participate.

participant
A follower who engages with the group and tries to make an impact.

activist
A follower who engages with the group and acts with considerable passion and energy.

diehard
A follower whose feelings of support or opposition are extremely intense.

stages of change theory
A model that presents a series of stages representing differing degrees of behavioral change.

diffusion of innovation theory
A model that categorizes individuals based on their receptivity to innovation.

1. The apprentice's path is chosen by individuals who would like to become leaders and who are motivated by self-transformation and attention to personal goals.

2. The disciple's path is followed by those who want to learn from and act similarly to their teacher and who are motivated by being part of something larger than themselves.

3. The mentee's path focuses on personal growth and self-transformation, with an emphasis on relationships rather than personal goals.

4. The comrade's path emphasizes social support and connectivity to the community, and it appeals to followers who seek respect, commitment, and love from others.

5. The path of loyalty is followed by people who are personally loyal to the leader and whose primary motivation is commitment.

6. The dreamer's path is based on an idea or a vision, rather than a particular leader, and focuses on self-expression and accomplishment of personal goals.

7. The lifeway path is for followers who prefer to remain followers and who find both self-expression and satisfaction of personal goals in the follower role.

The seven paths, along with their corresponding goals and attributes, are shown in exhibit 10.2. Disciples seek to transform themselves, whereas followers on the path of loyalty and the lifeway path seek self-expression. For the dreamer and the apprentice, personal goals have primary importance. Relationships have primary importance for mentees and comrades. By understanding follower motivation, leaders can better respond to followers' needs and work with them to implement positive change. Leaders should be aware, however, that followers may choose more than one of the paths at different points or even simultaneously.[16]

If followers find that they are unable to make progress on their chosen path, their approach to followership or their level of engagement may change. For instance, if star followers are on the apprentice path and aspire to be leaders but are not given the opportunity to lead, they may become alienated followers. At the same time, if star followers are on the lifeway path and are not given an opportunity to lead, they likely will remain star followers, because leadership is not their goal.

 Effective Public Health Leaders . . .

. . . recognize that "followers are more important to leaders than leaders are to followers."
—Barbara Kellerman[1(p242)]

Similarities Between Followership and Leadership Attributes

Many of the attributes of good followers are similar to the attributes of good leaders.

EXHIBIT 10.2
Paths, Goals, and Attributes of Followers

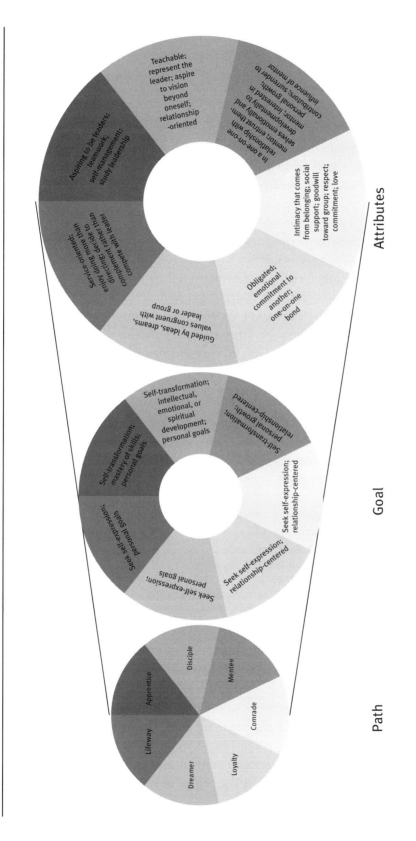

Path   Goal   Attributes

Source: Data from Kelley, R. E. 2004. "Followership." In *Encyclopedia of Leadership*, vol. 2, edited by G. R. Goethals, G. J. Sorenson, and J. M. Burns, 504–13. Thousand Oaks, CA: Sage.

They include being engaged and motivated by the public interest or by a common purpose that aligns with the organization's core values.[1,2] A bad follower is someone who does nothing and is not involved. However, just like good leadership, good followership depends on the situation. Good followers support leaders who are effective and ethical but oppose leaders who are ineffective and unethical.[1,2] Thus, they must be able to assess situations using personal and organizational values and distinguish ethical behavior from unethical behavior and effective leadership from ineffective leadership. These abilities correspond to the principle-centered thinking emphasized by Covey,[14] as well as to the concepts of self-awareness and social awareness, which are part of emotional intelligence.[10] This kind of followership places a high level of responsibility on the follower, and it requires a degree of independent, critical thinking that not every follower possesses.[16]

Both followership and leadership depend heavily on many of the traits identified by Kellerman,[1] Chaleff,[2] and Kelley,[16] as well as on emotional intelligence and trust. Covey and Link[18(p25)] write: "Trust is an enabling and empowering catalyst that is woven through every part of a strong, civilized society. But most of us are not even aware of it, or our dependence on it, until we lose it." Covey's[14] book *The 7 Habits of Highly Effective People* considers additional traits that can simultaneously be applied to leaders and followers (see exhibit 10.3), and his habits are organized based on the differences between dependent, independent, and interdependent individuals. A dependent person does not take initiative or personal responsibility; an independent person has a sense of confidence, accepts personal responsibility, and is able to achieve personal success; and an interdependent person recognizes the need to work cooperatively with others to achieve organizational or group outcomes. Independence and interdependence are necessary for both good followership and good leadership.

Leadership Application Case: The Performance Rating

The Leadership Application Case at the beginning of this book provides realistic scenarios for the application of key leadership concepts covered in the text. See the section marked "Chapter 10 Application" for the scenario and discussion questions that correspond with this chapter.

Leader–Follower Interactions

Leadership and followership can be thought of as reciprocal systems. Leadership has traditionally been regarded as the more active system, though the active nature of followership is increasingly being recognized.[19] Both leaders and followers must take responsibility for the leader–follower relationship and, ultimately, for the success of the organization. Organizations are most likely to be successful when their tasks and goals match the values and priorities

Habit	Description
Be Proactive	Being proactive involves taking both initiative and personal responsibility. Individuals who are proactive realize that they have the power to choose their words and actions and are willing to take responsibility for both their successes and their shortcomings.
Begin with the End in Mind	This habit involves focusing efforts on things that align with a personal vision, and it includes being self-aware about personal and professional goals and values. This self-awareness leads to action based on the goals and values identified.
Put First Things First	This habit involves organizing and focusing on the most important priorities that will make a positive difference. It incorporates proactivity (Habit 1) and a personal vision (Habit 2) that result in choosing to spend time, energy, and resources on those areas of greatest importance.
Think Win–Win	This habit emphasizes the need to find solutions that provide a beneficial outcome to everyone involved in the situation. This approach often identifies alternative solutions to a problem that may not have been considered by individual parties. Cooperation is necessary to achieve the mutually satisfying result.
Seek First to Understand, Then to Be Understood	This habit involves actively listening in order to effectively communicate. Through this approach, individuals attempt to fully understand prior to presenting their own ideas. Active listening can change the delivery of ideas and lead to better relations and communication.
Synergize	Synergy happens when people work together to find collective solutions or actions that are greater than any individual's contribution. This approach is demonstrated when the individuals involved believe that more insight and learning will result in better outcomes. High levels of communication, trust, and cooperation are necessary to achieve synergy.
Sharpen the Saw	This habit provides the foundation for the other six habits and involves a process of reflection and renewal. Through this reflection and renewal, a person can find balance in the physical, social/emotional, mental, and spiritual aspects of life. The process involves the ability to continuously learn, commit, and take action.

EXHIBIT 10.3
Covey's Seven Habits of Highly Effective People

Source: Data from Covey, S. R. 1989. *The 7 Habits of Highly Effective People*. New York: Simon & Schuster.

of both leaders and followers and when leader and follower personalities are compatible.[11] Many challenges within organizations are heightened by a lack of self-awareness or social awareness on the part of both leaders and followers.[10]

Followers have considerable impact on what the leader will be able to accomplish.[11] The rise of Adolf Hitler is commonly used as an example of an individual using leadership for evil purposes. However, Hitler would not have been able to take power and carry out his campaign of violence if he did not have willing followers who were receptive to his leadership.[20] The need for leaders and followers to work together is evident in every field, and examples in public health are commonplace. Comprehensive smoke-free policies at the city, county, or state level, for instance, could not be successful without both engaged followers willing to support implementation and effective leaders who understand how to engage followers in the process. Both leaders and followers are critical to establishing public health policy in any setting, and they should share credit for success when they do so.

A variety of factors can influence the effectiveness of leader–follower interactions. For instance, timing is an important consideration when leaders and followers introduce new ideas, communicate information, or even solve problems.[21] When a follower needs to push for an idea or suggestion, leaders are likely to be more receptive when they have their doors open and are in a good frame of mind than when they are in the middle of a stressful situation. Just as followers should consider timing as it relates to leaders, leaders should do the same as it relates to followers. Mutual respect with regard to timing is important for leader–follower interactions.

Consider This

"Followers and leaders both orbit around the purpose; followers do not orbit around the leader."
— Ira Chaleff[2(p13)]

Given the importance for both leaders and followers to orbit around the purpose of the organization, why do so many followers orbit around the effective public health leader?

The Cultural Framing of Leadership and Followership

Leadership and followership interact in complex cultural settings. In addition to interacting regularly with each of their followers, leaders also serve as mediators between their own leaders and the followers.[11,22] Factors that influence leader–follower interactions, as well as their individual and collective outcomes, include the following: (1) the leader's traits and skills; (2) the follower's traits and skills; (3) the leader's vision and behavior; (4) the follower's identification with the leader and resulting actions; (5) the leader's personal and cultural values and self-concept; (6) the follower's personal and cultural values and self-concept; and (7) intervening variables that are structural, role-based, and relational.[22] The first two items on that list—the traits and skills of the leader and the follower—have already been discussed at length in this chapter. The leader's vision is the differentiating factor between leaders and followers.[23]

Ultimately, if followers are not willing to follow the leader's vision, the leader becomes ineffective.

Motivation comes from both internal and environmental factors,[24] and the follower's identification with the leader is closely related to traits and skills, the leader's vision, personal and cultural values, and the self-concepts of the leader and the follower.[22] Both positive and negative correlations can exist between leadership style preferences and follower characteristics. For instance, a relationship-oriented leadership style is positively correlated with followers' desire for interpersonal relations, security, and participation in work but negatively correlated with followers' emphasis on achievement, risk taking, self-esteem, and structure.[25] Similarly, a task-oriented leadership style is positively correlated with followers' needs for achievement, structure, extrinsic work value (e.g., pay, benefits, work hours), and security at work but negatively correlated with risk taking and interpersonal relations.[25] Satisfaction for both leaders and followers occurs when motivation and personality are matched, such as when a highly motivated follower is paired with a participative leader; dissatisfaction is likely when such qualities are mismatched.[11]

Lord, Brown, and Freiberg[26] emphasize the role of **self-concepts**—essentially, the identities people have based on their beliefs about themselves—in leader–follower interactions. A person's self-concept can be defined at the individual, interpersonal, or collective level, and neither a follower nor a leader is able to focus on multiple levels of identity at the same time. Leadership is most effective when it is tailored to the level at which the follower chiefly identifies. At the individual level, the self-concept focuses on the person's traits and skills, which may be the same as or different from those of other individuals. When a follower's self-concept is focused at this level, the leader can achieve positive interactions by emphasizing performance feedback, contingent rewards, and fairness among followers. At the interpersonal level, the self-concept emphasizes relationships with others. When a follower's self-concept is chiefly at this level, the leader can be effective by developing the leader–follower relationship, mentoring the follower, and emphasizing shared values. At the collective level, the self-concept emphasizes identification with the team or organization and is concerned with the well-being and functioning of the group. When followers identify primarily at this level, the leader can encourage them by focusing on team-based leadership, a common vision and framework, and group identity. The manner in which the leader figures out what motivates or resonates with the follower and then provides the most effective leadership style resembles the situational leadership approach discussed in chapter 4.[9]

Individuals' self-concepts can change over time, and they can be influenced by a variety of events and experiences. Thus, identities are more accurately viewed as processes than as static entities.[27] A leader can influence a follower's self-concept, and vice versa, and transitions may occur as leaders and followers work together over an extended period in a particular organization. Often,

self-concept
The identity constructed from the beliefs people have about themselves at the individual, interpersonal, or collective level.

collectivistic values
Cultural views concerning the leader's/follower's relationship to the organization/work, family orientation, and general society.

followers tend to focus initially on the interpersonal level and then, over time, shift their focus to the collective or individual level.[28] Because of the changing nature of identity, leaders may sometimes have difficulty gauging the current level of a follower's self-concept at a particular point in time.

Leader–follower interactions are also affected by **collectivistic values** concerning the leader's/follower's relationship to the organization/work, family orientation, and general societal views.[22] Such views can affect the level of participation and action by both leaders and followers, as well as the degree to which followers participate in the leader's vision. If followers have an individualistic culture, a leader's attempts to focus on the collective may be considered incongruent; in such cases, a leader who focuses on the individual is more likely to be accepted and considered effective.

Leader–follower interactions also can be framed in terms of the outcomes, both individual and collective, with which the participants are concerned. Individual outcomes for leaders typically include reaffirmation of their status as a leader, self-efficacy, self-enhancement, and growth.[22] Followers, too, are concerned with the outcomes of self-efficacy, self-enhancement, and growth. The focus on status distinguishes leaders from followers, although status may be important to followers who strive to become leaders. Examples of collective outcomes for both leaders and followers include group and individual performance, worker satisfaction, work conditions, affirmation of social structure (e.g., hierarchy, roles for leaders and followers), interpersonal relationships, organizational commitment, and mutual growth.[22,26]

The nature of leader–follower interactions is also affected by the type of organization in which the interactions take place. If an organization is strongly hierarchical, leaders who depend on interpersonal interactions for decision making are likely to become frustrated. Conversely, if an organization is more decentralized, leaders who want to be seen as authority figures may become frustrated by their inability to control decisions and outcomes.[22]

Followership Continuum
A model in which followers can move (in either direction) across five levels of performance: employee, committed follower, engaged follower, effective follower, and exemplary follower.

The Followership Continuum

The performance of an individual follower, a team of followers, or an organization is significantly affected by changes in leaders, organizational structures, systems, processes, roles, responsibilities, and priorities. Both leaders and followers need to be able to accurately diagnose and categorize performance patterns of followers to ensure quality performance. Blackshear's[29] **Followership Continuum** provides a tool to help guide this process.

The Followership Continuum, illustrated in exhibit 10.4, identifies five stages of followership that reflect different levels of performance[29]:

- Employee (Stage 1): During this stage of followership, individuals begin working as new employees with their organization, team, or unit. At this stage, they receive the benefit of monetary compensation for the completion of work.
- Committed follower (Stage 2): In this stage, followers affirm the mission, idea, or purpose of the organization and work toward achieving it.
- Engaged follower (Stage 3): Entering this stage, committed followers decide to become active supporters who are willing to take on responsibilities beyond their current level; thus, they reach the level of engagement.
- Effective follower (Stage 4): At this stage, followers are both competent and reliable. They become known as the people who are always going to perform effectively and produce the results the organization desires.[21]
- Exemplary follower (Stage 5): Followers at the exemplary stage are those who have the ability to function as leaders but who have instead chosen to support others as leaders. Such followers are able to lead themselves.

The model maintains that follower performance is not constant, and so followers can move in either direction along the continuum, toward negative or positive performance outputs. Individuals' progression toward exemplary followership can be facilitated or hindered by a variety of internal, leadership-related, and structural influences. Facilitating influences might include personal satisfaction, ambition, initiative, competence, or rewards and recognition. Hindering influences might include lack of motivation or commitment, lack of interest in the job or organization, lack of respect or recognition, or lack of communication.[29]

The Followership Continuum can help leaders "take the pulse" of their organization.[29] Ideally, it should be used as one of many components that provide a thorough assessment and help facilitate desired outcomes. It is intended to be applied in a cyclical process—beginning with assessment, then moving on to intervention and implementation, and finally returning to assessment—to maintain or improve productivity and overall performance.

Expectations and Perceptions of Leaders Toward Followers

Mutual trust is an essential component of the leader–follower relationship.[13,24] Leaders expect followers to have motivation, the willingness to accept responsibility, appropriate education and experience for the job, a high level of activity,

EXHIBIT 10.4
Followership
Continuum

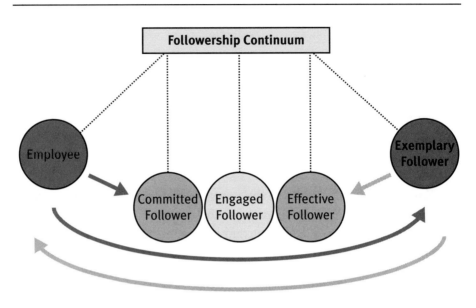

Source: Data from Blackshear, P. B. 2003. "The Followership Continuum: A Model for Increasing Organizational Productivity." *Public Manager* 32 (2): 25–30.

a broad perspective, and both self-awareness and social awareness.[11] They also want followers to be positive, innovative, and dedicated to staying current within the field of work.[13,30] Followers are perceived as high performers when they seek opportunities for personal and professional development and serve as a resource for leaders.[13,21,30] Such followers are self-managed, committed to the organization and its purpose, competent, and willing to learn from others.[11,21,24] A key aspect of learning from others involves the ability to collaborate.[13]

Effective followers are expected to be courageous, honest, and credible; they should be willing to tell the truth even if doing so means disagreeing with the leader.[24] They should come prepared for meetings and be respectful of the leader's time; one model recommends that followers spend ten minutes in preparation for every one minute of meeting time with the leader.[21] Followers can improve their interactions with leaders by being honest about what they need as followers; by taking partial responsibility for transforming the leader–follower relationship; by focusing on support, rather than criticism, of leaders; by helping leaders with their weaknesses; and by showing appreciation for leaders' support and positive behavior.[13,21]

Expectations and Perceptions of Followers Toward Leaders

The expectations and perceptions that followers have of their leaders in many ways mirror those that leaders have of their followers. Followers expect their leaders to be honest, motivated, forward thinking, inspiring, and competent.[13] They want leaders who have personality characteristics compatible with their own, who have demonstrated positive past performance,[19] and who can create a culture and an environment where people are encouraged to be the best they can be.[13] Followers' perceptions of a leader may be influenced by how the leader obtained the leadership role: Typically, followers express more positive opinions, show greater support, and have higher expectations for leaders who were elected than for those who were appointed.[19]

One of the most important expectations that followers have of leaders is effective communication, which leaders can exemplify through friendliness, active listening, receptiveness to ideas and suggestions, and recognition of followers' efforts.[11,13] Leaders are expected to clearly communicate the organization's mission, vision, goals, and objectives as they relate both to individuals and to the overall team. Followers expect leaders to provide role clarity and coaching; to offer honest, constructive feedback on performance; and to respect followers as individuals capable of independent, critical thinking.[11,13,30]

Effective leaders can accurately assess the ability, performance, and motivation of followers; provide feedback and reinforcement in a timely manner; and adapt their leadership style to meet followers' needs and increase the likelihood of successful performance.[9] Followers' performance tends to improve when leaders have high expectations of their followers. Effective leaders also seek to minimize the perceived power differences between themselves and their followers, thereby making themselves more accessible and open to feedback from followers.[11] In many cases, such leaders choose to devolve some of their power to followers, and the followers are prepared to accept it based on the leader's prior investment in their development and coaching.[21]

In public health, followers expect their leaders to serve as role models.[5,11] However, leader–follower interactions are enhanced when followers see leaders as they are rather than as followers think they should be. Followers should be willing to help leaders with their weaknesses.[13,21]

Role Ambiguity and Specialization

As noted earlier in the chapter, everyone is a follower, at least some of the time. People may engage in both leader and follower roles simultaneously, or they may exchange roles depending on particular settings and times.[11] For instance, a public health practitioner might lead a state coalition toward goals and objectives in a strategic plan while at the same time following a superior's direction. This same practitioner might lead in grant writing and work-plan development but follow in matters involving policy-related requests by the legislature. Knowing when to lead and when to follow is an important skill, as is knowing which leadership and followership styles are appropriate for a given situation. Typically, leaders who use a follower-driven leadership style—such as situational leadership, which focuses on the follower and the larger purpose of the organization[9]—can

Consider This

"Leadership and followership are fundamental roles that individuals shift into and out of under various conditions. Everyone—leaders included—is a follower at one time or another."

—Richard L. Daft[13(p198)]

Why do public health leaders often have difficulty recognizing that they are followers in certain situations?

transition into follower roles more readily and more seamlessly than leaders who focus primarily on what they need and how they can personally benefit.

The Leadership–Teamship–Followership Continuum

Townsend and Gebhardt's[31] **Leadership–Teamship–Followership Continuum** highlights the ambiguity and changing nature of the leader and follower roles. The continuum identifies four specific roles—two focused on leadership and two on followership—but recognizes that both leaders and followers may occupy places in between the defined roles. Like the Followership Continuum discussed earlier, the Leadership–Teamship–Followership Continuum emphasizes the movement of individuals to different positions along the continuum depending upon the situation, opportunity, and organization.

The four roles are (1) Leadership (with a capital L), (2) leadership (with a lowercase l), (3) active followership, and (4) passive followership. People in the capital-L Leadership role are responsible for the organization's overall direction and decision making, whereas those in the small-l leadership role work to influence others to action but might not make all the decisions. People in active followership roles work closely with leaders and provide ideas, suggestions, and questions that may influence leaders' decisions. Passive followers, meanwhile, do not engage the leaders, think critically, or participate in decision making; they simply perform the minimum amount of work required.[31]

Teamship is the place where the four roles meet and individuals work together to accomplish a shared goal. Within the team, individuals possess different levels of expertise relevant to particular situations, and variations in this expertise can cause the lines between leadership and followership roles to become blurred. A key aspect of the Leadership–Teamship–Followership Continuum is that all people in the organization use their gifts, skills, and abilities in a way that helps them in their individual roles while also supporting others in their roles. Leadership, followership, and teamship are regarded as behaviors rather than organizational positions, and people rely on many of the same skills to be effective in each role.[31]

Follower- and Leader-Specific Roles

People often transition into and out of leadership and followership roles or act as both leaders and followers simultaneously, and many of the attributes of leaders and followers are similar. Both leaders and followers, for instance, should

Leadership–Teamship–Followership Continuum
A model that describes the way individuals occupy—and move between—various roles of leadership and followership in a team environment.

teamship
The act of working together as a team within standards of behavior that each person within the team environment understands.

have their own personal vision, as suggested in Covey's[14] second habit, "Begin with the End in Mind." However, certain roles and attributes are more specific to followers and others more specific to leaders.

Effective followers, in particular, are expected to be humble and willing to follow[13,29]; fully accountable for their actions yet willing to give up some autonomy and authority[2]; mindful and willing to act, even if actions involve challenging authority[13]; supportive of the leader and the organization's mission, vision, and purpose[2,16,29]; courageous in opposing the leader if the leader behaves unethically or ineffectively[1,2]; valuable in ways that complement the leader and other followers in serving stakeholders[2,13]; useful as a resource for the leader and the organization[13]; flexible and adaptable in the midst of change[2,29]; cooperative[13,30]; and dependable.[13]

Leaders, meanwhile, are expected to be forward-thinking, with the ability to create and facilitate a vision[13,32]; inspiring to the people who work toward that vision[13,32]; clear, decisive, and timely in providing direction and feedback to followers[30]; capable of providing clarity of roles, responsibilities, goals, and objectives, both individually and collectively[13,30,33]; committed to developing, supporting, and empowering followers to realize their full potential[13]; able to use their power to achieve a common purpose[1,2]; willing to give some of their power to followers who are properly prepared for it[21]; and capable of serving as role models.[5,11]

Shared Influence

Although followers tend to have less formal authority than leaders, they still have influence.[1] Leaders influence followers to action and in return are influenced by followers.[13,19,26] Such influence can be positive or negative for either party, and it is most prevalent among active leaders and followers.[34] The amount of shared influence depends on the attributes of the leader or the follower, their motivation and common interest, and their mutual trust and willingness to listen.[11] When leaders and followers have trust, they are better able to communicate, collaborate, innovate, and improve business and efficiency.[18] The ability to share influence also improves when leaders and followers have high levels of self-confidence and self-worth.[2]

The organizational climate—particularly with regard to openness, desire for

Consider This

"Being mindful of learning opportunities when they arise—and spontaneously seizing them as a way to practice new abilities—offers ways to improve more quickly. Life is the laboratory for learning."
—Daniel Goleman[10(pp140–41)]

How do effective public health leaders make their organization part of life's laboratory for learning?

Effective Public Health Leaders . . .

. . . understand that "leadership and followership are mutual activities of influence and counterinfluence."
—Bernard M. Bass[11(p431)]

learning and growth, and empowerment of individuals to contribute—has a significant impact on the level of shared influence.[5,11] Shared influence is most prominent when the leader and the follower are focused on a common purpose or goal; it becomes less prominent when either party becomes more focused on self-interest.[2] In team settings where leaders and followers contribute within their areas of expertise, knowledge and competence can be more important in determining one's influence than formal position.[1]

Integrating Followership with Leadership Theories

Of the major leadership theories and concepts, the ones with the greatest consideration for followership are transactional leadership, leader–member exchange theory, authentic leadership, transformational leadership, situational leadership, and emotional intelligence.

Transactional Leadership, Leader–Member Exchange Theory, and Followership

Transactional leadership (discussed in chapter 7) emphasizes responsiveness and the giving and receiving of benefits between the leader and follower, thus suggesting an active role for followers.[11,19] Under a transactional approach, leaders can foster good followership by providing clear expectations about performance, explaining how followers can meet those expectations, providing criteria for performance measurement, offering feedback related to those objectives, and providing appropriate rewards when objectives are met.[11] Perceptions about the quality of the follower's performance determine the degree to which the leader supports or reprimands the follower. The leader is more likely to reprimand the follower if poor performance is perceived to be a result of internal causes, such as the follower's competence or effort, than if the performance is perceived to be a result of causes outside the follower's control.[11] The willingness of followers to comply with performance feedback is a measure of successful leadership.[11]

Leader–member exchange theory (discussed in chapter 6) emphasizes the role of the follower as a part of a dyadic relationship with the leader. Under this theory, the leader and the follower work together to determine the quality of their relationship as it develops over time. At first, the leader–member dyad is focused on material benefits, but as the relationship develops, the focus shifts toward social and psychological benefits, potentially resulting in a higher level of mutual trust.[12]

Authentic Leadership and Followership

Authentic leadership emphasizes the need for leaders to be transparent and trustworthy, to have integrity and high moral standards, and to be true to themselves and to others.[5] It focuses largely on the leader's own actions, self-awareness, and self-acceptance, but it also requires consideration of the follower and attention to the relationship between the leader and follower. One model of authentic leadership suggests that major and personal life events spur the development of self-awareness and self-regulation, which in turn improve the ability to align decisions and actions with values, thereby serving as a catalyst for authentic behavior. Authentic leadership highlights the need for followers to personally identify with the leader, to socially identify with the group in relation to the leader, and to have attitudes that are shaped by the hope, trust, and positive emotions exhibited by the leader.[35] When used effectively, authentic leadership can serve as the basis for transformational leadership. Under authentic leadership, followers often show improved commitment, engagement, performance, job satisfaction, and willingness to give extra effort, and they are less likely to withdraw from the group.[35]

If an organization has an inclusive, ethical, caring, and strength-based climate, the positive role-modeling of authentic leadership can lead to authentic followership. Authentic followership, in turn, leads to trust, engagement, sustainable performance, and a well-functioning workplace.[5] Both leaders and followers can model behavior that encourages authenticity by the other.

Transformational Leadership and Followership

Under transformational leadership (discussed in chapter 7), leaders pursue objectives that have a higher purpose, treat followers with respect, and help followers meet high-level needs such as achievement, self-esteem, self-fulfillment, and self-actualization.[6] Transformational leadership theory tends to assume that transformation occurs primarily because of the leader's actions,[22] but research suggests that the relationship between the leader and the follower plays an important role. The leader–follower relationship helps both parties achieve more through idealized influence, inspirational motivation, intellectual stimulation, and individualized consideration.

Transformational leadership involves a complex relationship between the leader and follower, and several factors related to the leader, the follower, and their interactions must be considered. Such factors include the leader's exhibited behavior, expected behavior, mood, emotional intelligence, and ability to hide intentions; the follower's mood, emotional intelligence, level of involvement, and extent of experience with the leader; and the prior interactions that have occurred between the two. Another key aspect involves the distinction between authentic transformational leadership, which is based on a sincere organizational focus, and pseudotransformational leadership, which is manipulative and self-serving. When authentic transformational leadership occurs, followers have a positive emotional response to the leader, and higher-quality leader–follower relationships result. These relationships, in turn, have a positive impact on follower motivation, work effectiveness, job performance, commitment, satisfaction, and clarity of roles and responsibilities.[1] The ability of followers to discern the intentions and potential effectiveness of leaders depends largely on emotional intelligence.

A military study by Dvir and Shamir[8] further demonstrates the impact that followers can have on transformational leadership. The researchers sought to investigate whether followers' development level (specifically, their level of self-actualization needs, acceptance of the organization's moral values, group focus, critical and independent thinking, active engagement, and self-efficacy) would predict transformational leadership. The results indicated that the development level of direct followers, who interacted closely with the leader, did not predict transformational leadership but that the development level of indirect followers, who had more distant interactions, did. Proposed explanations for the differences between the two follower groups considered the possibilities that direct followers might have been seen as a threat to the leader, that direct followers might have had sufficiently high developmental levels and did not require transformational leadership, and that direct followers might have been disillusioned from having observed the leader's behavior more closely than indirect followers had.

Situational Leadership, Emotional Intelligence, and Followership

Under situational leadership (discussed in chapter 4), the leader considers the situation and the follower's needs and then determines the appropriate leadership style. To effectively implement situational leadership, leaders must possess three primary competencies. The first is the ability to diagnose the situation, which involves defining the task, understanding followers, and having the social awareness to accurately assess the situation.[9] The second competency is the ability to adapt, which involves self-awareness, self-management, and relationship management.[9,10] The third competency is the ability to communicate with followers and tailor leadership behavior appropriately.[9] (This third competency is closely linked to Goleman's[10] ideas on relationship management and Kouzes and Posner's[36] guidelines for enabling others to act.) To engage in situational leadership, leaders must be self-aware, self-managed, socially aware, and willing and able to manage relationships—all of which are key components of emotional intelligence.[10] In addition, they must be proactive and seek first to understand others prior to being understood—which are two of Covey's[14] seven habits of highly effective people.

A key step in determining how to lead an individual or a group is assessing follower readiness. Readiness combines the follower's demonstrated ability with the follower's willingness to accept, understand, and perform a task.[9] Readiness varies depending on the specific task involved: A follower or a group that has a high level of readiness for one task will not necessarily have the same level of readiness for another. In addition, the leader should assess the follower based on the ability that the follower currently demonstrates rather than on the ability that the leader thinks the follower should possess or used to possess[9] (consistent with Covey's[14] principle of seeking first to understand others). Leaders who are assessing readiness must recognize the difference between enthusiasm and ability, and they must be able to discern between insecurity and lack of willingness or motivation.[9] Leaders should also be sure to focus on what the follower needs rather than what the follower wants.

In the situational leadership model (shown in exhibit 4.3), four quadrants correspond with leadership styles—S1 to S4—that have varying levels of task behavior and relationship behavior.[9] Task behavior involves directing, organizing, setting goals, establishing timelines, and specifying tasks to be completed, whereas relationship behavior involves communicating, supporting, facilitating interactions, providing feedback, and actively listening. The selection of an appropriate leadership style depends on the leader's ability to correctly diagnose follower readiness or developmental level.

Emotional intelligence is a key aspect of leaders' abilities to understand their followers, build strong interpersonal relationships, and lead effective teams.[37,38] Leaders with high levels of emotional intelligence are aware of social contexts, demonstrate empathy and sensitivity to followers' emotions, regulate their own emotions, and understand the relationships between emotions.[28] For instance, a leader who has a high level of emotional intelligence is not surprised when a follower's initial reaction to a change or restructuring is one of anxiety or fear, even if the leader has assured followers that their jobs are secure.[39] The quality of the leader–follower relationship can serve as an indicator of both the leader's effectiveness and the follower's motivation for being successful in the organization.[37]

> ### Check It Out
>
> For further discussion of emotional intelligence, visit Daniel Goleman's page at www.danielgoleman.info/daniel-goleman-how-emotionally-intelligent-are-you/.

The Integrative Model of Leadership and Followership

Bjugstad and colleagues[24] have combined elements of situational leadership and Kelley's followership model to create an integrative model that effectively aligns leadership and followership styles. The model's four leadership styles, based on the quadrants of the situational leadership model, are (1) telling/directing, (2) selling/coaching, (3) participating/supporting, and (4) delegating. The four followership styles, based on Kelley's types, are (1) alienated, (2) passive, (3) conformist, and (4) exemplary. The styles are shown, along with recommended leader and follower behaviors, in exhibit 10.5.

The telling/directing style of leadership relates to conformist followers, who are willing to do whatever is asked of them, are extremely supportive of the leader, and do not use critical thinking. The selling/coaching style relates

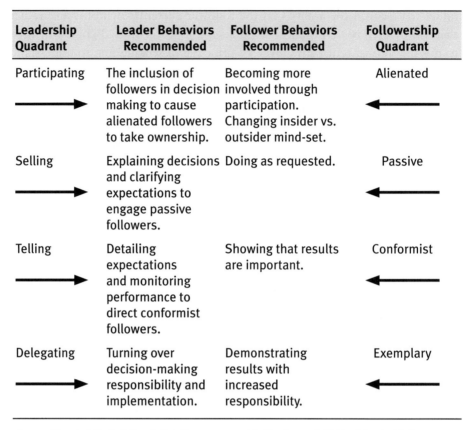

Source: Bjugstad, K., E. C. Thach, K. J. Thompson, and A. Morris. 2006. "A Fresh Look at Follower-ship: A Model for Matching Followership and Leadership Styles." *Journal of Behavioral and Applied Management* 7 (3): 304–19. Used by permission.

to passive followers, who are not highly engaged or supportive of the leader and who do not use critical thinking. Participating/supporting relates to alienated followers, who are critical, independent thinkers, but who are not supportive of the leader or have become disillusioned. Delegating relates to exemplary or star followers, who are able to excel without significant relationship or task behavior.

Effective leaders in any field should take followership into account when determining a leadership approach, but the need to do so is especially pronounced in public health. Restructuring, changes in leadership, and budget cuts are common in public health, and the workforce faces constant pressure to accomplish more with fewer resources. Under such circumstances, a leader's ability to focus on followership, understand followers' emotions, and make appropriate adjustments is critical for success.

Case Study: Global Polio Eradication

In 1988, the World Health Organization (WHO) launched the Global Polio Eradication Initiative (GPEI) with the aim of eliminating polio worldwide.[40] The new initiative followed a successful Pan American Health Organization campaign in Latin America and the Caribbean, which led to the region becoming polio free in 1991.[41] At the time GPEI began, polio was endemic in 125 countries and resulted in the paralysis of more than 350,000 children each year.[40]

By 2011, as such organizations as the WHO, Rotary International, the US Centers for Disease Control and Prevention, the United Nations Children's Fund, and the Bill and Melinda Gates Foundation were all working to complete the eradication of polio, issues of leadership arose in GPEI. In October of that year, a report by the Independent Monitoring Board of the Global Polio Eradication Initiative[42(p18)] found significant flaws in GPEI's leadership and stated that the initiative would succeed only if "its vast array of individuals are motivated, organized, well-linked, and well-led." The report emphasized that "people are the crucial ingredient" in the program and that, for a change-management program such as GPEI to be successful, leaders must pay attention to human factors rather than overemphasize technical elements. The report found that GPEI was in grave danger of failing in this regard.

The report posed the following questions[42(p18)]:

- How can it be that individuals known to be tired and ineffective are allowed to remain in key leadership positions?
- How can it be that front-line positions in some countries remain so underrewarded that they are not attractive to the kind of workforce that the GPEI needs?
- How can it be that some people are not held accountable for poor performance?
- How can it be that some vaccinators are not paid the money that they are promised?
- How can it be that some team leaders are not capable of quality assuring the work they are supervising?

Following the Independent Monitoring Board's report, the Polio Eradication and Endgame Strategic Plan 2013–2018 was developed, and leadership of GPEI was reinvigorated. By 2016, only 37 wild polio virus

(continued)

cases were reported worldwide, and they occurred only in Pakistan, Nigeria, and Afghanistan.[40] The strategic plan envisions a world free of polio by 2018.

Discussion and Application Questions

1. In your opinion, why is leadership important for change management?
2. How does an effective public health leader balance followers' needs for effective leadership with the technical requirements of a project such as GPEI?
3. As a key leader in GPEI, how would you engage your followers in an effort to reverse the findings of the Independent Monitoring Board?
4. How important is effective public health leadership to the polio eradication effort? How can the effort's leaders and followers effectively work together?

Summary

Just as good leaders are important for organizational success, so too are good followers. Good followers are those who share a common purpose with the leader, believe in what the organization is trying to accomplish, and work energetically toward organizational goals. Followers possess distinct characteristics and play an active role in the leader–follower relationship. Leadership and followership have a number of attributes in common, and a significant crossover exists between the two. After all, everyone, including leaders, is a follower at certain times.

Followers differ in their level of critical thinking, in the degree to which they are active and positive or passive and negative, and in their level of support and willingness to challenge leaders. Based on these differences, a number of basic follower types emerge. Kelley distinguishes between star or exemplary followers, who think independently while maintaining positive energy and active engagement; sheep or passive followers, who tend to have negative energy, are passive in their engagement, and do not think critically; alienated followers, who think critically but exude a negative energy or are passively engaged; and yes-person/conformist followers, who have positive energy but are highly dependent and do not think critically. Kellerman, meanwhile, identifies five groups based on increasing levels of engagement: isolates, bystanders, participants, activists, and dichards. Kelley also identifies seven paths, or goals, that motivate followers: the apprentice's path, the disciple's path, the mentee's path, the comrade's path, the path of loyalty, the dreamer's path, and the lifeway path. Many of the attributes of good followers are similar to the attributes of good leaders. For instance, both leaders and followers in public health should be engaged and motivated by the public interest or by a common purpose aligned with the organization's core values.

Both leaders and followers must take responsibility for the quality of the leader–follower relationship. Key factors in this relationship include the leader's traits and skills, the follower's traits and skills, the leader's vision and behavior, the follower's identification with the leader and resulting actions, the leader's personal and cultural values and self-concept, the follower's personal and cultural values and self-concept, and intervening variables based on roles and structures.

The Followership Continuum is a useful model that depicts various levels of follower performance. It maintains that follower performance is not constant and that followers can move back and forth between five levels: employee, committed follower, engaged follower, effective follower, and exemplary follower. Another model, the Leadership–Teamship–Followership Continuum, highlights the ambiguity and changing nature of both leader and follower roles. The continuum identifies four specific roles—two focused on leadership and two on followership—but recognizes that the lines between leadership and followership roles can become blurred.

Of the major leadership theories and concepts, the ones that most incorporate followership include transactional leadership, leader–member exchange theory, authentic leadership, transformational leadership, situational leadership, and emotional intelligence. An integrative model that combines elements of situational leadership and followership offers a method for aligning leadership and followership styles.

Discussion Questions

1. Why do public health practitioners need to understand followership?
2. What are Kellerman's five types of followers, and how do they relate to one another?
3. Compare and contrast the attributes of followership with those of leadership.
4. Which follower attributes are most important to you? Which are least important?
5. Describe the seven paths of followership. Which of the paths do you prefer, and why?
6. What are the key factors that affect leader–follower interactions? Which of those factors do you feel are most and least important?

7. How do good followers interact with ethical and/or competent leaders? How do they interact with unethical and/or incompetent leaders?
8. What factors are likely to facilitate followers' movement along the Followership Continuum?
9. What are the key leadership theories that focus on followers? Which ones do you prefer, and why?
10. For deeper thought: As an effective public health leader, discuss why you prefer to be either a leader or a follower.

Web Resources

Goleman, D. 2015. "How Emotionally Intelligent Are You?" Published April 21. www.danielgoleman.info/daniel-goleman-how-emotionally-intelligent-are-you/.

McCallum, J. S. 2013. "Followership: The Other Side of Leadership." *Ivey Business Journal.* Published September/October. http://iveybusinessjournal.com/publication/followership-the-other-side-of-leadership/.

Peterson, G. 2013. "Leadership 310: The Four Principles of Followership." *Forbes.* Published April 23. www.forbes.com/sites/garypeterson/2013/04/23/the-four-principles-of-followership/.

References

1. Kellerman, B. 2008. *Followership: How Followers Are Creating Change and Changing Leaders.* Boston: Harvard Business School Press.
2. Chaleff, I. 2009. *The Courageous Follower: Standing Up to & for Our Leaders,* 3rd ed. San Francisco: Berrett-Koehler.
3. Kotler, P., N. Roberto, and N. Lee. 2002. *Social Marketing: Improving the Quality of Life.* Thousand Oaks, CA: Sage.
4. Collins, J. 2005. *Good to Great and the Social Sectors: Why Business Thinking Is Not the Answer.* Boulder, CO: Jim Collins.
5. Gardner, W. L., B. J. Avolio, F. Luthans, D. R. May, and F. Walumbwa. 2005. "Can You See the Real Me? A Self-Based Model of Authentic Leader and Follower Development." *Leadership Quarterly* 16 (3): 343–72.
6. Johnson, C. E. 2009. *Meeting the Ethical Challenges of Leadership: Casting Light or Shadow.* Los Angeles: Sage.
7. Daft, R. L. 2016. *Management,* 12th ed. Mason, OH: South-Western.

8. Dvir, T., and B. Shamir. 2003. "Follower Developmental Characteristics as Predicting Transformational Leadership: A Longitudinal Field Study." *Leadership Quarterly* 14 (3): 327–44.

9. Hersey, P., K. H. Blanchard, and D. E. Johnson. 2008. *Management of Organizational Behavior: Leading Human Resources*, 9th ed. Upper Saddle River, NJ: Pearson Prentice Hall.

10. Goleman, D., R. Boyatzis, and A. McKee. 2013. *Primal Leadership: Unleashing the Power of Emotional Intelligence*. Boston: Harvard Business School Press.

11. Bass, B. M. 2008. *The Bass Handbook of Leadership: Theory, Research, and Managerial Applications*, 4th ed. New York: Free Press.

12. Howell, J. M., and B. Shamir. 2005. "The Role of Followers in the Charismatic Leadership Process: Relationships and Their Consequences." *Academy of Management Review* 30 (1): 96–112.

13. Daft, R. L. 2017. *The Leadership Experience*, 7th ed. Boston: Cengage Learning.

14. Covey, S. R. 1989. *The 7 Habits of Highly Effective People*. New York: Simon & Schuster.

15. Coyne, K. P., and E. Coyne. 2007. "Surviving Your New CEO." *Harvard Business Review* 85 (5): 62.

16. Kelley, R. E. 2004. "Followership." In *Encyclopedia of Leadership*, vol. 2, edited by G. R. Goethals, G. J. Sorenson, and J. M. Burns, 504–13. Thousand Oaks, CA: Sage.

17. Edberg, M. 2007. *Essentials of Health Behavior: Social and Behavioral Theory in Public Health*. Sudbury, MA: Jones & Bartlett.

18. Covey, S. M. R., and G. Link. 2012. *Smart Trust: The Defining Skill That Transforms Managers into Leaders*. New York: Free Press.

19. Hollander, E. P. 1992. "Leadership, Followership, Self, and Others." *Leadership Quarterly* 3 (1): 43–54.

20. Himmelfarb, M. 1984. "No Hitler, No Holocaust." *Commentary* 77 (3): 37–43.

21. Maxwell, J. C. 2005. *The 360 Degree Leader: Developing Your Influence from Anywhere in the Organization*. Nashville, TN: Thomas Nelson.

22. Erez, M., and P. C. Earley. 1993. *Culture, Self-Identity, and Work*. New York: Oxford University Press.

23. Drucker, P. F. 1993. *Managing for the Future*. New York: Penguin.

24. Bjugstad, K., E. C. Thach, K. J. Thompson, and A. Morris. 2006. "A Fresh Look at Followership: A Model for Matching Followership and Leadership Styles." *Journal of Behavioral and Applied Management* 7 (3): 304–19.

25. Ehrhart, M. 2001. "Predicting Followers' Preferences for Charismatic Leadership: The Influence of Follower Values and Personality." *Leadership Quarterly* 12 (2): 153–79.

26. Lord, R., D. J. Brown, and S. J. Freiberg. 1999. "Understanding the Dynamics of Leadership: The Role of Follower Self-Concepts in the Leader–Follower Relationship." *Organizational Behavior and Human Decision Processes* 78 (3): 167–203.

27. Collinson, D. 2006. "Rethinking Followership: A Post-structuralist Analysis of Follower Identities." *Leadership Quarterly* 17 (2): 179–89.

28. Lord, R., and R. J. Hall. 2005. "Identity, Deep Structure and the Development of Leadership Skill." *Leadership Quarterly* 16 (4): 591–615.

29. Blackshear, P. B. 2003. "The Followership Continuum: A Model for Increasing Organizational Productivity." *Public Manager* 32 (2): 25–30.

30. Bossidy, L. 2007. "What Your Leader Expects of You." *Harvard Business Review* 85 (4): 58–65.

31. Townsend, P. L., and J. E. Gebhardt. 2003. "The Leadership–Teamship–Followership Continuum." *Leader to Leader* 2003 (29): 18–21.

32. Goethals, G. R., G. J. Sorensen, and J. M. Burns (eds.). 2004. "Follower-Oriented Leadership." In *Encyclopedia of Leadership*, vol. 2, 494–99. Thousand Oaks, CA: Sage.

33. Bergmann, H., D. F. Russ-Eft, and K. Hurson. 1999. *Everyone a Leader: A Grassroots Model for the New Workplace*. Hoboken, NJ: Wiley.

34. *Psychology Today* Staff. 1992. "In Praise of Followers." *Psychology Today* 25 (5): 10.

35. Avolio, B. J., W. L. Gardner, F. O. Walumbwa, F. Luthans, and D. R. May. 2004. "Unlocking the Mask: A Look at the Process by Which Authentic Leaders Impact Follower Attitudes and Behaviors." *Leadership Quarterly* 15 (6): 801–23.

36. Kouzes, J. M., and B. Z. Posner. 2007. *The Leadership Challenge*, 4th ed. San Francisco: Jossey-Bass.

37. Goethals, G. R., and G. L. J. Sorensen. 2006. *The Quest for a General Theory of Leadership*. Northampton, MA: Edward Elgar.

38. Gardner, L. 2002. "Examining the Relationship Between Leadership and Emotional Intelligence in Senior Level Managers." *Leadership and Organization Development Journal* 23 (2): 68–78.

39. George, J. 2000. "Emotions and Leadership: The Role of Emotional Intelligence." *Human Relations* 53 (8): 1027–55.

40. Global Polio Eradication Initiative. 2017. *Annual Report 2016.* Accessed August 8. http://polioeradication.org/wp-content/uploads/2017/08/AR2016_EN.pdf.

41. Center for Global Development. 2017. "Case 5: Eliminating Polio in Latin America and the Caribbean." Accessed August 7. www.cgdev.org/page/case-5-eliminating-polio-latin-america-and-caribbean.

42. Independent Monitoring Board of the Global Polio Eradication Initiative. 2011. *Report: October 2011.* Published October. www.who.int/immunization/sage/3_GPEI_IMB_report_Oct2011_nov11.pdf.

11

TEAM LEADERSHIP FOR PUBLIC HEALTH

James W. Holsinger Jr.

Learning Objectives

Upon completion of this chapter, you should be able to

- describe the characteristics of effective teams and work groups,
- identify the various types of teams,
- distinguish between Tuckman's stages of team development,
- discuss Tuckman's use of the stages of team development to produce highly effective teams,
- employ situational leadership styles based on the team's performance readiness,
- differentiate between helpful and hindering team leadership behaviors,
- illustrate the characteristics of team excellence through Hill's team leadership model, and
- identify the five dysfunctions of a team and suggest leadership approaches to resolve them.

Focus on Leadership Competencies

This chapter emphasizes the following Association of Schools and Programs of Public Health (ASPPH) leadership competencies:

- Describe alternative strategies for collaboration and partnership among organizations, focused on public health goals.
- Engage in dialogue and learning from others to advance public health goals.
- Demonstrate team building, negotiation, and conflict management skills.
- Use collaborative methods for achieving organizational and community health goals.

(continued)

- Collaborate with diverse groups.
- Develop teams for implementing health initiatives.
- Develop capacity-building strategies at the individual, organizational, and community level.

It also addresses the following Council on Linkages public health leadership competencies:

- Collaborates with individuals and organizations in developing a vision for a healthy community.
- Provides opportunities for professional development for individuals and teams.

Note: See the appendix at the end of the book for complete lists of competencies.

Introduction

team
A group of interdependent individuals pursuing a common purpose.

Effective public health leaders must be able to skillfully manage their one-on-one leader–follower interactions, yet they also must recognize that most of their day-to-day leadership occurs in **team** or group situations. Teams and groups are entities unto themselves, and they possess a variety of characteristics and dynamics that leaders must be able to navigate. Leaders in public health rarely work alone, and organizational success depends on the ability of their teams and groups to serve as fully functioning units. Effective teams benefit public health organizations, as well as public health practitioners, by producing higher productivity, allowing for greater flexibility and speed, improving quality, providing for a flatter organizational structure, and increasing employee satisfaction and involvement, thereby reducing employee turnover.[1]

A *team* can be defined as a group of interdependent individuals collectively pursuing a common purpose.[2,3] Katzenbach and Smith[4(p45)] define the term more specifically as "a small number of people with complementary skills who are committed to a common purpose, performance goals, and approach for which they hold themselves mutually accountable," whereas Clawson[5(p230)] states that teams are "cohesive groups of people mobilized around a common goal." The various definitions of *team* have three main components: (1) the size of the group, which typically ranges from 3 to 20 members[6]; (2) work being done together on a regular basis, whether temporarily (e.g., on a project with specific starting and ending dates) or permanently (e.g., as an established part of a public health organization); and (3) a common goal shared by the team members.

Not every work group is a team. An effective team is distinguished by several key characteristics related to internal functioning or its organizational context[5]:

- A team possesses shared leadership and accepts team accountability.
- A team has a distinctive purpose and engages in shared work.
- A team uses direct, collective measures to accomplish real work, often through open-ended meetings.
- A team uses direct, collective measures to reward team members, and real work is the basis for team effort.
- Team members are able to manage their future, particularly as the group evolves over time.

Effective leadership is critical for team success, and ineffective leadership might well be the primary reason for team failure.[7,8] Leaders strongly influence team cohesion, drive, and the selection and attainment of team goals, and their relationship to the team has a marked impact on individual members. Followers tend to react differently to leaders in group settings than in one-on-one settings.[9]

Team leadership can be concentrated with a formal, assigned leader, or it can be shared among the various team members. Shared or distributed team leadership is known as **team capacity**. Such leadership incorporates the leadership skills of all the team members,[10] and it appears to have significant advantages over team leadership by a single individual.[11] Teamwork among peers, collaborators, and constituents in public health is extremely powerful, particularly in times of crisis. Unfortunately, however, true teamwork may be all too uncommon.

team capacity
Shared or distributed team leadership that incorporates the leadership skills of all the team members.

Types of Teams

Teams can be categorized into four main types: (1) functional work teams, (2) cross-functional teams, (3) self-managed teams, and (4) top executive teams. Virtual teams—those in which team members are not in close proximity to one another—may sometimes be considered a fifth type, though all types of teams may have some virtual characteristics.

Functional Work Teams

Functional work teams consist of individuals who have different responsibilities but who work together to perform a common function. Such teams often work together for long periods and have a high level of stability in team membership. Leaders of functional work teams usually have a high level of

functional work team
A type of team in which members have different responsibilities but work together to perform a common function.

authority, and members have little autonomy in determining the team's mission and objectives or the composition of the team. Team members have low to moderate autonomy in developing their own work procedures.

Cross-Functional Teams

cross-functional team
A type of team in which members from various functional subunits have responsibility for a particular project.

Cross-functional teams consist of members from various functional subunits who have responsibility for a particular project. Such teams are common in public health organizations, and they often include collaborators from outside organizations and members of constituent groups. Cross-functional teams are responsible for planning and carrying out complex functions,[12] and they aim to improve the coordination of work among the involved subunits of the organization.[13] Cross-functional teams emphasize cooperation and problem solving. The duration of each team's existence is variable, as is the stability of its membership. The authority of the team leader is moderate to high, and the team members have low to moderate autonomy in addressing their mission and objectives. Members do, however, have significant autonomy in their work procedures.

A public health organization may have several, or more, cross-functional teams in operation at any given time, since such teams are often transient in nature. If some team functions become more important than others, team membership may change as a result. Cross-functional teams tend to be highly diverse, and they rely heavily on the expertise of their members. Such teams are formed to solve problems, and the problems often require individuals with a variety of skills. The diversity in membership tends to enhance creativity and allows for a broad functional viewpoint, making the teams better able to accomplish their missions.

 Check It Out

To read more about the various types of teams in the workplace, go to www.capsim.com/blog/what-different-types-of-teams-are-in-the-workplace/.

As the practice of public health evolves to meet the demands of emerging health issues, leaders will increasingly activate and empower transdisciplinary public health teams. Haire-Joshu and McBride[14] have developed a model for these transdisciplinary teams that incorporates individual, team, organizational, and interorganizational efforts to address public health issues. Critically, the model emphasizes the transcendence of public health activities, and thus effective public health leadership, above and across public health and related disciplines.

self-managed team
A type of team in which much of the leader's authority and responsibility is turned over to the team members.

Self-Managed Teams

Self-managed teams are those in which much of the leader's authority and responsibility is turned over to the team members, making the teams semi-autonomous in nature. Such teams are often developed to produce a specific service or product or to handle technical problems or concerns. The members of self-managed teams, unlike members of cross-functional teams, usually have been chosen for their functional similarity and thus are not highly diverse. Self-managed teams possess a high level of autonomy for determining their work procedures. However, their mission, scope of work, and budget are established by a parent organization, and their authority beyond the immediate scope of work is variable. Self-managed teams tend to be stable and may exist for a long time.

Key advantages of self-managed teams include autonomy, a strong commitment to the team's work, and feelings of team empowerment.[15] Cross-training among team members can further increase job satisfaction, while also providing for flexibility within the team. A key disadvantage, however, is that self-managed teams can be difficult to establish effectively, particularly in situations where competent leadership and support are lacking. Failure to resolve interpersonal conflicts among members can lead to distrust, a lack of cooperation, and each team member functioning independently.[16] A self-managed team that is not implemented successfully may become an abject failure.

top executive team
A team that possesses a high level of autonomy in determining its mission and objectives, as well as in determining how it will function.

Top Executive Teams

Top executive teams are in a class all by themselves. Such teams possess high levels of autonomy in determining their mission and objectives, as well as in determining how they will function. Their team leader has high authority. Such teams often exist for extended periods with strong stability among team members, who possess a significant amount of diversity in their backgrounds. Top executive teams are especially important in large public health organizations. Continuity in membership allows such teams to plan for the future to improve the health of the community.

Consider This

"Not finance. Not strategy. Not technology. It is teamwork that remains the ultimate competitive advantage, both because it is so powerful and so rare."
—Patrick Lencioni[17(pvii)]

In your experience as a public health leader, why is teamwork so rare?

Virtual Teams

Virtual teams have members who are separated from one another geographically and rarely meet together face to face. The use of virtual teams has expanded dramatically as a result of the Internet, cellular telephones, videoconferencing, social media, and other advancements, to the point that telecommuting is now a common form of work engagement. Since virtual teams are not limited by geographic boundaries, their membership tends to be fluid in nature. They often include members from a variety of organizations and cultural backgrounds, spread across time zones or even on different continents. The most common form of virtual team is cross-functional in nature.

virtual team
A type of team in which members correspond chiefly through telecommunications technologies and rarely meet face to face.

In public health, the need for practitioners to cooperate with constituents and other collaborators has heightened the importance of virtual teams.

Coordination among public health agencies at the national, state, and local levels demands the use of such teams, particularly in the development of emergency plans for natural and human-made disasters. Virtual teams can be used for one-time tasks or for continuing arrangements that require planning or execution over large geographic areas. Fortunately, the flexibility afforded by the virtual setting helps organizations build teams with the most qualified individuals.

Team Life Cycles

Leaders looking to engage in effective team-building strategies in their orga-nizations first need to be aware of group dynamics and the ways that teams develop and change over time. Teams and small groups, whether short-term or long-term in nature, progress through a series of stages, each of which is marked by certain characteristics. Leaders who lack an understanding of these complexities are likely to be unsuccessful in organizing, guiding, and maintain-ing effective teams.

Tuckman's stages of team development
A sequence of four developmental stages—forming, storming, norming, and performing—through which teams and small groups progress; later versions of the model included additional stages of informing and adjourning.

Tuckman[18] developed a model for the team life cycle in 1965 after review-ing 50 studies on team development. **Tuckman's stages of team development**, as originally proposed, were (1) forming, (2) storming, (3) norming, and (4) performing. In 1977, Tuckman and Jensen[19] reconsidered the model and added an additional stage, adjourning. In subsequent years, other investigators[20] have considered additional stages in team development, including an informing stage that precedes forming. The stages of development are described at length in the sections that follow.

Before Stage 1: Informing

The **informing stage** precedes Tuckman's first stage of development, forming, although some investigators would include it as part of that stage. The inform-ing stage begins the team development process by notifying people of their membership in a team or small group. Such notification may be delivered in a face-to-face meeting or in writing, or even via e-mail. Informing may occur simultaneously to all individuals on a new team, or it may occur only to specific newcomers as members of an existing team are rotated or replaced.

informing stage
The stage at the start of the team development process in which people are notified of their membership in the group and informed about the group's mission.

The chief priority of the informing stage is to ensure that all new mem-bers receive the necessary information concerning the group, its mission, and its members. Some individuals being notified of their membership may already know about the team and its mission, and they may even know or have worked with some of the team members in the past. Even so, each member of the team must receive clear-cut, unambiguous guidance and direction. Failure to provide this information to each member raises the risk that individual members will develop different interpretations about the team's prospective work, which can be counterproductive in both the short and long term. A period of two to three weeks between notification of team membership and the team's first organizational meeting is usually considered appropriate.

Obviously, leaders should consider a number of factors when determining which individuals to assign to a team. The knowledge and skills that a person brings to the task are especially important, as is the person's desire to be a team member. A lack of skill relevant to the task or a disinterest in the team's activity will likely result in the individual being an unproductive team member. Whenever possible, the convening authority should consider the compatibility of team members and the quality of their working relationships to ensure that the team will function effectively.

Stage 1: Forming (Awareness)

Tuckman's first stage, the **forming stage**, is a stage of awareness and discovery, and it occurs when the new, immature group is beginning its orientation. During this stage, team members remain somewhat passive as they explore the team and learn what is expected of them as team members. Members tend to be overtly friendly and supportive toward one another, particularly if they do not already know one another, and they search for mutual support among members. A certain amount of testing occurs at this stage, as team members feel one another out and evaluate members' interest in the team and their commitment to team goals. A certain amount of conflict during the forming stage can help reduce the risk of **groupthink**, which occurs when a tendency to think and make decisions as a group discourages individual creativity and responsibility. This conflict can also give team members experience in conflict resolution, which can help prepare the team to resolve the problems it will encounter as it moves forward. The desired outcome of the forming stage is a commitment to and an acceptance of the team as a whole and its members.

forming stage
The stage of team development in which a new group is beginning its orientation and developing awareness.

groupthink
A tendency to think or make decisions as a group, to the point that individual creativity and responsibility are discouraged.

Stage 2: Storming (Conflict)

The **storming stage** represents a fractionating of the team and its work, as various members resist one another and advance conflicting ideas. It occurs when members lose their sense of obligation to the group and instead consider the accomplishment of the task as the overriding priority.[21] As members vie for leadership and attempt to control the group's direction, the goals and agendas of individuals may become more important than those of the team. Team members often show frustration or even hostility toward those who fail to support their preferred ideas or concepts. Communication between members is incomplete, and arguments and personal diatribes are common. Team members become confused and dissatisfied, and work output is low.

During the storming stage, team leaders must try to maintain team productivity while at the same time building the group's competence. Leaders should work to clarify the roles, purposes, and procedures within the team while creating an environment in which disagreements can be acknowledged

storming stage
The stage of team development in which team members resist one another and advance conflicting ideas.

and openly addressed. They should encourage all team members to engage in active listening and be attentive to one another's viewpoints. Desired outcomes of the storming stage include the clarification of roles and concepts, the development of an environment conducive to the generation of new ideas, an improved ability to manage disagreements, and a stronger sense of belonging. However, ineffective leadership during this time can prevent the team from moving beyond storming, thus causing it to disintegrate and fail in its mission.

When a team enters the storming stage, leaders from outside the group often have a tendency to intervene to influence the group and its processes. However, both leaders and team members should recognize that storming is a normal stage of development and that professional disagreements and frustration during this stage can be healthy and even necessary for the team to reach its full potential. Thus, the stage should not be micromanaged, and the conflict resolution process should not be rushed or cut short.

Stage 3: Norming (Cooperation)

norming stage
The stage of team development in which the team becomes more cohesive and functions according to agreed-upon roles and concepts.

The **norming stage** is a period of cohesion in which the team becomes a sharing group.[22] Once the team has moved beyond the storming stage, members discard their own agendas, seek the clarification of roles and concepts, and develop a sense of belonging. The various team roles have been clearly identified, and both formal and informal leaders work closely together to achieve the team's goals. The individual team members now have an appreciation for the differences within the team, and they find themselves more deeply involved in group decision making. They recognize that group success is also a source of their own personal power and authority, and they regard collaboration as a means for reaching their goals. Often, individuals who were disruptive during the storming stage exhibit less dissatisfaction during the norming stage, and they come to accept their roles (even though some roles will change over the life of the team). Members increasingly engage in the open exchange of ideas, information, and even personal feelings as they become accustomed to working with one another. At this stage, team members have agreed on rules for working together, ways of sharing information and resolving conflicts, and the processes and tools they will use to get the job done.[23] The expected outcomes of the norming stage include both heightened individual involvement and mutual support among team members. At this stage of the process, the team is prepared to accomplish the task assigned to it.

The norming stage can be somewhat bewildering for leaders, as they often will not fully understand the team's approach to developing its work processes. After all, the team's approach incorporates input from a number of creative and innovative individuals, and the task at hand is typically one that could not be done within normal organizational structures. During the norming stage, leaders should maintain a sense of humor, support good interpersonal communication, promote the exchange of feedback within the team, and provide affirmation for team members as they work toward the team's goal. Leaders should also encourage entrepreneurship, networking, and coalition building related to the team's task.

During the norming stage, leaders may need to consider removing or replacing team members who fail to norm with the rest of the team. Replacing a team member can be difficult and time-consuming, since the entire team may have to repeat the team-building process to acculturate the new member. Thus, many leaders find that dropping an ineffective team member and moving forward with a smaller team is preferable to trying to bring in a replacement.

 Effective Public Health Leaders . . .

. . . recognize that "no leader can be successful without the ability to manage resources and lead small groups."

—Gerald R. Ledlow and M. Nicholas Coppola[21(p166)]

Stage 4: Performing (Productivity)

The theme of the **performing stage** is interdependence. By this point in the process, team members have developed new ideas and approaches for completing their tasks, and they understand that they can achieve more as a team than they could have accomplished alone. Truly, they recognize that the whole of the team is greater than the sum of its parts. Individual members contribute to the group's work and achieve the desired end result while at the same time valuing the ideas and contributions of other team members.[22] The team has learned to work together in a collaborative fashion, performing a variety of tasks in parallel, rather than serial, fashion. Members find satisfaction in their achievements and feel a deep sense of pride—to the point that no member wants to be left out. Continued success in reaching major milestones sustains the momentum and enthusiasm. Team members continue to be challenged, but they are achieving significant results as their work is coming to completion.

During the performing stage, leaders should ensure that all team members share in the group's productivity and accomplishments, both of which produce a feeling of satisfaction and pride. Leaders can support team members through problem solving and decision making, use mentoring to foster productivity and achievement, and show appreciation for the team members' accomplishments. Team leaders must not take credit for the team's work; rather, they should share in the team's sense of accomplishment. The team's achievements and collective wisdom should engender a high level of trust and support between leaders and followers.

performing stage The stage of team development in which the team achieves results and develops a sense of pride through interdependence and collaborative work.

Stage 5: Adjourning (Moving On)

Once the team's assigned task has been accomplished and brought to a successful conclusion, the **adjourning stage** begins. At this point, the team has served

adjourning stage The stage in the team life cycle in which the team dissolves and its members transition to new challenges.

its purpose and opened new directions for the organization, and the team's members and leaders are ready to move on to new challenges. A successful team may be reconstituted for a new task, or its members may move to new team assignments or individual opportunities. In public health in particular, high-performing teams often will have learned valuable lessons and produced new and innovative approaches to key processes. Ensuring that this knowledge is retained in the organization's memory, so that it can serve as best practices for future teams, is an important final task in the team's life cycle.

Advancing Through the Stages of Development

Effective public health leaders support their teams through Tuckman's stages of development and help bring team members to the point where they are working toward a common goal in a highly effective manner.[23] Glacel[24] provides a cogent approach for advancement through the stages, and her ten key principles are shown in exhibit 11.1. Her tenth point might be the key to all team-building processes: Time must be allocated for forming, storming, norming, and performing. Time is also crucial during the informing stage and the adjourning stage. Of all the stages of development, the storming stage is especially critical, given that ineffective leadership at that point can stop the team's advancement and lead to failure in its assigned task.

Tuckman's stages outline essential steps in the development of highly productive and efficient teams, and they apply regardless of how old or large

---

EXHIBIT 11.1

Principles for Advancing Through the Stages of Team Development

1. Teams start the formation stages over at each meeting.
2. Any change in team membership means a new beginning to team formation issues.
3. Honest and real feelings expressed by team members help stimulate new ideas.
4. The team has more information and knowledge than is usually revealed.
5. Responsibility falls on all team members to bring people into discussion and to listen to ideas opposite from their own.
6. Talking about the team task is easy; talking about the process or working together is difficult.
7. Face-to-face meetings are needed for confronting difficult issues and reaching closure.
8. The team should reflect on team processes at every meeting.
9. Teams can get a lot done away from work.
10. Allocate time for forming, storming, norming, and performing.

Source: Data from Glacel, B. P. 1997. "Getting Teams to *Really* Work." *Innovative Leader* 6 (6): 11–20.

the organization may be.[20] Other team development models have been proposed,[25] but Tuckman's continues to stand the test of time.

Applying Situational Leadership to Develop Effective Teams

Hersey, Blanchard, and Johnson[26] have provided an application of situational leadership specific to the development of effective teams. As described in chapter 4, situational leadership involves efforts to match one's leadership style (S1–S4) with followers' developmental levels (D1–D4). However, leadership models that are effective in developing individual followers will not necessarily be effective when working with teams. Interactions among members bring added complexity to the team setting, and leaders must possess a high level of skill, particularly with regard to providing proactive leadership and receiving appropriate feedback from team members.

The application of situational leadership for team development emphasizes the alignment of goals with various group performance readiness levels (R1–R4). Under Hersey, Blanchard, and Johnson's[26] approach, *leadership* can be understood as behavior that occurs when a person attempts to influence the behavior of another person or a group, and a *group* can be defined as two or more people who interact in such a manner that the group must exist in order for each member's needs to be met. To function effectively, a group or team must have a defined purpose and clear-cut objectives and goals; without them, members will not have norms for group behavior. A team's progress toward its goals is a useful measure of its effectiveness.

Key Situational Leadership Questions

To apply the situational leadership model to effective team development, the leader asks five key questions, as shown in exhibit 11.2. The first question—"What objectives do we want to accomplish?"—seeks to identify the team's specific task and clarify the relevant outcomes, objectives, and milestones. If the team's objective is not clearly defined, the leader cannot possibly determine the team's performance readiness level or the appropriate leadership style to employ. The second question—"What is the team's performance readiness in the situation?"—aims to diagnose the team's level of performance readiness in relationship to the team's specific objective. The third question—"What intervention should the leader make?"—is the point where the leader determines the appropriate leadership style based on the needs of the team. Once a leadership intervention has occurred, the fourth and fifth questions—"What was the result of the leadership intervention?" and "What follow-up, if any, is required?"—lead to an assessment of whether the intervention is achieving

EXHIBIT 11.2
Situational
Leadership
Team-
Development
Questions

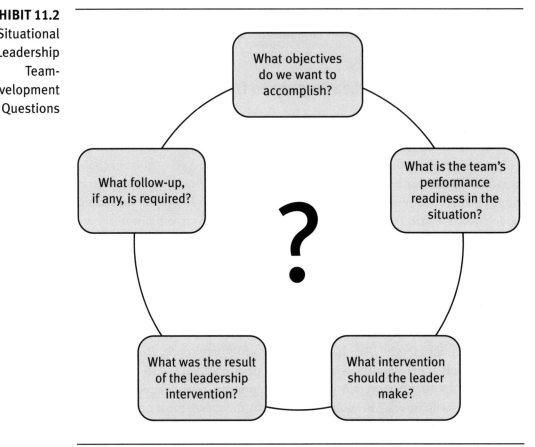

Source: Data from Hersey, P., K. H. Blanchard, and D. E. Johnson. 2008. *Management of Organizational Behavior: Leading Human Resources*, 9th ed. Upper Saddle River, NJ: Pearson Prentice Hall.

the expected results. If a gap exists between the results and expectations, an additional leader intervention is necessary, with the cycle repeating itself.[26]

Team Performance Readiness Levels

The levels of team performance readiness in the situational leadership application correspond with Tuckman's stages of team development. To determine the team's readiness level, the leader must assess both the team's ability and its willingness. Ability encompasses knowledge, skill, and experience, whereas willingness represents commitment, motivation, and confidence. In keeping with situational leadership's emphasis on the context or situation, the leader's diagnosis of the team's readiness level should be specific to the team's stated objective.

A team at the lowest level of performance readiness, R1, tends to be uncertain and insecure, and it might be unable or unwilling to engage in the task at hand. The team is in Tuckman's forming stage, and it requires clarification of the objective. The uncertain and chaotic manner in which the team functions might be said to resemble a game of "pick-up sticks."[26] As the team advances from R1 to R2, it is "coming around."[26] However, the team is entering Tuckman's storming stage, which brings dissonance within the team. Teams at this point often become divided, with members competing for recognition and influence. The team as a whole is still unable to engage in the team's task, but members are becoming more confident and willing. At R3, the team has reached Tuckman's norming stage and is now "coming together."[26] Adjustments are being made, and team cohesion is developing. Experts and informal leaders are emerging within the team, and modest accomplishments are being reached. Still, the team remains somewhat insecure and unwilling to function as a group. The R4 level is the point where the team acts "as one."[26] The team has entered Tuckman's performing stage, and it is willing and able to engage in the team's task. The team shows confidence and synergy as it performs well with clearly established functional roles. Having weathered the storms of R2, the group has become self-managing and is on its way to becoming a high-performing team. Key indicators of the four performance readiness levels are summarized in exhibit 11.3.

Although the performance readiness levels describe the team as a whole, certain members of the team may occupy different levels individually. If certain members lag behind the group's level of readiness, leaders should apply situational leadership as it pertains to individuals (see chapter 4) to help those members develop. Leaders may also involve other members of the team in efforts to assist individuals with lower levels of readiness.

Readiness Level	Tuckman Stage	Task Ability	Indicators
R1	Forming	Unable and insecure or unwilling	"Pick-up sticks," uncertain chaos, need for goal and objective definition
R2	Storming	Unable but confident or willing	"Coming around," intrateam dissonance, competition for recognition and influence
R3	Norming	Able but insecure or unwilling	"Coming together," team cohesion, emergence adjustment
R4	Performing	Able and confident or willing	"As one," functional role related-ness, self-managing team, esprit, performance synergy

EXHIBIT 11.3
Indicators of Team Performance Readiness

Source: Data from Hersey, P., K. H. Blanchard, and D. E. Johnson. 2008. *Management of Organizational Behavior: Leading Human Resources*, 9th ed. Upper Saddle River, NJ: Pearson Prentice Hall.

Team Leadership Styles

Once the team's performance readiness level has been assessed, the leader is ready to determine the specific leadership style to employ. When the group is at the R1 level, the leader's role focuses on structuring the group and defining the task. The appropriate leadership style, therefore, is S1, which in this case can be described as the "defining" style. The leader's chief concern is to focus the team to meet its objective, and the leader's communication is primarily one-way in nature. In the S1 style, the leader is clearly up front and in a position of control, in some respects standing outside the group itself.

When the team reaches the R2 level of readiness, the leader moves to the S2 style of leadership. At this point, the leader is becoming the center or hub of the group and has responsibility for clarifying the team's work, as well as the team members' roles and responsibilities. A key challenge involves moving the team past the storming stage, which is a point where many teams fail. Communication is now two-way and multidimensional, not only between the leader and team members, but also between team members themselves. At this stage of a team's life together, the leader answers the question of "why."

For a team at the R3 level of readiness, the leader employs the S3 style of leadership, which can be termed the "involving" style. The leader is now in an unequal position vis-à-vis the rest of the team, serving both as a contributing member of the team and as the team's leader. From an operational point of view, the leader's role diminishes as the team progresses through the norming stage. The leader involves all team members in the project and provides them with support, and the team, with the leader's guidance, sets its own goals and direction. Communication becomes clearly multidirectional, with the leader participating as an integral member.

Finally, the team readiness level of R4 corresponds with the leadership style of S4. The leader at this point empowers the team and delegates work, while offering less input and oversight. The leader is now distant from the daily work of the team and serves mainly to facilitate the team's work and connect the team to the rest of the organization. Effective public health team leaders, at this stage of their team's readiness, have effectively worked themselves out of a job.

Helping and Hindering

The four leadership styles represent varying degrees of task (directive) behavior and relationship (supportive) behavior, and the style chosen by the leader can either help or hinder the team's efforts. For leaders to be effective in the team setting, they need to adapt their roles and styles to fit the situation at hand and the needs of the team.

The S1 style of leadership is high in task behavior and low in relationship behavior, and it is applied during Tuckman's forming stage of team development. Use of the S1 style can be helpful to the team when the leader assists the team in getting started, clarifies the team's purpose, defines team goals, and maintains the team's direction. A hindering S1 style is aggressive in nature, with dominating leaders who criticize team members, exhibit an attacking personality, and use name calling as a means of control.

The S2 style, which is used during the team's storming stage, is high in both task behavior and relationship behavior. A helpful S2 approach is persuasive in nature, provides guidance and encouragement, and aims to coach the team toward the norming stage. The leader asks questions to uncover the issues at the center of the team's storming and assists the team members in developing resolutions. At the same time, the leader advocates for the team and its members, particularly with the outside organization. In contrast, a leader using a hindering S2 approach is manipulative, often presenting statements as questions, developing selective interpretations of data and personalities, and keeping the team off balance by jumping from one topic to another without reaching a conclusion.

The S3 style is high in relationship behavior and low in task behavior. A helpful leader using this style engages the group and facilitates each member's involvement in an effort to build commitment to the team's goal. Problem solving comes to the forefront of the leader's efforts, and the leader provides additional support by summarizing and synthesizing the team's work. A hindering leader at this stage tends to be dependent in nature, will agree to everything and anything, and avoids making decisions. Closure will be difficult to come by. Such a leader often seeks sympathy, uses sarcasm with other team members, and expresses feelings of futility, resignation, or helplessness.

When the team reaches its full potential in the performing stage, the leader adopts the S4 style, which is low in both task and relationship behaviors. A helpful approach at this stage will emphasize monitoring and observing. The leader uses a listening approach in interactions with team members, shows interest in the work product by taking notes or recording interactions, and attends to the needs of the team and its members. A hindering S4 approach is based on avoidance. The leader withdraws both psychologically and physically, reflecting both boredom with the project and a desire to escape the team.

Variation on the Model

Blanchard, Carew, and Parisi-Carew[27] offer a variation of the situational leadership approach in which the stages of group development are labeled *orientation*, *dissatisfaction*, *resolution*, and *production* (matching Tuckman's stages) and the leadership styles are labeled *directing*, *coaching*, *supporting*, and *delegating*. In their model, productivity, or team competence, increases steadily from the beginning of the orientation stage through the end of the production stage. Team morale, or the team's commitment to the task at hand, begins on a high note during orientation but plummets during the dissatisfaction stage. The drop in commitment signals the need for the leader to adopt a coaching style that is high in both directive and supportive behaviors. As the team rebounds from its "slough of despond," morale and commitment rebound, and they continue to increase through the rest of the team's lifetime. Regardless of the differences in details and terminology between versions, the situational leadership model has proved to be a valuable tool for effective public health leaders in team settings.

Hill's Team Leadership Model

Hill's team leadership model
A model that focuses on the leader's role in ensuring team effectiveness by diagnosing team problems and taking appropriate steps to correct them.

Hill's team leadership model is based on "the functional leadership claim that the leader's job is to monitor the team and then take whatever action is necessary to ensure team effectiveness."[28(p366)] Leaders, therefore, are considered to be firmly in charge of effective team performance. The model seeks to provide guidance to leaders as they diagnose team problems and take appropriate steps to correct them. It functions at three levels: initial leadership decisions, leadership actions, and indicators of team effectiveness.

To drive effective team performance, the leader develops a mental model of the situation at hand. This mental model is based on the leader's observation of the team's function, and it includes not only the team's task but also the environmental and organizational situation. The leader conceptualizes the team's problem and determines possible solutions, given environmental and organizational considerations. To respond appropriately, the leader must have flexibility in behavior and a variety of skills that are appropriate to the needs of team members. The problem can be solved if the leader's behavior matches the situation's complexity and meets the team's needs. Leadership behavior under Hill's model can be considered a team-based problem-solving process: The leader uses analysis of the situation, both internal and external, to select and implement appropriate team behaviors to achieve the team's goals.[28] Zaccaro, Rittman, and Marks[7] point out that leaders must exercise discretion in determining which team problems should be addressed and in deciding which solution to pursue, particularly when a number of possible solutions are present.

Leadership Decisions

The first level of Hill's[28] model focuses on leadership decisions, with specific attention to a series of questions that leaders ask themselves when deciding on an appropriate strategy. The questions are as follows:

1. Should I monitor the team or take action?
2. Should I intervene to meet task or relational needs?
3. Should I intervene internally or externally?

Hill[28(p374)] phrases the first question in full as, "Should I continue monitoring these factors, or should I take action based on the information I have already gathered and structured?" To answer the question, the leader considers the team's situation and decides between continuing to monitor the problem and taking action to resolve the problem. Monitoring, in this instance, involves diagnosing, analyzing, and forecasting the problem. If the leader takes action, such action must help the team.

The model's second decision question focuses on whether the team needs the leader's assistance in meeting either task or relational needs.[28] To answer this question, the leader needs to consider both task and maintenance perspectives. Task leadership functions include making decisions, solving problems, making plans, and reaching objectives, whereas maintenance functions involve engaging team members at a personal level, working to solve interpersonal problems, and satisfying team members' needs. Task and maintenance functions are closely interrelated, and both person-focused and task-focused behaviors are associated with teams that are perceived to be effective.[29,30] A well-maintained team will have strong relationships that enable team members to work together effectively to meet the requirements of the task. A failing team will have members who take out their frustrations on one another and thus accomplish little or nothing.

The model's third question focuses on whether the intervention should occur internally, within the group, or externally, in the outside environment.[28] The leader's analysis of the situation must look at both internal and external aspects, and the leader must be able to balance internal and external concerns when responding to a problem.

The leader's answers to the questions combine with the internal/external nature of the problem to point toward certain resolutions. If the leader chooses to monitor the problem and the problem is internal, the team's deficiencies should be diagnosed. If the leader chooses to monitor the problem and the problem is external, environmental changes should be forecast. If the leader decides to act and the problem is internal, remedial action is necessary. If the leader decides to act and the problem is external, the leader needs to prevent deleterious changes from damaging the team and its task.

The quality of a leader's decisions depends on the accuracy of the leader's mental model, and this model must be based on a careful scan of both the internal and external environments. The leader must carefully analyze and interpret the gathered information and develop a clear understanding of the team's current level of functioning. Feedback from team members is also valuable, since they too can participate in

Effective Public Health Leaders . . .

. . . consider the situation and take the required action.[28]

monitoring. Once information has been gathered and interpreted, an essential aspect of leadership is **action mediation**—the process by which the leader and the group select an appropriate course of action and create an organizational system for making high-quality decisions.[31]

Leadership Actions

action mediation
The process by which the leader and the group select an appropriate course of action and create an organizational system for making high-quality decisions.

The next level of Hill's model focuses on leadership actions, both internal and external.[28] Internal leadership actions include a variety of task and relational behaviors aimed at clarifying goals, obtaining team member agreement, and reaching team objectives. Important internal relationship actions include training team members (both formally and informally), assessing team member performance, encouraging or confronting individual members as needed, and coaching the team to achieve high performance. Other internal leadership actions include managing process improvement efforts, adjusting team member roles as needed, improving coordination, and obtaining information to guide decision making. The use of collaborative methods that involve all team members can help build esprit de corps, increasing team commitment and improving the team's ability to manage conflict. The team leader can also lead by example, modeling expectations for team members.

External leadership actions relate to the environment outside the team, and they may involve networking or connecting with other organizations to influence environmental conditions or gather information. Surveys, performance indicators, and other tools can help the leader assess the environment and better understand the impact of environmental conditions on the organization. Key environmental information should be shared with the team. The leader also should effectively represent the team to the outside world and buffer the team from outside distractions.

Team Effectiveness

The final level of Hill's model focuses on team effectiveness, and it includes two critical functions: performance and development. The characteristics of team excellence identified by Larson and LaFasto,[30] shown in exhibit 11.4, provide a framework for considering team effectiveness, and they closely align with the conditions of group effectiveness identified by Hackman and Walton.[32] These characteristics can function as performance standards, which the leader can use to assess the team's achievement and identify areas of ineffectiveness.

Effective teams have a clearly defined goal that motivates and elevates the team members. Such teams also have a results-driven structure that improves the likelihood that the goal will be reached. Effective teams consist of team members who are competent and trust one another. The composition of the team—having both the right number of team members and possessing diversity in knowledge, skills, and abilities—plays a major role in team effectiveness. A

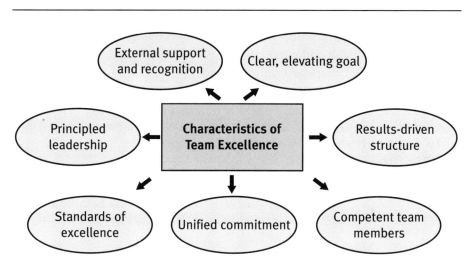

EXHIBIT 11.4
Characteristics
of Team
Excellence

Source: Data from Larson, C. E., and F. M. J. LaFasto. 1989. *Teamwork: What Must Go Right/What Can Go Wrong.* Newbury Park, CA: Sage.

group of individuals who lack unified commitment is not a team; it is simply a group of individuals. Thus, a collaborative climate is essential. Effective teams have standards of excellence that reflect team norms, help the team function, and urge all team members to perform at their best. Such standards should be clear to all members and concrete in nature. Team effectiveness also requires external support of the team by the parent organization, as well as recognition of the team's work.

A final characteristic of team excellence is principled leadership. An effective team leader is perceptive, objective, and analytical; above all, the leader must be a good listener with the requisite diagnostic skills. Team effectiveness is a direct outgrowth of good team leadership, and the leader therefore is at the center of Hill's model. However, as Zaccaro, Rittman, and Marks[7] point out, team excellence can also have an impact on leader effectiveness. The chief priority of the team leader is to determine the critical systems and structures of an effective team and to focus attention on them for possible intervention.[33] Appropriate rewards for the work of a highly effective team are always warranted.

Strengths and Weaknesses of Hill's Model

Hill's model has a number of strengths that make it useful to leaders pursuing continuous team analysis and improvement. It takes into account the complex aspects of team leadership, and it places the team in its organizational context, considering both internal and external factors. In doing so, the model provides guidance for both leaders and team members in assessing the team's performance, finding and fixing team problems, and taking appropriate action to enhance team effectiveness. The model's weaknesses include the fact that it, like many other leadership models, has not been thoroughly tested. Training in the model is difficult and potentially overwhelming, and it does not always answer the difficult questions facing the leader.

Clearly, team leadership is complex, and leaders, particularly in public health, have to address a variety of problems that lack simple solutions. The principles of Hill's model, even with its shortcomings, are highly valuable. Leaders must be able to objectively diagnose team difficulties and problems, and they must be able to take appropriate action (or inaction) to help the team meet its goals.[28] Effective public health leadership occurs when the leader will do whatever is required to meet the needs of the team and its members.

Leadership Application Case: The Big Blow-Up

The Leadership Application Case at the beginning of this book provides realistic scenarios for the application of key leadership concepts covered in the text. See the section marked "Chapter 11 Application" for the scenario and discussion questions that correspond with this chapter.

Dysfunctions of a Team

Lencioni[17] has approached the topic of team performance by examining the various forms of dysfunction that hinder team efforts. He argues that human beings are dysfunctional by nature and that teamwork is therefore rare and elusive. The behaviors of effective teams may seem uncomplicated in theory, but they are exceedingly difficult to master and put into practice. For a team to be successful, it must overcome the behavioral tendencies that breed dysfunction.

The Five Dysfunctions

five dysfunctions of a team
A model that identifies five forms of dysfunction that arise in team settings: absence of trust, fear of conflict, lack of commitment, avoidance of accountability, and inattention to results.

Lencioni[17] identifies **five dysfunctions of a team**:

1. Absence of trust
2. Fear of conflict
3. Lack of commitment
4. Avoidance of accountability
5. Inattention to results

The first dysfunction, absence of trust, arises from team members who are unwilling to appear vulnerable. Trust cannot develop if team members are not willing to be open about their weaknesses and mistakes. This failure to build trust leads directly to the second dysfunction, fear of conflict. Team members who do not trust one another are unable to engage in open dialogue and debate, and their discussions become cryptic and guarded. Without the benefit of healthy conflict within the team, the third dysfunction arises—lack of commitment. Since the team's decisions were not reached through vigorous and open discussion, the team members do not fully agree with or commit to those decisions (even though they may appear to do so). When the team members fail to commit to the team's decisions and do not engage wholeheartedly in the team's process, the fourth dysfunction, avoidance of accountability, emerges. If commitment to the team's action plan is lacking, even the most dedicated team members will be unwilling to hold other members accountable for behaviors that undermine the team's integrity. This failure to hold one another accountable leads to the fifth dysfunction, inattention to results. Team members start putting their own needs (e.g., ego needs, need for recognition, need for career advancement) ahead of the needs of the team, and the goals and objectives of the team are forgotten. Under Lencioni's model, each dysfunction feeds into the next; thus, once a single dysfunction is allowed to occur, teamwork evaporates.[17]

What, then, are the behaviors of the members of a cohesive team? According to Lencioni,[17(pp189–90)] members (1) "trust one another," (2) "engage in unfiltered conflict around ideas," (3) "commit to decisions and plans of action," (4) "hold one another accountable for delivering against those plans," and (5) "focus on the achievement of collective results." Lencioni finds that such behaviors, while simple in theory, require a level of discipline and persistence that is difficult to produce.

Addressing the Dysfunctions
Moving Beyond Absence of Trust

Lencioni[17(p195)] explains: "Trust is the confidence among team members that their peers' intentions are good, and that there is no reason to be protective or careful around the group. In essence, teammates must get comfortable about being vulnerable with one another." To team members who are used to being competitive with their peers, the idea of being comfortable with one's vulnerability may at first seem foreign. However, for a team to become highly effective, its members must be willing to be vulnerable and know that their vulnerabilities will not be used against them. If trust does not develop, the team will likely waste a significant amount of time and effort with unproductive behaviors, while at the same time struggling with low morale and high turnover.

A team can move beyond this dysfunction if members commit to sharing experiences over time, understanding one another's attributes, and building credibility with one another through work

Check It Out

For information about using the Myers-Briggs Type Indicator with Lencioni's five dysfunctions of a team model, go to www.cpp.com/pdfs/mbti-lencioni-guide.pdf.

accomplishments. A variety of experiential exercises and personality/behavior profiles, including the Myers-Briggs Type Indicator (discussed in chapter 3), can assist with this effort. Leaders can further foster trust by appearing vulnerable themselves. Doing so requires courage, but without taking this risk themselves, leaders cannot expect to create a team environment that engenders trust. Only genuine vulnerability on the part of the leader will be effective; anything else will come across as false and be counterproductive in building trust.

Moving Beyond Fear of Conflict

In many instances, particularly in the work environment, conflict is perceived negatively, which allows fear of conflict to take hold. However, a distinction must be made between productive conflict, which develops through people's differing ideologies and opinions, and interpersonal conflict, which often is mean-spirited and involves ad hominem attacks. Whereas interpersonal conflict can leave the team with a residue of hurt feelings, productive conflict spurs creativity, helps teams reach excellent solutions in the shortest possible time, and contributes to the growth both of individual team members and of the team itself. In short, it builds teams that are ready, willing, and able to tackle the next significant issue. Such productive conflict is only possible, however, if trust has developed among team members and with the team leader. Only through trust can team members engage in significant, open debate over the issues and objectives that face them.

To overcome dysfunction, team leaders and members alike must recognize that the proper kind of conflict is beneficial and should not be avoided. When conflict occurs, leaders may become concerned that they are losing control of their teams, or they may feel a need to intervene to protect certain team members. In many cases, such an intervention by the leader will interrupt healthy conflict and prevent members from resolving their issues in a natural manner. Leaders therefore must show restraint, exercise sound judgment, and encourage natural conflict resolution that will help the team to thrive. Effective leadership in this area is especially important given that inability to advance through Tuckman's storming stage is a common cause of team failure.

Moving Beyond Lack of Commitment

Team commitment occurs when members have engaged in productive conflict, voicing their own opinions and perspectives, and have come to recognize that the decision-making process has benefitted from each team member's ideas.[17] Commitment consists of two behaviors: clarity and buy-in. The decision must be clearly expressed and understood, and all team members, even those who opposed the decision, need to get on board once the decision has been made. If and when an impasse occurs and consensus cannot be reached, the team leader needs to be authorized by the group to make the final decision. Interestingly, consensus does not produce commitment; instead, commitment develops when all team members feel they have been heard and have had their thoughts considered.

The need for certainty can be an impediment to team member commitment. Whereas dysfunctional teams often try to delay their decisions in an attempt to gain both time and certainty, highly effective teams are able to unite around a decision and commit to the determined course of action, even when they have little or no assurance that the decision is correct. They know that an optimum level of certainty is possible in any given situation, and they resist paralysis by analysis. The team leader must be able to move forward based on the team's decision, even if the decision turns out to be erroneous. A flawed decision is better than no decision at all, and a decision that turns out to be the wrong one can usually be modified so that the team can work effectively.

Moving Beyond Avoidance of Accountability

Accountability is a difficult concept in team settings. Team members should not be held accountable for accomplishing tasks they have not been trained to accomplish, nor for outcomes that have not been discussed by the team,[17] but they must be held accountable for meeting standards, maintaining expectations, and achieving goals. At times, team members' efforts to hold one another accountable can lead to difficult conversations or even threaten to rupture valued personal relationships. However, lack of accountability can just as easily lead to resentment within the group, spurred by the dissipation of standards and failure to meet expectations.

Accountability within the team can be improved through clear standards and goals, regular progress reviews, and the existence of peer pressure. The team leader should ensure that the team itself—not just the leader—holds all members accountable. Accountability will be insufficient if the leader is the only source of discipline. However, in instances where the team fails to hold a member accountable, the leader must be the final authority.

Moving Beyond Inattention to Results

If team members are not held accountable for the results of their work, they will prioritize their own needs and their own career advancement above the good of the team. A focus on team member status or the feeling of simply being part of the team will not sufficiently motivate members toward team success. Team results are outcome based, and a failure to attend to those outcomes leads to team failure. If a leader focuses on anything in place of the team's results, the members will take note and respond accordingly. To avoid this dysfunction, team leaders must exhibit selfless behavior and empower the team members to stay focused on the team's results, not their own.

Case Study: Fighting Infant Mortality in Memphis[34]

Memphis, Tennessee, is a city rich in culture and history, but it is also plagued by chronic health problems and health disparities. In 2003, the infant mortality rate in Shelby County, which includes Memphis, was 14.9 per 1,000 live births—more than twice the national rate of 6.9 for the same year. Not only was it the worst rate among US counties with more than 12,000 annual births; it also was worse than 82 countries listed in the CIA World Factbook, ranking just behind Latvia (14.59) and just ahead of Sri Lanka (15.22).

Yvonne Madlock, who was director of the Shelby County Health Department at the time, recognized the urgent need to address the problem, and she coordinated a communitywide effort by public health and governmental officials, healthcare and business leaders, and citizens. The effort focused on the social determinants of health underlying the infant mortality problem—including education, income, and living conditions—and it sought to improve prenatal care, reduce teen pregnancies, and provide supportive resources to new and expectant mothers.

Health department officials and their collaborators identified several contributing factors, including premature birth, low birth weight, and birth defects, which, in turn, were antecedently linked to poorer or no prenatal care, drug use and smoking during pregnancy, and lack of insurance. To combat these factors, Madlock and her team implemented home visitation programs in which health and nutrition counselors visited expectant and new mothers to advise them on proper diet and self-care. The counselors emphasized the importance of attending doctor's appointments, taking medicine, and avoiding alcohol, tobacco, and other harmful substances. They also provided information about minimizing the risk of sudden infant death syndrome, which was a leading contributor to infant mortality in the county. Lactation specialists helped ensure higher rates of breastfeeding after birth, and health department staff worked to make sure that low-income new and expectant mothers had insurance coverage. The health department also launched a mobile application—B4BabyLife—that put parenting tips conveniently at users' fingertips.

Such a collaborative effort took immense interpersonal and organizational leadership. By 2015, the infant mortality rate for Shelby County had fallen to 8.2 deaths per 1,000 live births. Despite that significant improvement, the rate remained well above the national average, and a significant disparity existed between the African American population (12.4 deaths per 1,000 live births) and other population groups. Thus, health officials acknowledged that much more work needed to be done and that continued engagement from a broad team of health department employees, stakeholders, collaborators, and constituents was essential.

Discussion and Application Questions

1. What strategies did health department officials use to identify and address health concerns?
2. In what ways does the county's approach provide an example of effective public health leadership?
3. What challenges does this approach present to public health leaders?
4. As the new director of the Shelby County Health Department, what actions would you take to further address the county's high rate of infant mortality?

Summary

A team is a group of interdependent individuals collectively pursuing a common purpose. Teams can be characterized into four main types: (1) functional work teams, in which members have different responsibilities but work together to perform a common function; (2) cross-functional teams, in which members from various functional subunits have responsibility for a particular project; (3) self-managed teams, in which much of the leader's authority and responsibility is turned over to the team members; and (4) top executive teams, in which members possess a high level of autonomy in determining the team's mission and objectives. Virtual teams, in which members rarely meet face-to-face, may sometimes be considered a fifth type.

Teams and small groups progress through a series of stages, each of which is marked by certain characteristics that the leader should strive to understand. Tuckman described a sequence of four developmental stages—forming, storming, norming, and performing—through which teams and small groups progress; later versions of the model have added the stages of informing and adjourning. The informing stage occurs when people are notified of their membership in the group and informed about the group's mission, and the forming stage occurs when the groups is beginning its organization. Storming occurs as various members advance conflicting ideas, and norming occurs as the team becomes more cohesive. The performing stage is the point where the team achieves results through interdependence and collaborative work. With the adjourning stage, the team dissolves, and its members move on to new challenges.

The principles of situational leadership can be effectively applied to team settings using a model developed by Hersey, Blanchard, and Johnson. Under this approach, the leader uses a series of questions to assess the team's performance readiness level (R1–R4), and then the leader uses that assessment to select an appropriate leadership style (S1–S4). The four leadership styles represent varying degrees of task (directive) behavior and relationship (supportive) behavior.

Another approach, Hill's team leadership model, focuses on the leader's role in ensuring team effectiveness by diagnosing team problems and taking appropriate steps to correct them. It functions at three levels—initial leadership decisions, leadership actions, and indicators of team effectiveness—and takes into account the complex aspects of team leadership and the organizational context (both internal and external).

Lencioni approaches the topic of team leadership by examining five common dysfunctions in team settings: absence of trust, fear of conflict, lack of commitment, avoidance of accountability, and inattention to results. Under Lencioni's model, each dysfunction feeds into the next; thus, once a single dysfunction is allowed to occur, teamwork evaporates. Moving beyond the dysfunctions is difficult, but it can be done if team members trust one another, engage in productive conflict, commit to team decisions and action plans, hold one another accountable, and focus on collective results.

Discussion Questions

1. Compare and contrast the various types of teams. Which do you think is most effective in public health practice?
2. Describe virtual teams. What is their usefulness in public health practice?
3. Describe Tuckman's stages of team development.
4. Compare and contrast the four performance readiness levels for teams under the situational leadership approach. Discuss the nature of a team's progression from R1 to R4.
5. In applying situational leadership for teams, what is the relationship between performance readiness levels and leadership styles?
6. How might the four situational leadership styles function to either help or hinder the team?
7. What are the differences between internal and external leadership actions in Hill's model of team leadership?
8. Compare and contrast the situational leadership model, as applied to the leadership of teams, with Hill's model of team leadership.

9. What are the five dysfunctions of a team? Explain their sequencing in Lencioni's model.

10. For deeper thought: In your opinion, which of the team dysfunctions is the most problematic in public health? Defend your decision.

Web Resources

Boundless. 2017. "Stages of Team Development." Accessed July 31. www.boundless. com/management/textbooks/boundless-management-textbook/groups-teams-and-teamwork-6/building-successful-teams-53/stages-of-team-development-270-1614/.

Capsim. 2015. "What Different Types of Teams Are in the Workplace?" Published July 14. www.capsim.com/blog/what-different-types-of-teams-are-in-the-workplace/.

CCP, Inc. 2017. *Using the Myers-Briggs Instrument with Lencioni's 5 Dysfunctions of a Team Model.* Accessed July 31. www.cpp.com/pdfs/mbti-lencioni-guide.pdf.

SelfAwareness.org. 2013. "Situational Leadership and Developing Great Teams." Published September 29. www.selfawareness.org.uk/news/situational-leadership-and-developing-great-teams.

Singh, K. J. 2012. "What Is the Nature of the Teams?" *MBA Official.* Published September 12. www.mbaofficial.com/mba-courses/human-resource-management/human-resource-planning-and-development/what-is-the-nature-of-the-teams/.

References

1. Glassop, L. I. 2002. "The Organizational Benefit of Teams." *Human Relations* 55 (2): 225–49.

2. Zaiger Roberts, V. 1994. "The Organization of Work: Contributions from Open Systems Theory." In *The Unconscious at Work: Individual and Organizational Stress in the Human Services,* edited by A. Obholzer and V. Zaiger Roberts, 28–38. London, UK: Routledge.

3. Mallory, C. 1991. *Team-Building.* Shawnee Mission, KS: National Press Publications.

4. Katzenbach, J. R., and D. K. Smith. 1994. *The Wisdom of Teams.* New York: Harper Business.

5. Clawson, J. G. 2006. *Level Three Leadership: Getting Below the Surface,* 3rd ed. Upper Saddle River, NJ: Pearson Prentice Hall.

6. Orsburn, J. D., and L. Moran. 2000. *The New Self-Directed Work Teams: Mastering the Challenge.* New York: McGraw-Hill.

7. Zaccaro, S. J., A. L. Rittman, and M. A. Marks. 2001. "Team Leadership." *Leadership Quarterly* 12 (4): 451–83.

8. Stewart, G. L., and C. C. Manz. 1995. "Leadership for Self-Managing Work Teams: A Typology and Integrative Model." *Human Relations* 48 (7): 747–70.

9. Bass, B. M. 2008. *The Bass Handbook of Leadership: Theory, Research, and Managerial Applications*, 4th ed. New York: Free Press.

10. Day, D. V., P. Gronn, and E. Salas. 2004. "Leadership Capacity in Teams." *Leadership Quarterly* 15 (6): 857–80.

11. Solansky, S. T. 2008. "Leadership Style and Team Processes in Self-Managed Teams." *Journal of Leadership and Organizational Studies* 14 (4): 332–41.

12. Yukl, G. 2013. *Leadership in Organizations*, 8th ed. Upper Saddle River, NJ: Prentice Hall.

13. Ford, R. C., and W. A. Randolph. 1992. "Cross-Functional Structures: A Review and Integration of Matrix Organization and Project Management." *Journal of Management* 18 (2): 267–94.

14. Haire-Joshu, D., and T. D. McBride (eds.). 2013. *Transdisciplinary Public Health: Research, Education, & Practice*. San Francisco: Jossey-Bass.

15. Kirkman, B. L., and B. Rosen. 1999. "Beyond Self-Management: Antecedents and Consequences of Team Empowerment." *Academy of Management Journal* 42 (1): 58–74.

16. Langfred, C. W. 2007. "The Downside of Self-Management: A Replication and Interpretation in Strategic Persistence and Reorientation." *Academy of Management Journal* 50 (4): 885–900.

17. Lencioni, P. 2002. *The Five Dysfunctions of a Team: A Leadership Fable*. San Francisco: Jossey-Bass.

18. Tuckman, B. 1965. "Developmental Sequence in Small Groups." *Psychological Bulletin* 63 (6): 384–99.

19. Tuckman, B., and M. A. C. Jensen. 1977. "Stages of Small-Group Development Revisited." *Group & Organization Studies* 2 (4): 419–27.

20. Coppola, M. N. 2008. "Leveraging Team Building Strategies." *Healthcare Executive* 23 (3): 70–74.

21. Ledlow, G. R., and M. N. Coppola. 2018. *Leadership for Health Professionals: Theory, Skills, and Applications*, 3rd ed. Sudbury, MA: Jones & Bartlett Learning.

22. Study.com. 2017. "Stages of Group Development: Forming, Storming, Norming, Performing & Adjourning." Accessed February 6. http://

study.com/academy/lesson/stages-of-group-development-forming-storming-forming-performing-adjourning.html.

23. Project-Management.com. 2016. "The Five Stages of Project Team Development." Published November 25. https://project-management.com/the-five-stages-of-project-team-development/.

24. Glacel, B. P. 1997. "Getting Teams to *Really* Work." *Innovative Leader* 6 (6): 11–20.

25. Rickards, T., and S. Moger. 2000. "Creative Leadership Processes in Project Team Development: An Alternative to Tuckman's Stage Model." *British Journal of Management* 11 (4): 271–83.

26. Hersey, P., K. H. Blanchard, and D. E. Johnson. 2008. *Management of Organizational Behavior: Leading Human Resources*, 9th ed. Upper Saddle River, NJ: Pearson Prentice Hall.

27. Blanchard, K. H., D. Carew, and E. Parisi-Carew. 1990. *The One Minute Manager Builds High Performing Teams*. Escondido, CA: Blanchard Training and Development.

28. Hill, S. E. K. 2016. "Team Leadership." In *Leadership: Theory and Practice*, 7th ed., edited by P. G. Northouse, 366–96. Los Angeles: Sage.

29. Kinlaw, D. C. 1998. *Superior Teams: What They Are and How to Develop Them*. Hampshire, UK: Grove.

30. Larson, C. E., and F. M. J. LaFasto. 1989. *Teamwork: What Must Go Right/What Can Go Wrong*. Newbury Park, CA: Sage.

31. Barge, J. K. 1996. "Leadership Skills and the Dialectics of Leadership in Group Decision Making." In *Communication and Group Decision Making*, 2nd ed., edited by R. Y. Hirokawa and M. S. Poole, 301–42. Thousand Oaks, CA: Sage.

32. Hackman, J. R., and R. E. Walton. 1986. "Leading Groups in Organizations." In *Designing Effective Work Groups*, edited by P. S. Goodman, 72–119. San Francisco: Jossey-Bass.

33. Hackman, J. R. 2002. *Leading Teams: Setting the Stage for Great Performances*. Boston: Harvard Business Review Press.

34. Sainz, A. 2014. "Fighting Infant Mortality Still Tough in Memphis." *Washington Examiner*. Published February 6. www.washingtonexaminer.com/fighting-infant-mortality-still-tough-in-memphis/article/2543559.

POWER AND PUBLIC HEALTH LEADERSHIP

James W. Holsinger Jr.

Learning Objectives

Upon completion of this chapter, you should be able to

- develop your personal definition of *power* and compare it to the definitions provided;
- distinguish between hard power and soft power;
- compare and contrast power, authority, and influence;
- use the expanded French-Raven taxonomy to discuss the seven kinds of power;
- analyze the key differences between position power and personal power;
- identify the situational leadership styles associated with the various kinds of power;
- compare and contrast the social exchange theory and the strategic contingencies theory for the acquisition of power;
- understand the various influence tactics;
- compare and contrast the 11 proactive influence tactics; and
- employ the four guideline questions for determining ethical action.

Focus on Leadership Competencies

This chapter emphasizes the following Association of Schools and Programs of Public Health (ASPPH) leadership competencies:

- Develop strategies to motivate others for collaborative problem solving, decision-making, and evaluation.
- Collaborate with diverse groups.
- Demonstrate team building, negotiation, and conflict management skills.

(continued)

- Describe alternative strategies for collaboration and partnership among organizations, focused on public health goals.
- Influence others to achieve high standards of performance and accountability.

It also addresses the following Council on Linkages public health leadership competency:

- Modifies organizational practices in consideration of changes.

Note: See the appendix at the end of the book for complete lists of competencies.

Introduction

Lord Acton[1] famously asserted that "Power tends to corrupt, and absolute power corrupts absolutely." In recalling this quote, people all too often leave out the words "tends to" and simply state that "power corrupts." In reality, power does not need to be a source of corruption, and leaders in public health have an obligation to use it for the good of their followers and their organization. As John Gardner[2] and others[3,4,5] have noted, leadership and power are closely intertwined. People often speak of power in terms of an agent who possesses it and a target person who is affected by it. For the purposes of our discussion, the agent who possesses power is the leader, and the target person is the follower.

Power can be defined in a variety of ways, and several definitions are provided in exhibit 12.1. Most of those definitions have two main elements in common: potential and influence. The word *potential* recognizes that power may or may not be used, and *influence* reflects the leader's ability to affect the beliefs, attitudes, and actions of followers. For our purposes, we will define *power* as the capacity or potential of a leader to influence one or more followers to achieve goals or outcomes desired by the leader in a specific situation.

James MacGregor Burns[4] wrote that all leadership is dependent on the leader's use of power to influence followers and to accomplish the task at hand. In considering both leadership and power, he understood both as relationships. Power collapses without the essentials of motive and resources. Max Weber[6(p152)] wrote that "'Power' (*Macht*) is the probability that one actor within a social relationship will be in a position to carry out his own will despite resistance, regardless of the basis on which this probability rests." Analysis of power within its context and with attention to individuals' motives and constraints is more difficult than the study of raw power itself; thus, true understanding of the nature of power has remained elusive.

EXHIBIT 12.1
Definitions of
Power

The force that can be applied to work

—Bernard M. Bass

The ability to get what one wants

—Michael Parenti

The ability to get things done

—Rosabeth Moss Kanter

The ability to cause or prevent change

—Rollo May

The potential ability to influence behavior, to change the course of events, to overcome resistance, to get people to do things they would not otherwise do

—Jeffrey Pfeffer

The absolute capacity of an individual agent to influence the behavior or attitudes of one or more designated target persons at a given point in time

—Gary Yukl

The potential ability of one person in an organization to influence other people to bring about desired outcomes

—Richard L. Daft

Influence potential—the resource that enables a leader to gain compliance or commitment from others

—Paul H. Hersey, Kenneth H. Blanchard, and Dewey E. Johnson

The capacity or potential to influence

—Peter G. Northouse

The ability to make something happen

—James G. Clawson

Sources: Bass, B. M. 2008. *The Bass Handbook of Leadership: Theory, Research, and Managerial Applications*, 4th ed. New York: Free Press; Parenti, M. 1978. *Power and the Powerless*. New York: St. Martin's Press; Kanter, R. M. 1993. *Men and Women of the Corporation*, 2nd ed. New York: Basic Books; May, R. 1972. *Power and Innocence: A Search for the Sources of Violence*. New York: Dell; Pfeffer, J. 1994. *Managing with Power: Politics and Influence in Organizations*. Boston: Harvard Business School Press; Yukl, G. 2013. *Leadership in Organizations*, 8th ed. Upper Saddle River, NJ: Prentice Hall; Daft, R. L. 2015. *The Leadership Experience*, 6th ed. Mason, OH: South-Western; Hersey, P. H., K. H. Blanchard, and D. E. Johnson. 2008. *Management of Organizational Behavior: Leading Human Resources*, 9th ed. Upper Saddle River, NJ: Pearson Prentice Hall; Northouse, P. G. 2016. *Leadership: Theory and Practice*, 7th ed. Los Angeles: Sage; Clawson, J. G. *Level Three Leadership: Getting Below the Surface*, 3rd ed. Upper Saddle River, NJ: Pearson Prentice Hall.

Power is most often ascribed to political figures, military commanders, and senior governmental officials; however, it clearly plays a major role in the practice of leadership across a variety of settings, including public health. Power should be viewed not as a thing but as a collective attribute. It is based on relationships that exist between leaders and followers, and it relies on the behaviors of both. Leaders who possess power draw not only on their own motivations but also on those of their followers. Both leadership and power are based on the achievement of a purpose or purposes, but leadership may, in fact, be more limited in nature than power. All leaders may actually or potentially possess power, but not all individuals with power are leaders. Leadership requires that the use of power be intertwined with the goals and needs of followers.

The leader–follower relationship is based on interactions between individuals who have different levels of power and motivation but are engaged in a common or joint purpose.[4] In this discussion, we will work under the premise that leaders who understand and utilize power will be more effective than those who do not, or prefer not to, use it.

Consider This

"Although leadership and the exercise of power are distinguishable activities, they overlap and interweave in important ways."

—John W. Gardner[2(p56)]

As you consider this statement, how do you think power and leadership overlap and interweave?

Power, Authority, and Influence

Power can be described in a variety of ways. It can be labeled "hard" or "soft," and it can be examined in terms of the authority it provides the leader or the influence it has on followers.

Hard and Soft Power

hard power
Power based on the leader's position within the organization and the authority vested in the leader; also called *position power*.

Power is usually divided into two categories: (1) **hard power**, also called *position power* or *formal power*, and (2) **soft power**, also called *personal power*. Hard power arises from the position the leader holds within the organization. It is based on the authority vested in the leader, and it allows the leader to issue orders or commands and administer rewards or punishments. Hard power is important for the functioning of most individuals in leadership positions. However, it is also a temporary entitlement that exists only while the person holds a particular position or office. Thus, leaders who possess hard power often live with the fear of losing it—and the more power they possess, the more they have to lose.[5] Effective leaders need to know how to acquire hard power, how to effectively and appropriately use it, and how to gracefully surrender it.

soft power
Power based on the leader's personality characteristics and the personal relationships the leader has with followers; also called *personal power*.

Soft power is based on the personality characteristics of the leader and the personal relationships that the leader has with followers. It stems from the key personal attributes that represent the leader's potential to accomplish the tasks assigned. It involves the use of persuasion to resolve conflicts, the development of shared interests to enhance the sense of community, and the integration of personal characteristics and internal capabilities with the requirements of the external world. Personal power belongs to the individual; unlike position power, it cannot be withdrawn. In the sixteenth century, Niccolo Machiavelli[7(p96)] posed the question of "whether it be better to be loved than feared, or the reverse." Love, in this quotation, represents soft or personal power, whereas fear represents hard or position power. Like Etzioni,[8] Machiavelli believed that leaders should aim to be both loved and feared; however, he concluded that "it is much better to be feared than loved if you cannot be both."[7(p96)] Under Machiavelli's reasoning, leadership relationships based on fear (hard power) will last longer because the followers are aware that they may have to suffer the consequences of their actions. Relationships based on love (soft power), on the other hand, are more volatile and may be quickly terminated, often without significant consequences. Nonetheless, Machiavelli also warned against taking fear (hard power) to an extreme, because doing so can result in hatred and negative actions in opposition to the leader's and the organization's best interests.

Soft power is essential in public health, and all public health leaders should strive to clearly understand the nature of their personal power. Leaders who can effectively influence followers through soft power can minimize their reliance on hard power, using it only in a supportive role when absolutely necessary.

Authority

Authority is an important aspect of hard power, and it comprises the advantages, duties, rights, and obligations linked to a person's position.[9] Leaders who possess authority are able to make decisions for the organization within a certain range, based on the scope of authority delegated to them by virtue of their position. They also can make certain requests of followers, and those requests must then be carried out. Effective leaders must make a point to use legitimate authority in an ethical manner.

Authority—both formal and informal—plays an important role in public health practice, as well as in virtually every other aspect of life. In analyzing authority, Weber[6] considered three types: (1) rational authority, (2) traditional authority, and (3) charismatic authority. **Rational authority** is based on legal authority associated with a specific role or office, and it is bound by the rules under which it is granted. **Traditional authority** is based on the values, attitudes, behaviors, and social norms that are ingrained in social systems, and it requires obedience and conformity from the group in which it is based. Both rational and traditional authority are formally conferred based on the individual's assignment to a specific role. Formal authority is especially notable

authority
The advantages, duties, rights, and obligations linked to a specific position within an organization.

rational authority
Legal authority associated with a specific role or office and bound by the rules under which it is granted.

traditional authority
Authority based on tradition, established values, and social norms.

in hierarchical organizations, where various levels of power and authority are delegated downward. Often in organizations, obedience to authority is deemed a moral imperative.

charismatic authority
A form of authority that is informally granted from below based on an individual's personal characteristics.

Charismatic authority, on the other hand, is a form of informal authority based on an individual's characteristics. This type of authority is bestowed from below, with no formal confirmation from the organization and without regard for the individual's formal role. It is highly personal in nature, and it stems from followers' recognition that the leader possesses exceptional qualities (e.g., skill, expertise, technical competence, experience). Individuals who possess charismatic authority may have no specific organizational power, yet they are nonetheless important assets. The organization can benefit greatly from their personal competence and the guidance and assistance they provide to others.

Locus of Control

locus of control
A concept reflecting the degree to which individuals feel they can control their life situations or are affected by outside forces.

Closely related to authority is the concept of **locus of control**, which was first considered in the middle of the twentieth century. One's locus of control can be described as either internal or external, and it is a qualitative measure of the degree of control one feels over experiences and events in life. In other words, it indicates whether people feel that authority resides with them internally or with external entities. People with a high internal locus of control feel that they are in control of their life situations and in control of the consequences of the decisions that they make. They view success or failure in their lives as a result of their own actions, which makes them more self-reliant and proactive in dealing with success or failure. People with a high external locus of control feel that external forces—whether other people, outside conditions, or simply luck—play a powerful role in determining their life situations. Such individuals tend to react to events as they occur, have less confidence in their own abilities, and rely on the judgment of people whom they perceive to be in authority.

influence
The way a leader affects a follower, particularly in terms of the impact of requests and decisions.

The study of locus of control with regard to leadership is limited, but it suggests that individuals whose locus of control is internal are more likely to develop as leaders than individuals whose locus of control is external. In addition, groups led by people with an internal locus of control appear to perform more successfully than those led by people with an external locus of control. An internal locus of control is often associated with leadership characteristics such as confidence and motivation, as well as with energy to complete the tasks at hand. Leaders with an external locus of control are more likely to feel insecure, and they may seek to compensate for these insecurities through the use of coercive power.[5] However, locus of control is only one of many important considerations for the development of effective leadership.

commitment
An outcome in which a follower agrees internally with a request or decision made by the leader and works to carry it out.

Influence

Influence is a key concept in the definitions of both *leadership* and *power*. In brief, it refers to the way the leader affects the follower. More specifically, it refers to the impact of the exchange that occurs when a leader makes a request or decision affecting a follower. This exchange can lead to any of three types of outcomes: commitment, compliance, or resistance. **Commitment** is an outcome in which the follower agrees internally with the leader's request or decision and makes every effort to effectively carry it out. **Compliance** is an outcome in which the follower carries out the wishes of the leader but is unenthusiastic, making little or no effort to perform effectively. Compliance commonly occurs when the leader fails to convince the follower of a task's importance or effectiveness, and it typically does not produce the most successful results. In the case of compliance, the leader's influence has affected the follower's behavior but not the follower's attitude. **Resistance**, the third type of influence outcome, occurs when the follower is opposed to the leader's request or decision and makes a minimal effort to carry it out. Resistance can take a variety of forms. Resisting followers might simply refuse to comply, or they might pretend to comply while actively and willfully trying to sabotage the effort. They might try to overturn the leader's decision by appealing to a higher authority, or they might make excuses for failing to comply.

To effectively influence the follower, the leader must consider the motives and perceptions of the follower in relation to the request or decision being made, as well as the situation within which the influence process is occurring. Kelman[10] identifies three influence processes: instrumental compliance, internalization, and personal identification. The three processes differ significantly from one another but can often occur simultaneously. In the **instrumental compliance** process, the follower completes a task or carries out a decision requested by the leader with the understanding that a tangible reward or punishment will occur based on the follower's action. The response is instrumental in nature in that the follower's compliance is based solely on the reward or punishment, and the follower is likely to do the minimum amount to obtain the reward or to avoid being punished. Instrumental compliance may also occur when the follower accepts being influenced by the leader in order to be perceived in a favorable light by the leader. In such cases, the follower receives satisfaction through the social effect of accepting the leader's influence. The second influence process, **internalization**, occurs when the follower commits to supporting and implementing the leader's request or decision because the tasks are desirable in and of themselves and compatible with the follower's personal beliefs and values. In such cases, the follower completes the tasks without regard to possible rewards or sanctions and derives satisfaction from the tasks' completion. **Personal identification**, the third process, occurs when the follower attempts to imitate the leader's behaviors and thus identifies with the leader's attitudes, goals, and objectives. Acceptance and esteem needs play a key role in motivating the follower to gain the leader's approval, and a desirable relationship between the follower and the leader typically results. The act of conforming produces satisfaction based on the follower's identification with the leader.

compliance
An outcome in which a follower carries out the leader's wishes but is unenthusiastic, making little or no effort to perform effectively.

resistance
A outcome in which a follower is opposed to the leader's request or decision and makes a minimal effort to carry it out.

instrumental compliance
An influence process that occurs when a follower completes a task requested by the leader with the understanding that a reward or punishment will result.

internalization
An influence process that occurs when a follower commits to a task requested by the leader because the task is deemed desirable in and of itself and compatible with the follower's beliefs and values.

personal identification
An influence process that occurs when a follower attempts to imitate the leader's behaviors and thus identifies with the leader's attitudes, goals, and objectives.

An Expanded French-Raven Taxonomy of Power

In 1959, French and Raven[11] developed a taxonomy of power, which identified five bases of power: legitimate power, reward power, coercive power, referent power, and expert power. The taxonomy expanded in 1965 when Cartwright[12] added ecological power, and it grew again in 1972 when Pettigrew[13] determined that control over information also served as a source of power. The expanded **French-Raven taxonomy of power**, therefore, consists of seven kinds of power, as shown in exhibit 12.2. These seven types can be divided into two categories: position power and personal power.[8,14] Position power and personal power may overlap, but they are generally considered independent of each other.[15]

Legitimate Power

Legitimate power is based on the titles, positions, or roles that people have as a result of their formal assignment within the organization.[3] The leader possesses the prerogatives that accrue to the position held, as well as the rights and responsibilities pertaining to it, and the followers must accept the leader's right to direct their activities and make decisions. According to Bass,[16(p282)]

EXHIBIT 12.2
The Expanded French-Raven Taxonomy of Power

Position Power	Personal Power
• **Legitimate Power:** Followers comply because they believe that the leader has the right to make the request and the follower has the obligation to comply.	• **Referent Power:** Followers comply because they admire or identify with the leader and want to gain the leader's approval.
• **Reward Power:** The follower complies in order to obtain rewards controlled by the leader.	• **Expert Power:** Followers comply because they believe that the leader has special knowledge about the best way to do something.
• **Coercive Power:** The follower complies in order to avoid punishments controlled by the leader.	
• **Information Power:** The leader has control over the flow of information.	
• **Ecological Power:** The leader has substantial control over the situation, including the physical environment, workflow and organization, and the technology utilized.	

Source: Data from Yukl, G. 2013. *Leadership in Organizations*, 8th ed. Upper Saddle River, NJ: Prentice Hall.

"legitimate power is based on norms and expectations that group members hold regarding behaviors that are appropriate in a given role or position." If followers feel that the leader holds attitudes that are appropriate to their norms, they are more apt to accept the leader's power as legitimate.

French and Raven[11] describe three possible sources of legitimate power: (1) cultural values that give leaders the right to employ power, (2) acceptance of a social structure in which certain positions bestow power, and (3) appointment of an individual to a position of power by an appropriate organizational entity. Most followers accept leadership based on legitimate power, but they tend to be more enthusiastic when leadership has a basis in expert power. Legitimate power produces an influence process that is largely based on the consent of the followers to be directed.[17] Followers' compliance is often based on their expectations of certain benefits in return,[18] their loyalty to the organization, their own expectations of obeying authority figures, or the perceived appropriateness of the task with regard to the core values of the organization or society at large. Yukl[9] offers guidelines for the use of legitimate authority. Among other things, he highlights the need for the leader to make requests clearly and politely, to not exceed their authority, and to follow the appropriate channels. Whenever a leader exercises legitimate authority, compliance should be insisted upon and verified.

Reward Power

Reward power is based on the ability of leaders to give appropriate rewards to followers. It typically stems from the authority a leader has over pay increases, bonuses, promotions, improved work schedules, expense accounts or budgets, and such perks as a reserved parking space or a more prestigious office.[9] Thus, reward power has a clear basis in the leader's formal authority. For reward power to exist, the leader must control the necessary resources, and followers must perceive that the leader has the ability to provide things that the follower would like to have.[3] Reward power suggests a *quid pro quo* relationship between the leader and the follower, and the leader must have the authority to carry out any promises made. If the leader lacks credibility, reward power will fail. Use of reward power can be enhanced when leaders understand each follower's motivating intangibles and use the most important rewards in a tailored approach for each individual.

A common pitfall in the use of reward power is the classic "rewarding A but hoping for B" error. As Kerr[19(p769)] so aptly puts it, "Numerous examples exist of reward systems that are fouled up in that behaviors which are rewarded are those which the rewarder is trying to *discourage*, while the behavior he desires is not being rewarded at all." Leaders may be surprised to discover that the behaviors being rewarded in their systems are not conducive to the organization's goals or are even antithetical to the goals' accomplishment. Leaders therefore must determine exactly which behaviors are being rewarded, and they need to make sure that those behaviors are in fact the ones they are seeking from their followers. Kerr[19(p782)] concludes: "For an organization to *act* upon its members, the formal reward system should positively reinforce desired behaviors, not constitute an obstacle to be overcome."

Yukl[9] offers succinct guidelines for the use of reward power. They highlight the need to offer a desired reward that is not only fair but also ethical, to promise only what can be delivered, to develop simple criteria to determine whether rewards have been earned, and to avoid manipulating followers.

Coercive Power

Coercive power can be used by leaders to punish followers or to recommend punishment based on the leaders' authority to do so. Traditionally, coercive power has been associated with military and political leaders; by comparison, other organizational leaders usually have far less authority to exact punishment. Coercive power has been on the wane particularly in governmental or quasi-governmental organizations such as public health departments.[20] In the United States, abusive coercive power is largely prohibited.

Nonetheless, coercive power is present when a leader has the authority to demote or terminate followers, refuse followers' pay increases, or criticize followers and their work. When a leader engages a follower and the follower fails to perform or respond, some consequences may be appropriate.[3] Use of coercive power varies depending on the situation at hand, the organizational context, and the degree of coercive power the organization authorizes for its leaders. In some cases, coercive power can help ensure discipline, but it is difficult to use and can have significant negative side effects, including anger or resentment among followers. Coercive power is almost impossible to use in a lateral fashion from peer to peer; when used in this way, it often results in retaliation or significant conflict. In public health, use of coercive power should be minimal. Its primary function should be to deter illegal or inappropriate behavior that damages the organization or its reputation (e.g., theft, embezzlement), threatens the safety of oneself or others, or shows willful disregard for orders or requests. Coercive power in an appropriate organizational context may result in compliance, but it is unlikely to produce commitment. Ultimately, coercive power is simply the negative side of position power.

Information Power

information power Power based on the leader's ability to control the flow of information that followers consider important.

Information power, which Pettigrew[13] added to the taxonomy in 1972, is a form of position power based on one's ability to control the flow information that other people consider important. People often say that "information is power," and certainly, in public health organizations, information can be a critical resource. Obviously, certain individuals within an organization will possess more information than others. However, effective public health leaders should be sensitive to their followers' needs for current and useful information, and they should seek to empower followers through the broad sharing of that information.[21] Kouzes and Posner[22] point out that information is worthless if it is not connected with the people who need to possess it; thus, leaders must ensure that they and all necessary team members are closely connected to information sources that help the organization accomplish its goals.

Leaders who possess information power have a heightened ability to influence followers' attitudes and perceptions, and they can also minimize followers' ability to dispute the leaders' own perceptions. Leaders should avoid using such influence improperly—for instance, they should not control the flow of information for the purpose of hiding their own errors or calling attention to their individual accomplishments. The unnecessary withholding of information can lead to distrust and other negative effects within the organization, and failure to appropriately distribute information can prevent the organization from being effective.

Given that access to information is often based on the organization's hierarchy, the release of information from leaders to followers must occur in such a manner that the organization will reach its goals. However, the growth of the Internet and social media has markedly increased the amount of information available, and the availability of this information is not always based on the organizational hierarchy. People can possess exclusive access to information—and thus information power—regardless of their formal position in the organization. As a result, information power may be directed not only from the top down but also upwardly and laterally.

Ecological Power

Ecological power is based on the leader's control of the physical work environment, technological systems, and organizational structure in which people work. It gives leaders the ability to influence performance by changing the context within which leaders and followers function. Architectural changes, for instance, might result in workflow redesign and new patterns of follower interaction, both with each other and with the leader. Likewise, altering the organizational structure can affect the way that followers view workplace opportunities and constraints, which in turn may influence their behavior and motivation.[12] Schein[23] finds that leaders can influence follower behaviors and attitudes by changing the organizational culture. Changing the culture is a difficult and time-consuming process, but it may be necessary if the existing culture is impeding leadership or creating a disconnect between the values of the followers and those of the leader. Ecological power is dependent on both the leader and the followers sharing an organizational values system.

ecological power
Power based on the leader's control of the physical work environment, technological systems, and organizational structure in which people work.

Referent Power

Referent power, one of the two types of personal power in the taxonomy, is based not on the position the leader holds but rather on the personal characteristics the leader demonstrates. When followers respect and admire the leader, they are far more likely to accept direction and carry out requests. Leaders gain referent power by demonstrating characteristics that produce loyalty and emotional attachment among followers and inspire followers to want to emulate them. Personal identification of the follower with the leader is the strongest form of referent power.[8]

The leaders most likely to engender referent power are those who are trustworthy, who show concern for followers' needs and feelings, and who both express and demonstrate a consistent set of personal and professional values. Character and integrity are essential for this type of power. Manipulation and exploitation of followers are counterproductive, as is flattery. When a strong bond exists between the leader and the follower, the leader usually has no need to exploit referent power; the leader can simply ask the follower to carry out a task. However, leaders should not use referent power for requests that are outside the limits of loyalty and cooperation in the work setting.

Yukl[9] summarizes several ways in which leaders can acquire and maintain referent power. They should demonstrate acceptance and regard for followers, avoid insincere forms of interaction, and support and defend followers when appropriate. Promises should be kept, and favors should be extended without the follower's request. Self-sacrifice on the leader's part can further demonstrate concern for the follower. Since imitation is the sincerest form of flattery, followers will often model themselves after leaders they admire. Leaders therefore should always seek to model appropriate behavior.

 Consider This

"Behaviour that's admired is the path to power among people everywhere."

—Anonymous[24]

Does admired behavior act as a form of influence? If so, why? If not, why?

Expert Power

Expert power, another form of personal power, is based on the leader's possession of task-relevant knowledge, skills, and attributes. Daft[21(p374)] writes: "When a leader is a true expert, subordinates go along with recommendations because of his or her superior knowledge." Possession of unique knowledge is common in leadership positions but may also occur at other levels of the organization, and it affects interactions among followers, peers, and superiors. Regardless of where it is found in the organization, expert power can influence other people's behaviors and affect key decisions made in the organization.

The amount of expert power a person possesses depends on the degree to which other people in the organization depend on the person's expertise for problem solving or task completion, the importance of the problems or tasks being addressed, and the degree to which the person's expertise is recognized and seen as reliable. In some cases, perception of expertise may be more important than reality. Leaders can acquire or expand expert power by learning technical skills, leading in a manner that builds credibility, developing practical experience, and pursuing additional education. Followers often come to depend on an expert leader and will often carry out the leader's wishes without requiring a rationale for doing so.

Yukl[9] offers several guidelines for the use of expert power. Leaders should remain confident and decisive, even in crisis situations, and they should clearly explain the rationale for their requests, providing evidence as appropriate. To avoid losing expert power, leaders must not make careless or inconsistent statements, lie or exaggerate to followers, or misrepresent the facts of a situation. Regardless of the leader's expertise, the follower's ideas and concerns should be not only heard, but also considered.

Using the Various Types of Power

Effective public health leaders should be prepared to use all seven forms of power depending on the situations they encounter. Position power will often be effective within the public health organization, particularly when dealing with employee followers, but it will not avail in all situations. Personal power—both referent and expert—will be essential when engaging with peers, constituents, and stakeholders. Regardless of the situation, effective public health leaders should only rarely use coercive power.

The concept of **dependency** is closely related to several of the power types included in the taxonomy. The more a follower depends on the leader, the greater is the leader's power.[25] Followers may become dependent on their leader for information or expertise, or for resources that the leader controls. A major area of dependency involves the follower's need to have a job and earn an income. This type of dependency can vary based on economic conditions: Followers tend to be less dependent on their leaders if job opportunities are plentiful, but they are likely to be more dependent if job opportunities are few. In a similar manner, leaders may become increasingly dependent on followers if they feel that replacing those followers will be difficult. According to Mintzberg,[26] three main characteristics affect dependency and power in organizations: importance, scarcity, and nonsubstitutability. When a leader controls resources that the follower considers highly important, and when those resources are considered scarce and have no substitutes, the follower's dependency increases, giving the leader greater power. On the other hand, when the leader controls resources that are considered unimportant or widely available, or when a suitable substitute is available, the follower's dependency and the leader's power decline.

dependency
A source of power based on the leader's control over something that the follower desires or depends on.

 Leadership Application Case: Gone by Midnight

The Leadership Application Case at the beginning of this book provides realistic scenarios for the application of key leadership concepts covered in the text. See the section marked "Chapter 12 Application" for the scenario and discussion questions that correspond with this chapter.

Power and Situational Leadership

Hersey, Blanchard, and Johnson[3] investigated the use of power in leader–follower relationships by applying the concepts of situational leadership (previously discussed in chapters 4 and 11) to the expanded French-Raven taxonomy. In doing so, they demonstrated a series of relationships that exist between follower readiness level (R1–R4), leadership style (S1–S4), and the type of power that drives each leadership style. Their model is illustrated in exhibit 12.3. To achieve results under the model, the leader needs to use the appropriate leadership style for a given follower readiness level, and that leadership style must be supported by the appropriate type of power.

Coercive Power and S1 Leadership

Followers at the R1 readiness level primarily require guidance and direction from their leaders, meaning that the appropriate leadership style is S1 (directing). The S1 style involves a high level of directive behavior and a low level of supportive behavior. Leaders who provide too much supportive behavior at this level risk coming across as permissive or making the error of "rewarding A but hoping for B." Under this model, the S1 leadership style is best supported by coercive power, based on the follower's perception that the leader has the authority to levy consequences if the follower fails to perform.[3] Such

EXHIBIT 12.3
Situational Leadership Applied to the French-Raven Power Framework

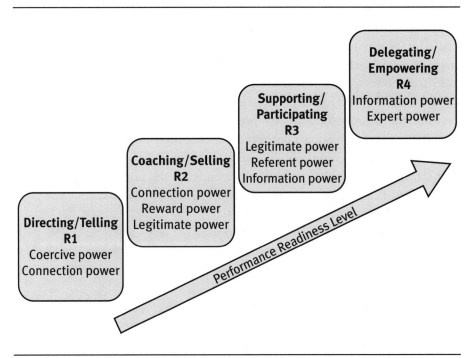

Source: Data from Hersey, P. H., K. H. Blanchard, and D. E. Johnson. 2008. *Management of Organizational Behavior: Leading Human Resources*, 9th ed. Upper Saddle River, NJ: Pearson Prentice Hall.

consequences may include reduction in pay, reprimand, transfer, demotion, or even termination from the job. Without the support of coercive power, the leader's efforts to influence the follower will not be successful. Leaders who rely on coercive power must be prepared to follow through on expected sanctions, or else their effectiveness will be lost. Leaders will also lose their effectiveness if sanctions are applied regardless of performance. As noted previously, coercive power should be used only rarely, and when it is used, it should be applied fairly and clearly based on performance.

Connection Power and S1/S2 Leadership

As the follower is beginning to advance from the R1 readiness level to R2, a high level of directive leadership behavior is still necessary, but supportive behavior must now be increased. The appropriate leadership styles at this point are S1 and S2 (coaching), and both of these styles will be most effective if the leader possesses connection power. **Connection power**, as explained by Hersey, Blanchard, and Johnson,[3] is based on the perceived association of the leader with influential people and organizations. To some extent, it is a component of ecological power, which is otherwise not part of this model. This power is driven by the fact that followers at the R1 and R2 readiness levels wish to avoid negative sanctions and hope to associate themselves with leaders who have strong connections with important people both within and outside the organization. Hersey, Blanchard, and Johnson are quick to note that the follower's *perceptions* of the leader's connections are what matter; real connections may not even be required.

connection power
Power based on the perceived association of the leader with influential people and organizations.

Reward Power and S2 Leadership

The R2 level represents a low to moderate degree of readiness, and the follower at this point requires a high level of both supportive and directive behavior from the leader. The S2 leadership style is appropriate at this level, and the leader's coaching is significantly enhanced when it is supported by reward power. Followers at the R2 level are willing to comply with the leader and develop new skills if they perceive that the leader has the authority to reward performance appropriately.[3] For use of reward power to be effective, the reward must be offered in a timely manner, it must be perceived as appropriate for the level of effort expended, and, most importantly, it must be something that the follower truly regards as a reward. Since the use of tangible rewards (e.g., money) is not always possible, leaders should know what types of intangible rewards most effectively motivate particular followers. Proper use of rewards at this stage helps reinforce the follower's growth in the direction desired by the leader.

Legitimate Power and S2/S3 Leadership

As the follower's readiness level moves from R2 to R3, the most appropriate leadership styles are S2 and S3 (supporting), both of which are supported by legitimate power. Legitimate power is based on the follower's perception that the leader is empowered—either by role, title, or position in the organization—to make certain decisions.[3] Once leaders have legitimized their power, they are able to gain follower compliance by virtue of their position within the organization. Thus, they can reduce the amount of directive behavior and increase the amount of supportive behavior, which is extremely helpful to leaders using either coaching or participating (supporting) leadership styles. The use of legitimate power tends to be more successful with R2 and R3 followers than it is with followers at the R1 and R4 levels. At R1, followers tend to have little interest in the leader's title, whereas R4 followers tend to be more interested in the leader's expertise and information.

Referent Power and S3 Leadership

Followers at the R3 readiness level are often insecure or may even be unwilling to perform the tasks assigned to them. Thus, a highly supportive S3 leadership style is needed to provide them with encouragement. Referent power, which is based on the perceived attractiveness of the leader's personal attributes, such as honesty and integrity, is key at this stage.[3] A leader who establishes trust, confidence, and a good rapport with followers is likely to be admired and seen as someone to be emulated. Followers at the R3 level do not require a large amount of direction but instead need support and communication from the leader; thus, the appropriate leadership style relies heavily on a strong leader–follower relationship. Leaders can use referent power to engage followers in a positive manner and to develop the confidence of followers who may be insecure.

Information Power and S3/S4 Leadership

At the R3 and R4 readiness levels, followers are performing at an above-average level, and the appropriate leadership styles are S3 and S4 (delegating), both of which can be undergirded by information power. Information power is based on the perception that the leader possesses or has access to important information.[3] Information power can exist with or without expertise; the key aspect is that the leader can control the flow of information to followers. Such control affords the leader a significant ability to influence the behavior of others. The movement of followers from R3 to R4 can best be facilitated by a leader whom followers perceive as able to clarify the requirements for a task and provide access to the necessary information. Followers at the R4 level are both willing and able, and leaders who use information power will be able to appropriately lead them.

Effective Public Health Leaders . . .

. . . recognize that "power is a matter of perception; use it or lose it!"
—Paul H. Hersey, Kenneth H. Blanchard, and Dewey E. Johnson[3(p163)]

Expert Power and S4 Leadership

Followers who have reached the R4 level of readiness are confident and competent for the task at hand, and they require little supportive or directive behavior from the leader. They, for the most part, are willing and able to function on their own, and they relate best to leaders who possess knowledge, skills, and ability—traits that highly motivated followers respect and consider important for completing the assigned task. Thus, leaders can achieve the best results with an S4 (delegating) leadership style supported by expert power. Expert power is based on the follower's perception that the leader possesses the appropriate experience, education, and expertise.[3]

Use of Power in Situational Leadership

From a situational leadership perspective, position power (i.e., coercive power, connection power, reward power, legitimate power, and information power) and personal power (i.e., referent power and expert power) interact to create an influence system that largely determines the public health leader's effectiveness. Position power is delegated to the leader from the organization based on the trust and confidence that exists between the leader and the delegating authority; thus, the leader earns position power on a daily basis by building and maintaining this trust and confidence. Personal power, on the other hand, is granted by followers based on the trust and confidence they have in the leader; thus, the leader earns it each day by building and maintaining effective follower relationships.

Perception is the key to power in situational leadership. The perceptions of followers determine the magnitude of the leader's personal power, whereas the perceptions of the appointing authority determine the magnitude of the leader's position power. The position power and the personal power that a leader possesses tend to affect one another. Often, a leader's ability to use position power (e.g., the ability to grant rewards) will create strong perceptions among followers that increase the amount of personal power the leader possesses. Likewise, a leader's ability to use personal power might lead the delegating authority to perceive that the leader is well liked, possesses expertise, and has good information, which in turn may lead the authority to grant the leader more position power. Leaders in public health have a limited amount of power, and this power must be sustained. Erosion of the bases of power will result in the loss of the leader's effectiveness.

The Acquisition of Power

Power is not static in nature. It can be acquired through a variety of means and may change over time based on the organization's situation or context. Of the various theories that describe how power is gained and lost, two of the most important are social exchange theory and strategic contingencies theory. Both theories demonstrate the usefulness of expertise as a way to gain power and authority.

Social Exchange Theory

social exchange theory
A theory that examines reciprocal influence processes that occur in small groups and determine how power and influence are gained or lost.

Social exchange theory examines the reciprocal influence processes that occur in small groups and determine how power and influence are gained or lost. From childhood, individuals begin to understand social exchanges; become aware of the benefits of those exchanges, whether psychological (e.g., respect, affection, love) or material (e.g., food, shelter, money); and develop an expectation that such social exchanges will be equitably or reciprocally handled.

Hollander[27,28] and Jacobs[17] have applied this theory to issues of leadership and power. Followers maintain certain expectations of the leadership role within their group, and their expectations are significantly influenced by the leader's loyalty and leadership competency. In determining the level of status and power to grant to the leader, group members consider the leader's probable contributions to the group's work. Such contributions may be related to the leader's good judgment, access to information, control of resources, or expertise. If the leader develops effective proposals that are successfully implemented, the level of trust between the leader and the followers will likely increase, resulting in enhanced status and influence for the leader. However, if the leader's proposals fail, followers may reassess their relationship with the leader, potentially resulting in a loss of the leader's status and power. In reassessing after a failure, followers will likely consider how much control the leader had over the terms of the failure, whether the leader showed incompetence or poor judgment, and whether the leader acted selfishly or irresponsibly. The followers' perception of these and other factors will determine the extent of the damage to the exchange relationship. The leader's loss of status and power will correlate with the degree of failure perceived by the followers; it may also be influenced by how much status and power the leader possessed at the beginning of the process.

strategic contingencies theory
A theory that examines how power is gained and lost by various parts of an organization and how such power distribution influences the organization's effectiveness.

Social exchange theory expects that leaders will be competent to deal with problems as they arise. Leaders who fail to deal with serious problems, who do not show initiative, or whose proposals are unsuccessful will forfeit their followers' influence and esteem.[9] In terms of the French-Raven taxonomy, social exchange theory emphasizes expert power rather than reward or referent power. Position power, which is delegated by the appointing authority, is less dependent on followers.

Strategic Contingencies Theory

Strategic contingencies theory focuses on how power is gained or lost by various parts of an organization and how such power distribution influences the organization's effectiveness, particularly when the context is fluid. Hickson and colleagues[29] proposed that the power of a unit or division within an organization depends on three factors: (1) the unit/division's expertise, especially when dealing with difficult problems; (2) the importance of the unit/division to the organization's workflow; and (3) the substitutability of the unit/division's expertise.

All organizations, at one time or another, must deal with critical issues or contingencies, which are usually situational or contextual in nature. To deal with these issues effectively, organizational units/divisions must have individuals who possess expert power. When a unit/division uses its expertise to deal with a critical issue, it will gain power if it effectively resolves the problem, and it will gain additional power if it is the only unit/division with the capability of resolving it. Thus, unique capability and nonsubstitutable expertise are key to determining the amount of power a unit/division has. The shadow side of this theory is that a unit/division occupying a dominant position in the organization might use that position to deny other units/divisions the opportunity to exhibit their own expertise.

In studying strategic contingencies theory, Salancik and Pfeffer[30] found that power allows leaders to deal with the critical issues of the organization but that the way power is developed and used leads the organization to "suboptimize" its performance. However, they conclude that if any criteria other than power were used as the basis for the organization's decisions, a worse result would occur. Saunders[31] also studied the theory and determined that organizations may benefit from moderating the relationship between power and the capacity for power and allowing leaders to consider the importance of power strategies within changing organizational contexts.

Influence Approaches

Power and influence are interrelated in complex ways, but they can nonetheless be regarded as separate functions.[9] Whereas power reflects one's ability to influence other people, **influence tactics** are the behaviors used by one individual to change the behaviors, opinions, or attitudes of another.[32] Yukl, Lepsinger, and Lucia[33] have developed a tool known as the Influence Behavior Questionnaire (IBQ) to measure the influence tactics used by leaders to influence followers. The IBQ distinguishes between four general types of influence tactics: impression management tactics, political tactics, proactive influence tactics, and reactive influence tactics.

Impression Management Tactics

Impression management tactics are behaviors used by individuals to influence the way they are perceived by others. Leaders may use impression management tactics to influence followers to like them or to favorably evaluate them.

influence tactics
Behaviors that are used by one individual to change the behaviors, opinions, or attitudes of another.

impression management tactics
Behaviors used by individuals to influence the way they are perceived by others.

Likewise, followers may use impression management tactics to influence the opinions of their leaders. Exemplification, ingratiation, and self-promotion are key elements in the impression management process. Exemplification behavior is used to exhibit loyalty and dedication, both to the organization's mission and to other individuals. Exemplification behaviors used by leaders typically seek to demonstrate consistency, selflessness, and commitment to the objectives of the group or organization. Exemplification behaviors used by followers may include working longer hours than are required or demonstrating positive behaviors when the leader is watching. Ingratiation behaviors aim to influence another person, whether a leader or follower, to see one's positive qualities, such as consideration, kindness, or friendliness. Such behaviors may involve offering praise, agreeing with the other person's opinions, laughing at the other's witticisms, or expressing interest in the other's personal life. Self-promotion is behavior designed to make a good impression on the other person, often by talking about one's own personal achievements and skills. The decoration of one's office with awards, certificates, and diplomas is a subtle but nonetheless effective means of self-promotion. Impression management tactics may also include intimidation behaviors, which rely on the perception that the power one possesses may be used to harm the other person should that person not perform as desired. Fear or respect is the desired endpoint of intimidation behavior; however, this tactic is a demotivator, not a motivator.

Leaders often use impression management to make followers see them as important, competent, in control, or all three. Typically, successes are celebrated, and failures are downplayed.[34,35] Leaders often claim credit for successes while shifting the blame for failures to the environment.[36] When problems arise, symbolic acts can be extremely important in influencing impressions. Often, simply the presence of the leader in a time of crisis serves as the most effective impression management tool. Conversely, the leader's absence during a crisis can have a strongly negative effect. Consider, for instance, the criticism faced by President George W. Bush when he flew over New Orleans in the aftermath of Hurricane Katrina but did not land, or by President Barack Obama when he decided to continue with vacation plans during the Gulf oil spill crisis in 2010.

Political Tactics

political tactics
Behaviors through which people acquire, develop, and use power, as well as other resources, in an attempt to gain desirable future outcomes.

The acquisition or use of power by a leader can be seen as a largely political process. Pfeffer[34] writes that politics is a means by which leaders are enabled to acquire, develop, and utilize power, as well as other resources, in an effort to gain desirable future outcomes, particularly when the possible outcomes are uncertain. Thus, **political tactics** comprise a variety of behaviors to influence decisions made by the group or organization or to obtain benefits for the group or an individual.

Daft[21] writes that political behavior can enhance the pursuit of organizational goals. However, in employing political tactics, leaders need to be conscious of the various frames of reference through which they can view the world. Early in their development, leaders may begin with a structural frame of reference, in which they see the organization as a machine and strive to make it run with machinelike precision. This framework emphasizes goals, systems, efficiency, and formal authority. As the leaders develop, they begin to see value in the human resources framework, in which the organization is viewed as a family to which they belong. Thus, the emphasis is shifted to people and relationships. A third frame of reference, the political frame, views the organization through the lens of power and schemes, and it emphasizes resource allocation, negotiation, and coalition building. Finally, to reach their full potential, leaders must also have a symbolic frame of reference, in which they see the organization as a theater through which they can harness followers' dreams and emotions. The symbolic framework emphasizes vision, culture, values, and inspiration. All four frames of reference are important, and attempts to lead while using only one or some of them will be incomplete. Effective use of political tactics requires more than just the use of the political framework; it requires the integration of all four.

> **Effective Public Health Leaders . . .**
>
> . . . will consistently use power for the good of their followers and the groups or organizations they lead.

Proactive and Reactive Influence Tactics

Proactive influence tactics have the objective of immediately engaging the follower in taking on a new task or implementing a change. When the follower deems the task or change to be appropriate, a simple request, based on the leader's legitimate power, may be sufficient. However, if the follower resists, the leader may have to take a proactive approach based on rational persuasion. Rational persuasion involves the use of logical arguments, explanations, and factual evidence to influence the follower for the purpose of reaching task objectives.[8] Sometimes, a brief explanation will suffice, but other times, a stronger form of persuasion, with more detailed arguments, will be necessary. The effectiveness of rational persuasion depends on the leader's perceived trustworthiness and credibility.

Yukl[9] and his colleagues identified and defined 11 proactive influence tactics, as shown in exhibit 12.4. In studying the various kinds of tactics, they determined that the four most effective were rational persuasion, consultation, collaboration, and inspirational appeals. As in so many instances involving leadership, the situation or context determines what kind of tactics a leader should employ. Obviously, the appropriateness of any given tactic will depend on the relationship between the leader and the person being influenced, particularly if this person is a subordinate, peer, or superior. Any type of tactic can and will fail if it is used in an unethical or inappropriate manner.

Reactive influence tactics are behaviors used by followers to oppose an unwanted influence attempt or to modify the leader's request to improve its

proactive influence tactics
Behaviors intended to immediately engage the follower in taking on a new task or implementing a change.

reactive influence tactics
Behaviors used by followers to oppose an unwanted influence attempt or to modify the leader's request to improve its acceptability.

EXHIBIT 12.4 Proactive Influence Tactics	Rational Persuasion	The agent uses logical arguments and factual evidence to show a proposal or request is feasible and relevant for attaining important task objectives.
	Apprising	The agent explains how carrying out a request or supporting a proposal will benefit the target personally or help advance the target person's career.
	Inspirational Appeals	The agent makes an appeal to values and ideals or seeks to arouse the target person's emotions to gain commitment for a request or proposal.
	Consultation	The agent encourages the target to suggest improvements in a proposal or to help plan an activity or change for which the target person's support and assistance are desired.
	Exchange	The agent offers an incentive, suggests an exchange of favors, or indicates willingness to reciprocate at a later time if the target will do what the agent requests.
	Collaboration	The agent offers to provide relevant resources and assistance if the target will carry out a request or approve a proposed change.
	Personal Appeals	The agent asks the target to carry out a request or support a proposal out of friendship, or asks for a personal favor before saying what it is.
	Ingratiation	The agent uses praise and flattery before or during an influence attempt, or expresses confidence in the target's ability to carry out a difficult request.
	Legitimating Tactics	The agent seeks to establish the legitimacy of a request or to verify authority to make it by referring to rules, policies, contracts, or precedent.
	Pressure	The agent uses demands, threats, frequent checking, or persistent reminders to influence the target to carry out a request.
	Coalition Tactics	The agent seeks the aid of others to persuade the target to do something, or uses the support of others as a reason for the target to agree.

Source: Reprinted from Yukl, G. 2013. *Leadership in Organizations*, 8th ed. Upper Saddle River, NJ: Prentice Hall. Used by permission of Pearson Education, Inc., New York.

acceptability. Such tactics are attempts to reverse influence, and, as such, they demonstrate the two-way nature of the influence process in leader–follower interactions. In using influence tactics, every individual, whether leader or follower, should be conscious of the types of tactics being used, understand the rationale behind the use of each type, and know the likely effects associated with each one. Leaders should be aware that negative influence tactics tend to produce negative results. Positive results are best achieved through influence tactics that develop followers' self-confidence and self-esteem.

Ethical Considerations for the Use of Power

Leaders have a responsibility to use power ethically in pursuit of the organization's goals. Clearly, however, power can be abused. With regard to power, the leader's integrity and personal motives play an important role in distinguishing between ethical use and unethical abuse.

Leaders can be separated into two categories based on the way they conceive of power and the way they use it. **Personalized leaders** have a significant need for personal power; tend to be impulsive, selfish, and lacking in self-control; and use power for their own interests rather than those of the group.[32] **Socialized leaders**, on the other hand, are more emotionally mature and use power to serve higher goals that benefit the organization, other leaders, and followers.[21] In short, socialized leaders care about others, whereas personalized leaders care about themselves. The personality traits commonly associated with personalized leaders—for instance, being nonegalitarian, exploitative, and self-aggrandizing—tend to be inimical to effective leadership. Socialized leaders exhibit the opposite traits—being egalitarian, supportive, and empowering—and are more ethical in their use of power.

All of the 11 proactive influence tactics listed in exhibit 12.4 can be used appropriately by leaders, or they can be abused. The tactics of rational persuasion and apprising, for instance, can quickly become abusive if the leader relies on lies and distortion. Similarly, inspirational appeals can turn destructive if they are based on fear or envy, and exchange and collaboration can be abused if a leader makes empty promises. Efforts by leaders to ingratiate themselves with their followers may simply be insincere. Effective leaders should make every effort to use proactive tactics in an ethical manner, with a focus on the goals of the group rather than personal gain. Deception and manipulation of others is always unethical.

Cavanaugh, Mobert, and Velasques[37] have developed a series of four questions to guide decisions about the ethical use of power:

1. Is the action consistent with the organization's goals, rather than being motivated purely by self-interest?
2. Does the action respect the rights of individuals and groups affected by it?
3. Does the action meet the standards of fairness and equity?
4. Would you wish others to behave in the same way if the action affected you?

The first question is the most important one because it clearly establishes whether the leader's self-interest or the interest of the group is paramount.

personalized leader
A leader who has a significant need for personal power and uses it selfishly and without self-control.

socialized leader
A leader who uses power to serve higher goals that benefit the organization, other leaders, and followers.

Thereafter, the questions address concerns about the rights of others, the standards of fairness and equity, and whether the leader would desire to be treated in a similar fashion. By applying these questions sequentially to a particular influence tactic, leaders can help ensure that the decision they reach is ethical. Leaders in public health have a responsibility—not only to their followers, but to the public, their constituents, their collaborators, and stakeholders—to use their power and influence responsibly to produce the greatest good for the communities they serve.

Case Study: SARS Outbreak in China[38,39]

Between November 2002 and July 2003, a form of pneumonia termed *severe acute respiratory syndrome* (SARS) infected more than 5,000 people in China, killing 349 of them. The outbreak is believed to have begun in southeastern China, bordering Hong Kong and Macau, and frontline Chinese health personnel were aware of the disease as early as mid-December 2002.

Health experts were sent to investigate the SARS outbreak in early January 2003. Reports began flowing up through governmental hierarchies by the end of the month, but action was delayed because the system lacked a sufficient number of authorized provincial health officials to read the reports. By early February, news of a "strange and deadly flu" had begun spreading via word of mouth and mobile phones, but the government's first formal press conference on the disease did not occur until the middle of the month. Even after the press conference, all reporting on the disease was filtered through provincial and national government bureaucracies. A news blackout continued throughout March and into April, and little information was shared with the World Health Organization until early April. The Chinese government's hesitation in sharing information contributed to widespread fear and misunderstanding, and economists began predicting that China's economy could be headed toward a recession. Finally, amid growing international and domestic pressure, the government launched a full-fledged effort to contain the disease.

At the start of the outbreak, China's massive governmental infrastructure seemed to be an impediment to the flow of information and the development of an effective response. However, once the appropriate resources were mobilized, the response was swift and effective. In mid-April, approximately five months after the outbreak began, the government officially listed SARS as a surveillance-level disease with a daily reporting mandate. Government media began daily publication of disease incidence by province, and government health agencies began providing information to healthcare workers about treatment of the disease. By the end of May, nearly 1,000 health officials and government workers had been disciplined for the slowness of their initial response to the outbreak.

Once the force of government got fully behind the public health effort, interdepartmental and interagency collaboration increased, effectively reengineering the government's response system for public health emergencies. Within two months, SARS was under control. The disease was eliminated in China by August 2003.

Discussion and Application Questions

1. In what ways were public health leaders in China particularly challenged by this epidemic?
2. How did the lack of an effective protocol initially hamper response to the SARS outbreak?
3. In the end, how might the SARS outbreak have actually helped China's public health response system?
4. In your opinion, how could public health leaders in China have more effectively dealt with the outbreak of SARS?
5. What form of power could Chinese public health leaders have used most effectively in combatting SARS?

Summary

Power can be defined in a variety of ways, but in this chapter we define it as the capacity or potential of a leader to influence one or more followers to achieve goals or outcomes desired by the leader in a specific situation. Power should be viewed not as a thing but rather as a collective attribute. It is based on relationships that exist between leaders and followers, and it relies on the behaviors of both.

Two concepts closely related to power are authority and influence. *Authority* refers to the advantages, duties, rights, and obligations linked to a person's position. The three main types of authority are rational authority, associated with a specific role or office; traditional authority, based on established values and social norms; and charismatic authority, based on the individual's personal characteristics. *Influence* refers to the impact of the exchange that occurs when a leader makes a request or decision affecting a follower. This exchange can lead to any of three types of outcomes: commitment, compliance, or resistance.

Power can be either hard or soft in nature. Hard power, also called *position power*, is based on the leader's position within the organization and the authority vested in the leader. Soft power, also called *personal power*, is based on the leader's personality characteristics and the relationships the leader has with followers. Within these two broad categories are the seven types of power in the expanded French-Raven taxonomy: (1) legitimate power, (2) reward power, (3) coercive power, (4) information power, (5) ecological power, (6) referent power, and (7) expert power. The first five types are forms of position power, whereas referent and expert power are forms of personal power. Effective public health leaders should be prepared to use all seven forms of power depending on the situations that arise, though coercive power should be used only rarely. Applying the concepts of situational leadership, Hersey, Blanchard, and Johnson have linked follower readiness levels with appropriate leadership styles and the types of power that should be used to support those styles.

Social exchange theory and strategic contingencies theory examine the ways that power can be gained and lost within organizations. Social exchange theory focuses on the reciprocal influence processes that occur in small groups and the ways that power can be gained or lost based on followers' perceptions of the leader's contributions. Strategic contingencies theory focuses on how power is gained or lost by various parts of an organization and how such power distribution impacts the organization's effectiveness.

Influence tactics are the behaviors used by one individual to change the behaviors, opinions, or attitudes of another. The four general types of influence tactics are impression management tactics, political tactics, proactive influence tactics, and reactive influence tactics. Regardless of the type of tactics used, leaders in public health have a responsibility to use their power and influence in an ethical manner. The ethical use of power distinguishes socialized leaders, who serve the higher goals of the organization, from personalized leaders, who use power selfishly and without self-control.

Discussion Questions

1. How do hard and soft power come together in the definition of *power*?
2. What is the role of authority in public health practice?
3. Identify and define the three outcomes of influence.
4. How do the three influence processes relate to one another?
5. What are the seven types of power in the expanded French-Raven taxonomy?
6. Which are the most effective types of power in the taxonomy?
7. How does the expanded French-Raven taxonomy relate to the follower readiness levels and leadership styles of situational leadership?

8. What are the two theories for the acquisition of power, and how do they relate to each other?

9. Define the four kinds of influence tactics, and explain how they relate to one another.

10. For deeper thought: As the leader of a public health working group, describe how you can abuse the various proactive influence tactics. Defend your answer.

Web Resources

Bal, V., M. Campbell, J. Steed, and K. Meddings. 2008. *The Role of Power in Effective Leadership*. Center for Creative Leadership. Accessed August 14, 2017. http://insights.ccl.org/wp-content/uploads/2015/04/roleOfPower.pdf.

Mind Tools. 2017. "French and Raven's Five Forms of Power: Understanding Where Power Comes from in the Workplace." Accessed August 14. www.mindtools.com/pages/article/newLDR_56.htm.

References

1. Online Library of Liberty. 2017. "Acton on Moral Judgements in History." Accessed February 6. http://oll.libertyfund.org/pages/acton-on-moral-judgements-in-history.

2. Gardner, J. W. 1990. *On Leadership*. New York: Free Press.

3. Hersey, P. H., K. H. Blanchard, and D. E. Johnson. 2008. *Management of Organizational Behavior: Leading Human Resources*, 9th ed. Upper Saddle River, NJ: Pearson Prentice Hall.

4. Burns, J. M. 1978. *Leadership*. New York: Harper & Row.

5. Beerel, A. 2009. *Leadership and Change Management*. Los Angeles: Sage.

6. Weber, M. 1947. *The Theory of Social and Economic Organization*. New York: Free Press.

7. Machiavelli, N. 1981. *The Prince*. London: Penguin Group.

8. Etzioni, A. 1961. *A Comparative Analysis of Complex Organizations*. New York: Free Press.

9. Yukl, G. 2013. *Leadership in Organizations*, 8th ed. Upper Saddle River, NJ: Prentice Hall.

10. Kelman, H. C. 1958. "Compliance, Identification, and Internalization: Three Processes of Attitude Change." *Journal of Conflict Resolution* 2 (1): 51–60.

11. French, J. R. P. Jr., and B. Raven. 1959. "The Bases of Social Power." In *Studies in Social Power*, edited by D. Cartwright, 259–69. Ann Arbor, MI: Institute for Social Research.

12. Cartwright, D. 1965. "Leadership, Influence, and Control." In *Handbook of Organizations*, edited by J. G. March, 1–47. Chicago: Rand McNally.

13. Pettigrew, A. M. 1972. "Information Control as a Power Source." *Sociology* 6 (2): 187–204.

14. Bass, B. M. 1960. *Leadership, Psychology, and Organizational Behavior*. New York: Harper.

15. Yukl, G., and C. M. Falbe. 1991. "The Importance of Different Power Sources in Downward and Lateral Relations." *Journal of Applied Psychology* 76 (3): 416–23.

16. Bass, B. M. 2008. *The Bass Handbook of Leadership: Theory, Research, and Managerial Applications*, 4th ed. New York: Free Press.

17. Jacobs, T. O. 1970. *Leadership and Exchange in Formal Organizations*. Alexandria, VA: Human Resources Research Organization.

18. March, J. G., and H. A. Simon. 1958. *Organizations*. New York: Wiley.

19. Kerr, S. 1975. "On the Folly of Rewarding A, While Hoping for B." *Academy of Management Journal* 18 (4): 769–83.

20. Katz, D., and R. L. Kahn. 1978. *The Social Psychology of Organizations*, 2nd ed. New York: Wiley.

21. Daft, R. L. 2015. *The Leadership Experience*, 6th ed. Mason, OH: South-Western.

22. Kouzes, J. M., and B. Z. Posner. 2007. *The Leadership Challenge*, 4th ed. San Francisco: Jossey-Bass.

23. Schein, E. H. 1992. *Organizational Culture and Leadership*, 2nd ed. San Francisco: Jossey-Bass.

24. SparkNotes. 2017. "Beowulf: Important Quotations Explained." Accessed February 6. www.sparknotes.com/lit/beowulf/quotes.html.

25. Emerson, R. E. 1962. "Power–Dependence Relations." *American Sociological Review* 27 (1): 31–41.

26. Mintzberg, H. 1963. *Power in and Around Organizations*. Upper Saddle River, NJ: Prentice Hall.

27. Hollander, E. P. 1958. "Conformity, Status, and Idiosyncrasy Credit." *Psychological Review* 65 (2): 117–27.

28. Hollander, E. P. 1980. "Leadership and Social Exchange Processes." In *Social Exchange: Advances in Theory and Research*, edited by K. J. Gergen, M. S. Greenberg, and R. H. Willis, 103–18. New York: Plenum Press.

29. Hickson, D. J., C. R. Hinings, C. A. Lee, R. S. Schneck, and J. M. Pennings. 1971. "A Strategic Contingencies' Theory of Intra-organizational Power." *Administrative Science Quarterly* 16 (2): 216–29.

30. Salancik, G. R., and J. Pfeffer. 1977. "Who Gets Power—and How They Hold On to It: A Strategic Contingency Model of Power." *Organizational Dynamics* 5 (3): 3–21.

31. Saunders, C. S. 1990. "The Strategic Contingencies Theory of Power: Multiple Perspectives." *Journal of Management Studies* 27 (1): 1–18.

32. Hughes, R. L., R. C. Ginnett, and G. J. Curphy. 1993. *Leadership: Enhancing the Lessons of Experience.* Homewood, IL: Richard D. Irwin.

33. Yukl, G. A., R. Lepsinger, and A. Lucia. 1992. "Preliminary Report on the Development and Validation of the Influence Behavior Questionnaire." In *Impact of Leadership*, edited by K. E. Clark, M. B. Clark, and D. P. Campbell, 417–27. Greensboro, NC: Center for Creative Leadership.

34. Pfeffer, J. 1977. "The Ambiguity of Leadership." *Academy of Management Review* 2 (1): 104–12.

35. Pfeffer, J. 1981. *Power in Organizations.* Marshfield, MA: Pittman.

36. Salancik, G. R., and J. Pfeffer. 1984. "Corporate Attributions as Strategic Illusions of Management Control." *Administrative Science Quarterly* 29 (2): 238–54.

37. Cavanaugh, G. F., D. J. Mobert, and M. Velasques. 1981. "The Ethics of Organizational Politics." *Academy of Management Review* 6 (3): 363–74.

38. World Health Organization. 2017. "Summary of Probable SARS Cases with Onset of Illness from 1 November 2002 to 31 July 2003." Accessed August 22. www.who.int/csr/sars/country/table2004_04_21/en/.

39. Abraham, T. 2007. *Twenty-First Century Plague: The Story of SARS.* Baltimore, MD: Johns Hopkins University Press.

MENTORING AND COACHING LEADERS IN PUBLIC HEALTH

James W. Holsinger Jr.

Learning Objectives

Upon completion of this chapter, you should be able to

- define the terms *mentoring*, *mentor*, and *mentee*;
- compare and contrast mentoring and coaching;
- analyze the mentoring functions that support individual development;
- explain the benefits of mentoring;
- describe the qualities and roles of a good mentor;
- discuss the steps for choosing a mentor;
- appraise the laws of mentoring;
- compare and contrast the Anderson and Shannon mentoring model and the situational leadership mentoring model;
- interpret the myths of mentoring;
- explain the four-step coaching process; and
- discuss the need for feedback in the coaching process and the ways a coach can provide it effectively.

Focus on Leadership Competencies

This chapter emphasizes the following Association of Schools and Programs of Public Health (ASPPH) leadership competencies:

- Engage in dialogue and learning from others to advance public health goals.
- Collaborate with diverse groups.
- Influence others to achieve high standards of performance and accountability.

(continued)

> - Prepare professional plans incorporating lifelong learning, mentoring, and continued career progression strategies.
>
> It also addresses the following Council on Linkages public health leadership competencies:
>
> - Contributes to continuous improvement of individual program and organizational performance.
> - Ensures use of professional development opportunities by individuals and teams.
>
> *Note: See the appendix at the end of the book for complete lists of competencies.*

Introduction

mentor
A person who provides guidance and shares experiences to help develop the abilities of another person.

mentoring
A support process that is based on concern for the professional success of an individual, is both personal and intimate, and requires face-to-face interaction.

mentee
A person who seeks wisdom and guidance from a mentor.

The term *mentor* has its origins in Homer's epic poem *The Odyssey*. In that work, while Odysseus fights in the Trojan War, his son Telemachus is entrusted to a friend whose name is Mentor. Mentor's job is to function as Telemachus's guardian and adviser—in other words, his **mentor**.

Mentoring is an important aspect of leadership, though specific definitions of the term vary. For the purposes of this chapter, we will define *mentoring* as a support process that is based on concern for the professional success of an individual, is both personal and intimate, and requires face-to-face interaction. Bell[1(p54)] explains that a mentor is "someone who helps someone else learn something that he or she would have learned less well, more slowly, or not at all if left alone." Cobb and colleagues[2(p372)] provide a more specific definition tailored to the academic setting, stating that mentors are individuals who "provide guidance, support, and feedback to facilitate personal and career development to help novices learn about the culture of the academy and expand opportunities for those traditionally hampered by social and institutional barriers." According to Ledlow and Coppola,[3(p394)] a mentor is "a person of greater knowledge or wisdom who shares his or her experiences to help develop the abilities of a person junior to the mentor," and a **mentee** is a person seeking wisdom and guidance from a mentor.

The terms *mentoring*, *coaching*, and *training* are often treated as synonyms, or at least as words whose meanings are intertwined. To properly understand leadership, however, each of these three terms should maintain its own identity. Normally, mentoring involves informal instruction in one-on-one interactions, which distinguishes it from training, which most often takes place in settings with multiple people. Mentoring also aims to assist individuals in developing their careers and their career choices, which distinguishes it from

coaching, which is more about helping a person do a particular job more effectively. Another terminology issue involves the use of the word *protégé*, which often appears in lieu of *mentee* to refer to the person being mentored. For our purposes, however, a **protégé** is a person involved in a long-term leader-development process designed for personal succession, with the intention that organizational responsibility and control will be transferred as the protégé advances. A protégé may, of course, be mentored, but the words *protégé* and *mentee* should not be regarded as synonyms.

Modern concepts of mentoring began to take shape in 1978, when Levinson and colleagues[4] considered the benefits and measures that we commonly associate with mentors and the people who receive mentoring. Since that time, a number of other authors have continued to develop those concepts. In 1988, Kram[5] listed a series of functions within the mentoring process that provide both career-related and psychosocial support for the mentee's development. The career-related functions of mentoring are specifically directed toward the person's job functions, and they assist the mentee in developing work capabilities, learning how things are done in the organization, and improving organizational standing. Such functions include sponsorship, protection, challenges, exposure and visibility, and coaching. The personal psychosocial functions of mentoring are highly personal, closely tied to behaviors and values, and directed toward the mentee's inner being. Such functions include role modeling, counseling, acceptance and confirmation, and friendship. The psychosocial aspects of mentoring address such issues as workplace behavior, desire for acceptance, identity clarification, feelings of competence, and professional effectiveness. Together, the career-related and psychosocial functions of mentoring prepare mentees to advance in their careers.[5]

Effective public health leaders develop followers through both mentoring and coaching. As noted, *mentoring* and *coaching* are not synonyms, but coaching can be considered as a part of the larger concept of mentoring. The two concepts differ in a number of ways. Mentoring focuses chiefly on the mentee's career development, whereas coaching is directed toward specific situations—for instance, correcting behavioral issues, improving performance, or developing skills to carry out new responsibilities. Mentoring tends to be a long-term relationship (though it may have defined time limits), whereas coaching is usually based on short-term requirements. Unlike mentoring, coaching might not be intimate in nature or require significant amounts of personal contact. In a coaching situation, the coach directs the individual's learning, and the individual's participation may be mandatory. In a mentoring situation, both the mentor and the mentee voluntarily agree

coaching
Instructing, training, and directing one or more people to learn specific skills or achieve a goal.

protégé
An individual receiving guidance in a long-term leader-development process designed for personal succession.

Consider This

"Mentoring is a brain to pick, an ear to listen, and a push in the right direction."

—John Crosby[6]

For an effective public health leader, how important is the job of mentoring followers?

to the relationship, and the mentee often takes charge of the learning process and initiates the interactions. Coaching relies heavily on telling and instructing, with appropriate feedback from the person being coached, whereas mentoring involves role modeling and advice from the mentor and careful listening on the part of the mentee. Finally, a coach is often a superior or direct supervisor, whereas a mentor usually is not in a hierarchical relationship with the mentee.[7]

Mentoring can help mentees to reach their full potential in whatever field the relationship is based. Although mentoring has traditionally occurred in informal relationships, many organizations, recognizing its usefulness, have now developed formal programs to pair mentors with mentees. A mentoring relationship can last a lifetime or exist for only a short period, depending on the needs of the mentee. Such relationships can have a substantial impact, given that they allow for genuine communication and encompass such elements as camaraderie, companionship, correction, and friendship.[8]

The Mentoring Experience

As the value of mentoring has become more widely recognized, its use has increased across a variety of fields, including public health.[9] Young public health practitioners come from a variety of disciplines, and effective mentoring relationships can help them manage their careers, develop leadership skills and qualities, and better serve their communities. Mentors are often older than mentees, but age is not the issue; the most important aspects of mentorship are the knowledge, skills, and experiences that the mentor brings to the relationship and shares with the mentee.[10] Typically, a mentee will have only one mentor at a time, although a person may engage with multiple mentors sequentially. Having more than one mentor simultaneously is unusual.

Benefits of Mentoring

In an effective mentoring process, all parties involved—the mentee, the mentor, and the organization at large—can be expected to benefit. Mentees benefit by developing professional abilities, enhancing their decision-making and problem-solving skills, and acquiring useful information and expertise.[11] They also gain an improved understanding of the processes by which the organization functions. As they develop, mentees can provide valued assistance to other team members, be assigned to more challenging and difficult tasks, and be considered for promotions and other career opportunities either within the organization or outside of it. Mentoring helps mentees better apply their intelligence while contributing to the success of the organization.[12] They learn about effective management and leadership, and they understand the importance of integrity and the appropriate use of power.[13]

Mentors often feel renewed through the process of imparting knowledge to others,[4] and they gain self-esteem and respect from peers as the people they have mentored contribute to the organization.[14] Effective mentors can build a legacy through the people they mentor, who over time become trusted colleagues. Mentors can benefit further through the retention of followers, increases in work satisfaction, and their own career development.[15] Efforts to develop followers can be particularly beneficial to mentors in organizations where mentorship is used as a criterion for evaluation and reward.[16]

Mentor Qualities and Roles

Effective mentoring depends largely on the qualities the mentor possesses and the roles in which the mentor engages the mentee.[17] Over time, the mentor's use of these qualities and roles changes as the mentoring relationship matures and as the mentee's abilities develop.[18] Carruthers[17] emphasizes three main areas of mentor qualities and roles: serving as a role model, being a trusted counselor, and maintaining confidentiality. Mentors must have the requisite experience to model appropriate behavior for the mentee. They should be proven leaders who are knowledgeable in the ways and culture of the organization. As trusted counselors, they must be able to offer guidance and advice, openly share resources, and provide the tools to help the mentee function effectively in the organization. At the same time, the mentor should be a friend to the mentee, part of a relationship built on trust and mutual respect. The mentoring relationship often becomes so close that the mentor and mentee demonstrate true affection for each other. Mentors should be open and accessible, skilled in active listening, and fully engaged in the mentoring experience. They must also respect the confidentiality of sensitive mentor–mentee exchanges.

Public health practitioners want mentors who will provide advice and assistance to guide their careers. However, the mentees themselves have the responsibility to fully engage in the mentoring experience by putting forth sufficient time and effort. Although some organizations have formal mentoring programs (discussed later in the chapter), the effectiveness of most mentoring experiences depends on the mentee's selection of a mentor in a largely informal process. Not all effective public health leaders will be good mentors, so the mentee should carefully think through the desired qualities of a potential mentor prior to making a decision.

Effective Public Health Leaders . . .

. . . know that what goes on within the mentor–mentee relationship stays within the relationship.

Developing the Mentoring Relationship

Establishing an effective mentor–mentee relationship is a complex process. Although some organizations match mentors with mentees in a formal program, the more common approach is for mentees to select their own mentors. At the start of this process, mentees must determine their own personal values and create a vision based on their own personal goals. Once they have done so, they can begin searching the organization for a person who has accomplished similar goals.[10]

Wickman and Sjodin[19] have developed a detailed approach to guide the process of choosing a mentor. It begins with the aspiring mentee setting at least one goal for the mentoring experience. Once the goal or goals have been identified, the individual identifies people in the organization who are goal-oriented achievers. Once the best candidates have been identified, the individual sets goals for meetings with each candidate, makes the necessary appointments, and prepares a series of questions with which to engage the prospective mentors. During each meeting, the aspiring mentee and the prospective mentor engage in a conversation in which they explore the other's life story and discuss personal goals. The individual uses follow-up questions to elicit more information and asks the prospective mentor for suggestions. Following each short trial meeting, the aspiring mentee sends the prospective mentor a thank-you note, evaluates the information gained from the meeting, and works to implement the prospective mentor's suggestions. Once the suggestions have been implemented and results have occurred, the aspiring mentee reports those results to the prospective mentor and evaluates the prospective mentor's response. Based on an evaluation of the process at this point, the individual determines whether the prospective mentor is an appropriate match. If the match is positive, the aspiring mentee reengages the prospective mentor and proposes a mentoring relationship.

This selection process may seem long and cumbersome, and effective mentoring relationships can in some cases be developed through less structured interactions. However, the tailored approach offered by Wickman and Sjodin ensures clear communication at the start of the relationship and often brings rich rewards.

Wickman and Sjodin[19] have also enumerated 16 laws of mentoring that can help guide the development of successful relationships:

1. The Law of Positive Environment
2. The Law of Developing Character
3. The Law of Independence
4. The Law of Limited Responsibility
5. The Law of Shared Mistakes
6. The Law of Planned Objectives
7. The Law of Inspection
8. The Law of Tough Love
9. The Law of Small Successes

10. The Law of Direction
11. The Law of Risk
12. The Law of Mutual Protection
13. The Law of Communication
14. The Law of Extended Commitment
15. The Law of Life Transition
16. The Law of Fun

Several of these laws are of particular importance. The Law of Positive Environment emphasizes that a positive environment is essential for an effective mentoring relationship; without a positive environment, many of the other laws would be impossible to carry out. The Law of Tough Love, which highlights the need to encourage independence in mentees, is often difficult for mentors to embrace, because the mentors recall times earlier in their own careers when they were being mentored and thus can relate to the mentee's experiences. Nonetheless, mentors cannot allow mentees to become overly dependent. The Law of Mutual Protection reinforces the importance of confidentiality. What transpires between a mentor and mentee—as long as it fully meets a strict ethical test—stays between the two. The Law of Communication emphasizes the open exchange of information, without which effective mentoring cannot occur. The Law of Extended Commitment reflects the fact that an effective mentoring relationship is an extended one, sometimes lasting a lifetime; for the relationship to be maximally effective, it cannot be of short duration. However, the Law of Life Transitions acknowledges that the relationship may be brought to a close when a mentor or mentee moves into a new stage of life. Certainly, such a time occurs when mentees are ready to try their wings and fly on their own. When this time comes, effective mentors provide a smooth transition, allowing the mentee to metamorphose into a trusted colleague.

An effective mentoring relationship is based on shared responsibility between two partners, both of whom benefit as the mentor helps develop the mentee's effectiveness within the organization. As Rowitz[10] so aptly states, the ultimate goal of the mentoring relationship is the mentee's independence. The product of good mentoring is exhibited when the mentee becomes sufficiently comfortable engaging change that reliance on the mentor gradually disappears.

Criteria for Selecting Mentors in Public Health

The Mid-America Regional Public Health Leadership Institute has developed a set of criteria for the selection of mentors in public health, and these criteria can be summarized and adapted as follows.[10] The person to be selected as a mentor should be a recognized leader in public health and should be willing to work with the mentee for at least one year, if not longer. The mentor must have the skills necessary to provide appropriate insight in discussions with mentees as the mentoring process progresses, as well as to support mentees in their professional growth and development. Individuals serving as public health mentors must have the support of their organization, to ensure that they have the time to mentor another person. The mentor should have at least 10 to 15 more years of public health experience than the person being mentored. Mentors often have local, state, and national level leadership credentials. A significant breadth of experience in a variety of public health settings, and with a variety of followers, is usually expected.

The Anderson and Shannon Mentoring Model

Anderson and Shannon mentoring model
A conceptualization of the mentoring process that incorporates mentoring dispositions, relationships, functions, and activities.

In 1988, Anderson and Shannon[20(p40)] published a conceptualization of mentoring with an extensive and all-encompassing definition of the term: "a nurturing process in which a more skilled or more experienced person, serving as a role model, teaches, sponsors, encourages, counsels, and befriends a less skilled or less experienced person for the purpose of promoting the latter's professional and/or personal development. Mentoring functions are carried out within a context of an ongoing, caring relationship between mentor and protégé [mentee]." Dimensions and components of the **Anderson and Shannon mentoring model** are presented in exhibit 13.1.

mentoring disposition
A characteristic attributed to a mentor that defines the mentor's actions in a certain situation.

The Anderson and Shannon model is based on three **mentoring dispositions** that define mentors' actions in certain situations. The first disposition is the opening of the mentor to the mentee. Mentors should be willing to allow mentees to see and understand their actions, and they should be willing to inform mentees of the rationales behind their decisions. Secondly, the mentor should have the disposition to engage with the mentee incrementally over time. The third disposition is the mentor's expression of interest in the professional and personal needs of the mentee. The nature of the mentor's dispositions provides the basis on which the mentoring relationship functions.

In the mentoring relationship, the mentor serves as a role model while at the same time nurturing the mentee and acting as a care giver. In serving as a role model, the mentor motivates the mentee to grow and develop professionally. Nurturing occurs when the mentor clearly perceives the mentee's ability, experience, and psychological maturity and, by doing so, is able to engage the mentee in appropriate activities to enable professional development. The mentor also engages in a continued caring relationship with the mentee.

Anderson and Shannon propose five functions in the mentoring process: teaching,

> ## Spotlight
>
> The Anderson and Shannon[20] mentoring model is based on their understanding (a) that mentoring is fundamentally a nurturing process, (b) that the mentor must serve as a role model to the protégé (mentee), and (c) that the mentor must exhibit certain dispositions that help define the process.

EXHIBIT 13.1
Anderson
and Shannon
Mentoring
Model

Dimensions	Components	Details
Mentoring dispositions	Opening ourselves	
	Leading incrementally	
	Expressing care and concern	
Mentoring relationship	Role model	X is a model for Y
	Nurture	X nurtures Y
	Care giver	X cares for Y
Functions of mentoring	Teach	Model, inform, confirm/disconfirm, prescribe, question
	Sponsor	Protect, support, promote
	Encourage	Affirm, inspire, challenge
	Counsel	Listen, probe, clarify, advise
	Befriend	Accept, relate
Mentoring activities	Demonstration lessons	
	Observations and feedback	
	Support meetings	

Source: Data from Anderson, E. M., and A. L. Shannon. 1988. "Toward a Conceptualization of Mentoring." *Journal of Teacher Education* 39 (1): 38–42.

sponsoring, encouraging, counseling, and befriending. The teaching function encompasses the mentor's efforts to inform the mentee and model appropriate professional activities. In carrying out this function, the mentor may on occasion prescribe the mentee's actions, but the mentor should clearly be open to questioning. The mentor and mentee should confirm or disconfirm what is being taught, to ensure that the mentee clearly understands the mentor's intentions. The sponsoring function occurs when the mentor serves as a kind of guarantor for the mentee. In so doing, the mentor exhibits three kinds of behavior: (1) protective behavior, which aims to protect the mentee from the environment and from the mentee's own actions; (2) supporting behavior, which occurs in the mentor's involvement with the mentee's project; and (3) promoting behavior, which may involve the introduction of the mentee to the mentor's network or the recommendation of the mentee for assignments and opportunities. The encouraging function includes efforts by the mentor to affirm, inspire, and challenge the mentee—all of which contribute to growth and professional development. The counseling function serves to develop the mentee's listening and problem-solving skills, as well as the mentee's willingness to probe the thinking of the mentor. The mentee should feel free to ask clarifying questions, and the mentor should be willing to provide advice. Ultimately, counseling should result in mentees solving their own problems. The befriending function requires that the mentor be willing to accept the mentee, relate with the mentee in an open and supportive manner, and develop a closeness that will sustain the mentoring process.

The mentoring activities in Anderson and Shannon's model encourage the mentee to implement the lessons that were learned through the five functions. The activities in Anderson and Shannon's model were initially directed toward the mentoring of teachers, but they are relevant to public health practice as well. One of the activities, demonstration lessons, involves efforts by the mentor to model and demonstrate techniques and behaviors. For example, a mentor can demonstrate how to lead a group by allowing the mentee to sit in on meetings. The mentee can shadow the mentor to observe a skillful practitioner at work. At the same time, the mentor can observe the mentee and provide valuable feedback to guide improvement. Regular mentor–mentee meetings allow the mentor to provide continued support. Mentoring activities should be purposely scheduled and not left to chance encounters. As the mentor and mentee engage in the process, they should identify other activities through which the functions of mentoring can be expressed.

Despite its many components, the entire Anderson and Shannon model is based chiefly on the three mentoring dispositions. Mentors who possess these dispositions will be poised to make a positive difference in the lives of the people they mentor.

 Consider This

"We make a living by what we get; we make a life by what we give."
—Sir Winston Churchill[21]

As an effective public health leader, in addition to mentoring, what can you give your followers?

The Situational Leadership Mentoring Model

The situational leadership model, as discussed in previous chapters, can be applied to a number of aspects of leadership, including the mentoring relationship.[22] Mentoring is based on a partnership that develops between the mentor and mentee, with the mentor serving not as a power figure but as a trusted adviser.

Stages and Phases in the Mentoring Partnership

Bell[1] describes four stages in the mentor–mentee partnership: (1) leveling the learning field, (2) fostering acceptance and safety, (3) giving learning gifts, and (4) bolstering self-direction and independence. In the first stage, two individuals, the mentor and the mentee, develop their relationship into a true partnership and build a rapport. By removing all aspects of command and power, the learning field is flattened. In the second stage, the mentor helps the mentee develop a feeling of acceptance. The mentor is receptive, listens attentively, and validates the mentee's feelings, building a relationship based not on sympathy but on empathy. The mentee should understand that the mentor was once in the same place as the mentee and thus understands the mentee's needs. In the third stage, the mentor gives the mentee the gifts of affirmation, focus, support, and even courage, while at the same time encouraging the learning process by providing feedback and advice. Ambiguity should be avoided, as it can leave the mentee confused rather than assisted. Finally, the fourth stage focuses on the mentee's development of self-direction and independence, enabling the mentee to eventually graduate from the mentoring relationship. The mentoring relationship should culminate with a sense of closure when maximum growth through the process has been reached, and it should evolve into a long-standing personal and professional friendship.

Kram[23] describes the mentoring relationship in four phases: (1) initiation, (2) cultivation, (3) separation, and (4) redefinition. She anticipates that the mentoring relationship will last approximately five years, with the first phase accounting for approximately 6 to 12 months. In the initiation phase, the relationship between the two individuals begins and continues to increase in importance to both the mentor and the mentee. The second phase, cultivation, lasts two to five years. Important psychosocial aspects of the second phase include role modeling and counseling, in addition to acceptance, confirmation, and friendship. The bond between the two partners deepens as the mentor and mentee interact closely in meaningful career-related activities. The third phase, separation, lasts for about two years, and it represents a turning point, as both the mentor and the mentee find that the mentoring relationship is losing value and is no longer needed in its present form. This separation leads to the fourth phase, in which the relationship is redefined and becomes more peerlike in nature. The redefinition phase lasts for an indefinite amount of time, and both the mentor and mentee should strive to ensure a positive ending to the relationship.

Bell's stages and Kram's phases are closely aligned. The first stage (leveling the learning field) and the first phase (initiation) are similar in nature, and the second and third stages (fostering acceptance and safety and giving learning gifts) correspond with the second phase (cultivation). The fourth stage (bolstering self-direction and independence) functions in much the same manner as the third phase (separation). The fourth phase (redefinition) serves to redefine the relationship for the future—a process that is assumed in Bell's fourth stage, where the mentoring relationship changes into a peer relationship. The sequences outlined in both Bell's model and Kram's model provide a basis for the mentee readiness levels used in the situational leadership approach.

Mentee Readiness Levels

The key to applying situational leadership to the mentoring process is under-standing the readiness of individuals to engage as mentees. Since most people will not have prior experience in mentoring relationships, they come to the process with little or no competence in the task of being mentored. At the same time, people who have selected a mentor will come to the process with a high degree of commitment, though they may feel insecure. Thus, the mentee begins at the first mentee readiness level, MR1, which focuses on initiation. As noted in Kram's model, the initiation phase is the point in the process where rapport between the mentor and mentee is beginning to develop. The MR2 mentee readiness level, cultivation, begins when the mentee is starting to gain some competence in the task of being mentored. At the same time, however, the mentee's commitment, which began on a high note, is waning, often because the mentee is not seeing progress from the relationship or feels unable to move forward. The MR3 level, acceptance, occurs when the mentee is able to move forward in developing the relationship with the mentor. Competence in the process continues to grow and is reaching a high point, while commitment is moving from low to variable. The mentee is able to accomplish the task but may again feel insecure following the difficult period of MR2. By the time the mentee reaches the MR4 level, independence, both competence in the task of being mentored and commitment to the process are high. The mentee is not only able but also confident in the relationship with the mentor.

Mentor Leadership Styles

As in other applications of situational leadership, the leader, or the mentor, must use leadership styles (S1–S4) that are congruent with the follower's, or the mentee's, level of readiness. The application of situational leadership for the mentoring process is modeled in exhibit 13.2.

When the mentee is at the MR1 level of readiness, the appropriate leader-ship style for the mentor is S1 (forming). Like the S1 approaches described in other situational leadership applications, the S1 style for mentoring is high in task behaviors and low in relationship behaviors. As the relationship is forming, the mentor and mentee need to develop the framework within which the two will function. This step occurs primarily at the first meeting between the two, when the ground rules for the relationship are developed. The mentor takes the lead in developing the ground rules, though the mentee, who has a strong sense of commitment at the MR1 level, also plays a key role. Despite the S1 style's normally low level of relationship behavior, the mentor does have to use some degree of supportive behavior to effectively begin the relationship-building process.

At the MR2 readiness level, the mentee's commitment tends to drop, and the appropriate leadership style for the mentor is S2 (guiding), which requires high levels of both task and relationship behaviors. At this point

	Forming	Guiding	Encouraging	Empowering	**EXHIBIT 13.2**
Mentor behaviors	(High task, low relationship)	(High task, high relationship)	(High relationship, low task)	(Low relationship, low task)	Situational Leadership Applied to Mentoring
	S1	S2	S3	S4	
	MR1	MR2	MR3	MR4	
	Initiation	Cultivation	Acceptance	Independence	
Mentee readiness	(Low competence, high commitment; unable and/or insecure)	(Some competence, low commitment; unable but confident)	(High competence, variable commitment; able but insecure)	(High competence, high commitment; able and confident)	

Sources: Adapted from Hersey, P., K. H. Blanchard, and D. E. Johnson. 2000. *Management of Organizational Behavior: Leading Human Resources*, 8th ed. Upper Saddle River, NJ: Prentice Hall; Blanchard, K. H., P. Zigarmi, and D. Zigarmi. 1985. *Leadership and the One Minute Manager: Increasing Effectiveness Through Situational Leadership*. New York: William Morrow; and Holsinger, J. W., Jr. 2010. *How to Develop Lay Ministry Within a Local Church*. Lewiston, MA: Edwin Mellen Press.

of the process, the mentor should aim to provide good coaching and foster acceptance and safety. Highly supportive behavior is apparent in the mentor's use of active and attentive listening. Bell[1(p54)] explains: "Great mentors who are effective at communicating acceptance don't speak as if they are testing a protégé, being judgmental, or acting as a parent. Great mentors show their acceptance through attentive, dramatic listening. When listening is their goal, they make it the priority; they don't let anything distract." Effective active listening requires complete absorption in the person speaking and the things the person is saying; thus, the mentor must listen to the mentee without an agenda. At this point of the process, Covey's[24] maxim to "seek first to understand, then to be understood" is key to the relationship. Mentees gain a sense of safety when mentors are receptive, validate their feelings, and identify with them empathetically. When mentees feel that they are being heard, they feel that they are valued. Being a great mentor requires being a great listener.

When the mentee reaches the MR3 level, the situational leadership model calls for the mentor to use the S3 (encouraging) leadership style. At this point in the relationship, mentees are becoming highly competent in the task of being mentored, and their commitment to the process is steadily increasing; however, they may still have some feelings of insecurity. The S3 leadership style is high in relationship behaviors and low in task behaviors. The mentor at this point provides strong supportive actions and gives the mentee many of the learning gifts described in Bell's model (e.g., affirmation, focus, support, courage). Now that the relationship has become stronger, the mentor can provide useful advice and effective feedback to the mentee. Advice, typically, is simply about giving information, whereas feedback is about assisting with blind spots. With that distinction in mind, Bell[1(p55)] describes potential obstacles at this point in the mentoring process: "The issue associated with advice is potential resistance; the issue with feedback is potential resentment." At times, the mentor may wish to ask the mentee if giving advice would be appropriate for a given situation; doing so may help minimize the likelihood of resistance. The ultimate goal of both advice and feedback is for the mentee to develop identification with the mentor.

When the mentee reaches the MR4 readiness level, the mentor should adopt the S4 (empowering) leadership style, which is low in both relationship and task behaviors. At this point, the mentor bolsters the mentee's self-direction and independence and brings the mentoring process and relationship to an end. Both the mentor and the mentee should make an effort to finish the task well and end the process on a high note. A simple event, such as a walk in a park, can help bring the mentoring process to closure. Since the relationship has become so intimate, ending it is not without emotion; however, as the mentoring relationship ends, a new relationship, between the two individuals as peers, develops. In some respects, the best assistance a mentor can give to a mentee is a strong ending to the mentoring relationship, closing with consideration, confidence, and compasssion.[1]

As demonstrated in several chapters of this book, leaders in public health can use situational leadership in a variety of ways. Since situational leadership is a contingency model of leadership, it considers not only the normal features of the leader–follower or mentor–mentee relationship but also outside influences, events, situations, and circumstances, all of which can contribute to mentoring. All of us experience events that strongly influence us, and many of these events are fortuitous or unexpected. Such events—even our crises—present us with opportunities. Effective mentors embrace the mentoring potential of their own life experiences as they interact with their mentees.[22]

Ensuring Effective Mentoring

Clearly, mentoring can make a meaningful difference in the life of the person being mentored. Leaders can use this tool to its fullest potential if they understand the truth behind the myths, avoid common pitfalls, and know the best ways to develop a formal mentoring program.

Dispelling the Myths of Mentoring

Exhibit 13.3 lists some of the common myths of mentoring, as identified by Sandler.[25] The first two myths—about mentoring being the best way to succeed and always beneficial—reflect the considerable value of mentoring, but they should not be regarded as absolute truths. Certainly, a close personal

---

EXHIBIT 13.3
Common
Mentoring
Myths

1. The best way to succeed is to have a mentor.

2. Mentoring is always beneficial.

3. The mentor should be older than the person being mentored.

4. A person can have only one mentor at a time.

5. Mentoring is all for the benefit of the mentee.

6. If you are seeking a mentor, you have to wait to be asked.

7. When a man mentors a woman, the chances are great that it will develop into a sexual encounter.

8. Men are better mentors for women.

9. The mentor always knows best.

Source: Data from Sandler, B. R. 1993. "Women as Mentors: Myths and Commandments." *Chronicle of Higher Education* 39 (27): B3.

relationship with a mentor can enhance the mentee's career, but it can also carry a significant disadvantage if the mentee comes to rely solely on a single person for career development. In such an instance, the time and emotional commitment required of the mentor–mentee relationship can cause the mentee to become isolated, thus foregoing the possibility of important relationships with others.

Although some experts[14] believe that a mentor should have 8 to 15 years more experience than the mentee, the myth that the mentor should be older than the mentee may fail to take into consideration the importance of other important factors, including interpersonal skills. A good mentor will be the person who exhibits the mentoring dispositions. The myth that people can have only one mentor at a time may seem reasonable, but sometimes multiple mentors are necessary or beneficial. Often, a mentee will have difficulty finding someone who possesses all the characteristics they desire in a mentor, so having more than one mentor might be the best way to meet the mentee's needs. Also, having multiple mentors can be a good way for mentees to expand their own networks—a considerable benefit given the importance of networking in public health.

Clearly, the idea that mentoring is solely for the benefit of the mentee is a myth. Mentoring should be seen as a two-way street, benefiting both the mentee and the mentor. Mentors benefit by gaining respect, self-esteem, and an improved reputation. They might also gain insight and information from the mentee about programs or problems with which the mentor is unfamiliar.[25] The idea that aspiring mentees have to wait to be asked is also untrue. Mentees can and do actively seek out mentors.

The myth about mentoring relationships leading to sexual encounters reflects a major pitfall that all mentors and mentees should avoid. The

Leadership Application Case: Is It All Over?

The Leadership Application Case at the beginning of this book provides realistic scenarios for the application of key leadership concepts covered in the text. See the section marked "Chapter 13 Application" for the scenario and discussion questions that correspond with this chapter.

mentoring relationship should be mutually professional and must not become sexual in nature. The myth that men are better mentors for women has an element of truth only insofar as men traditionally have been more likely to hold powerful positions in many organizations. In the practice of public health, however, women have long held positions of responsibility and authority; thus, women are readily available to engage in productive mentoring relationships with either men or women.

Finally, the idea that the mentor always knows best also is a myth. Mentors, like everyone else, sometimes make mistakes, and some have knowingly exploited their mentees. A mentor can err by setting goals for the mentee that are too high or too low, by offering advice that does not advance the mentee's goals, or by failing to recognize the point at which the mentee has grown past the need for mentoring. A mentor's failure to disengage at the appropriate time can have a negative impact on the mentee and cause the mentor–mentee relationship to terminate badly.

Avoiding Mentoring Pitfalls

Sandler[25] has also proposed certain rules to help mentors avoid common pitfalls and develop effective mentoring relationships. The mentoring process, whether informal or formal, should have the full engagement and support of organizational leaders. Leaders should not be afraid of mentoring, and they should not underestimate the knowledge they possess—not only about their own organizations, but also about the public health system as a whole. Knowledge of one's organization, networks, and contacts can all be placed at the disposal of the person being mentored. Mentors should not be concerned if they do not personally possess all the knowledge, skills, and abilities that their mentees aspire to possess; they can simply offer what they do possess to assist their mentees. If possible, mentors should include their mentees in informal activities to help broaden their understanding of the organization. For instance, mentees need to learn how to access the organization's systems to connect with others, attend conferences, and engage in special projects.

Effective mentoring can be significantly threatened by poor communication and a lack of clarity concerning boundaries and expectations. Mentors should therefore make sure that their mentees have a clear understanding of the amount of time and energy the mentors are willing to invest in the relationship. By doing so, the relationship will have appropriate ground rules, and mentees will know if they are expecting too much or too little. When communicating, mentors must offer constructive suggestions for improvement to their mentees, but their criticism should be provided privately, in a confidential and nonthreatening manner. Mentors should also seek to promote the accomplishments of their mentees; after all, the process is intended to enhance the mentee's career. Finally, although people often have an inclination to seek out individuals similar to themselves for mentoring relationships, mentors must be willing to cross boundaries of race, ethnicity, gender, class, and religion to support mentees' development.

Developing a Mentoring Model

Although some investigators have found that informal mentoring efforts tend to be more successful than formal programs,[26] formal efforts can nonetheless achieve meaningful results. To a large extent, how well a formal program functions depends on the training of mentors. Chao, Walz, and Gardner[27] write that formal mentoring programs can be further enhanced through voluntary participation by mentees, encouraging choice in the process; explanation of both pitfalls and benefits of the program; and clear delineation of the mentor and mentee roles, as well as the processes to be used.

> **Check It Out**
>
> For more information about how to develop a mentoring program, go to http://chronus.com/how-to-start-a-mentoring-program.

Ledlow and Coppola[3] have identified six critical elements in the development of a formal mentoring model, as shown in exhibit 13.4. All six elements respond to the needs of the people being mentored. First, a formal program must have clear strategic goals that are understood by all participants; without such goals, failure is likely. Second, all potential participants, both mentors and mentees, must clearly understand the program's method of selecting mentors. The third critical element is confidentiality between the mentor and mentee; without it, mentees are unlikely to participate. Fourth, a formal program must provide the requisite training to ensure that both mentors and mentees possess the skills necessary for a successful outcome. Fifth, both members of the relationship must understand the need to be politically astute. Finally, the organization must monitor and assess the program, considering both outcomes for mentees and the personal rewards for mentors.

Coaching

Coaching is an interactive process through which leaders and followers solve performance issues and develop the follower's capabilities.[7] As noted at the start of the chapter, coaching is not the same as mentoring, but it can be

EXHIBIT 13.4
Critical
Elements
for a Formal
Mentoring
Program

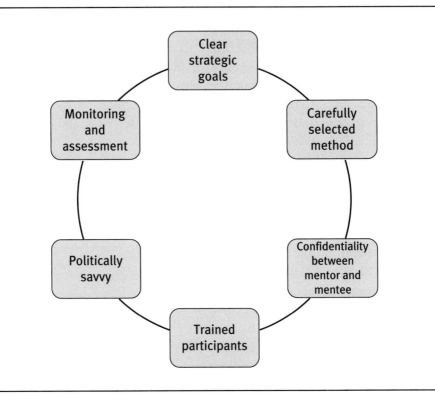

Source: Data from Ledlow, G. R., and M. N. Coppola. 2014. *Leadership for Health Professionals: Theory, Skills, and Applications*, 2nd ed. Sudbury, MA: Jones & Bartlett Learning.

considered part of the mentoring process. Coaching is all about improving the job performance of the person being coached and bridging the disparity between current performance and desired future performance.[10] Coaching has three main components—technical help, personal support, and individual challenge—that are held together by an emotional bond between the coach and the person being coached. For coaching to succeed, this emotional bond must be positive.

Benefits of Coaching

Effective coaching has a number of benefits both for individuals and for the organization, as shown in exhibit 13.5.[7] Coaching can help employees overcome performance problems and deal with their work assignments more effectively. It can help employees develop new skills and take on new responsibilities, which in turn can allow the coach (supervisor) to devote more time to other tasks. Coaching can lead to increased productivity, as followers gain important knowledge and information that enables them to work smarter. Through coaching, leaders can develop their followers and ensure that the followers possess the knowledge and skills necessary for promotion to higher-level jobs.

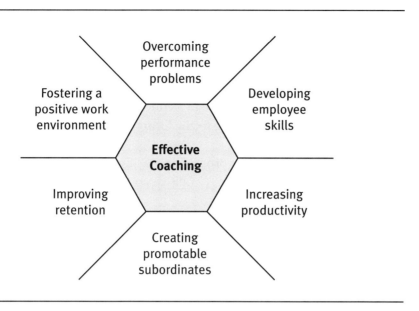

Source: Data from Harvard Business Essentials. 2004. *Coaching and Mentoring*. Boston: Harvard Business School Press.

EXHIBIT 13.5
Effective
Coaching

An effective, collaborative coaching process can help build loyalty and trust between leaders and followers.[7] When followers feel like valued employees, retention improves, and the organization spends less time and energy trying to fill vacant positions. Ultimately, coaching contributes to a positive work culture, with higher employee motivation and job satisfaction. Strong relationships between leaders and followers improve organizational results while also making the leader's job easier.

An effective performance management system helps leaders identify individuals who might benefit from coaching. Such a system can be used not only to appraise followers' work but also to identify new skills and knowledge that can enhance followers' work capabilities. When the performance management process reveals a problem, a clear opportunity for the leader arises. Early intervention through coaching can help the leader strengthen employees' skills and rectify problems caused by employee behaviors.

The Coaching Process

In considering the coaching process for public health, Rowitz[10] emphasizes several key points. The coach must observe the person being coached, often called the *coachee*, in action. The coach and the coachee should engage in a careful and thoughtful discussion about the issues involved, as well as the coaching process itself. Both parties need to clearly agree on the performance goals that they expect to reach through the coaching effort. The coaching methodology should be carefully explicated, and specific meeting times should be arranged. The coach and the person being coached should carefully analyze current performance and develop strategies and timelines to meet the agreed-upon goals. After the appropriate actions have been implemented, feedback and follow-up by the coach are essential. The coach should focus on progress and future performance rather than past mistakes, in keeping with Goldsmith's[28] concept of "feedforward" rather than feedback. Feedforward contributes to a climate of support while looking to the future with an emphasis on the organization's goals.

For closer analysis, the process of coaching can be broken down into four main steps: (1) preparation, (2) discussion, (3) active coaching, and (4) follow-up.

Preparation

Preparation, the first step in the coaching process, involves direct observation of the situation, the person to be coached, and that person's current skills—all of which need to be understood before the coaching relationship is initiated. The insights gained through observation can help ensure that the coach's efforts are appropriate, informed, relevant, and timely. The prospective coach should observe the individual both informally and formally, both during meetings and at the individual's work site. The coach should practice active listening and avoid making premature judgments based on incomplete knowledge. By comparing the person's observed performance with the requirements of the position, the coach can identify performance gaps and skill deficiencies—both of which can be addressed through the coaching process. During the observation stage, coaches should test their hypotheses by checking with trusted colleagues.

Once a problem has been observed and defined, the prospective coach needs to determine whether it can be resolved through coaching. Waldroop and Butler[29] have found that the likelihood that a change in behavior will occur depends largely on the degree to which the behavior is entrenched and by the frequency with which the behavior occurs. If a behavior is deeply ingrained, occurs frequently, and is part of the person's substance, changing it through coaching will be extremely difficult. If a behavior is infrequent or limited to a specific situation, changing it will be easier. However, for a change in behavior to occur through coaching, the person being coached must want to make the change. Assisting the person to arrive at that point is a key element in the coaching process.

Every step in the coaching process, including preparation, requires the involvement of both the coach and the person being coached. An excellent way to engage prospective coachees at this point is by having

Consider This

"Character-driven behaviors are like crabgrass: deeply rooted and difficult to weed out."
—James Waldroop and Timothy Butler[29(p113)]

Why do people have difficulty changing their character? Is the crabgrass analogy appropriate?

them complete self-appraisals of their work performance and then comparing the self-appraisals with the goals set forth in an earlier performance review. The self-appraisals can help determine the extent to which the goals have been reached, which goals have been exceeded, which goals are a struggle, and what obstacles are making goal progress difficult. The self-appraisal assists the coach in identifying coaching opportunities and also helps the coachee understand the need for coaching in particular areas.

Discussion

The second step in the coaching process, discussion, focuses on dialogue between the coach and the person being coached. The two should discuss the issues at hand, understand why the issues need to be addressed, and develop shared strategies for moving forward. Importantly, the dialogue should focus not on personal attitudes and motives but on actual observed behaviors. Criticism of an individual's attitudes or motives may be perceived as a personal attack, whereas comments about observed behavior are less closely tied to the individual's identity and self-worth.[7] When coaches describe behaviors, they must be truthful and frank, but also supportive. Once the coach has raised the relevant performance issues, the person being coached must be given the opportunity to respond. Mutual understanding is more likely to result from a two-way dialogue than from a monologue on the part of the coach.

To foster a more effective dialogue, coaches should use open-ended, probing questions that will elicit thorough and thoughtful responses. Simple yes-or-no questions are not as useful. Coaches should listen actively while maintaining eye contact and smiling as appropriate. They should carefully observe the person's body language and nonverbal cues, paying close attention to any emotions that might lurk behind the words. The coach may wish to focus on listening and note taking during the conversation and then evaluate the notes after the conversation is over. Paraphrasing and repeating the person's comments during the conversation can effectively demonstrate that the person is being heard.

As the discussion continues, the coach can make a determined effort to understand the causes behind the person's behaviors, while at the same time establishing a connection and encouraging collaboration. The endpoint of the discussion stage is to develop a plan for systematic performance improvement.

Active Coaching

The third step in the coaching process is the active coaching stage. Once the coach and the person being coached have reached a mutual agreement on the goals of the coaching process, they create an action plan. The action plan specifies how the two individuals will work together and how they will measure success as they move toward their goals. It typically includes a timeline for the work to be accomplished and details about the specific role the coach will play.

The action plan ensures that both individuals know exactly what is expected of the relationship. By involving the person being coached in the creation of the action plan, the coach can strengthen the individual's buy-in for the process. In some cases, depending on the situation and the goals, a formal action plan may not be necessary.

Once the action plan has been agreed upon, active coaching commences. The coach must be able to communicate ideas in a way that the person being coached not only grasps but also appreciates. People learn in different ways, and what works for one person might not work for another. Some individuals are "eye learners" who prefer to be given something to read, whereas others are "ear learners" who prefer to hear directly from the coach. Still others learn best through personal examples. Coaches should try to communicate in whatever manner best enhances the learning of the person being coached. Regardless of the approach used, active coaching requires that the coach and the coachee engage in two-way communication.

An effective coaching style balances telling and questioning. Such a balance allows the coach to provide effective advice about what to do and how to do it, while at the same time allowing the person being coached to think independently and engage the coach in a Socratic manner, enhancing the learning process. The questioning approach cannot be the sole means of coaching, or else the person being coached will fail to obtain the full measure of the coach's knowledge. Effective coaching usually begins with easier material and progresses to the more difficult, and complex processes are often taken in graduated steps. Such an approach will reduce the likelihood of failure in the coaching relationship.

Active coaching, like active listening, requires the coach to give and receive feedback in a two-way exchange of ideas. The coach can provide supportive communication in the form of both praise and positive feedback. Positive feedback goes farther than simple praise for a job well done; it recognizes some action that particularly merits positive attention, with the aim of enhancing the learning experience. A similar distinction can be made concerning communication that addresses the negative side of performance. Criticism makes the point that the person has done something wrong, but it provides little explanation; negative feedback, on the other hand, helps the person to understand why the action needs to be corrected. Feedback, whether positive or negative, supports a discussion between the two individuals and fills in details that often go unmentioned in simple praise or criticism. An effective coach needs to provide useful feedback while also being receptive to feedback from the person being coached. Such feedback demands the coach's undivided attention, as it can help the coach understand whether key teaching points have been understood.

Harvard Business School[30] has offered a series of guidelines for the use of feedback during the coaching process. Feedback should be given in a timely manner, and it should focus on both positive and negative aspects of performance.

It should be future oriented, directed at performance issues that can be corrected in the future, not at issues that have happened once and will not recur. Feedback should focus on the behavior of the individual being coached, not on the individual's character, attitude, or personality. Negative feedback that is interpreted as a personal attack can impede the coaching process or even destroy the coaching relationship. Feedback, to be effective, must be sincere, realistic, and specific. Generalizations usually have little effect if the person being coached does not receive sufficient information to guide a change in behavior. Feedback should be designed to make a difference in the life of the person being coached, while at the same time focusing on factors that can be controlled. Feedback concerning factors outside the person's control is typically useless.

Sergeant Joe Friday, in the television show *Dragnet*, famously said, "All we want are the facts, ma'am."[31] So it is with feedback. Opinions may be relevant, but they do not carry the same weight as facts. Specific, fact-based feedback helps the individual being coached to understand exactly what constitutes correct or incorrect behavior.

Follow-Up

The fourth step in the coaching process is follow-up, which seeks to ensure that the person who has received coaching remains on track for continued improvement. The coach should make sure that effective communication, clear understanding, and progress toward goals continue and that important teachings are reinforced. Opportunities for follow-up should not be left to chance; they should be an integral part of the coaching plan.

Case Study: Zika Outbreak in Miami[32,33]

Zika virus is disseminated to people primarily by *Aedes aegypti* mosquitoes, and it can be transmitted among people through sexual intercourse, blood transfusion, or laboratory exposure. The virus can also be passed from a mother to an unborn child. Fetal exposure to Zika can cause severe birth defects, including microcephaly. Microcephaly is a condition in which newborns' heads and often brains are significantly smaller than normal, often resulting in severe brain defects and other health problems, including eye defects, hearing loss, and impaired growth. Zika is also known to cause Guillain-Barre syndrome, in which a person's own immune system attacks nerve cells, leading to muscle problems and paralysis. At the time of this writing, no vaccine against Zika exists. Primary prevention mechanisms include protection against mosquito bites and the avoidance of unprotected sexual encounters.

(continued)

Zika virus was first identified in 1947 in Uganda, but human cases and outbreaks have historically been rare and located almost exclusively in Africa and Southeast Asia. In spring 2015, however, Zika outbreaks began occurring across Brazil and then in other Latin American and Caribbean nations. As outbreaks ravaged these countries, public health leaders and infectious disease experts in the United States predicted that America's ground zero for Zika would be in Miami, Florida. Miami-Dade County's mosquito-control division, operating annually on a $1.7 million budget, received an additional $300,000 in funding. However, even with those funds, the county's mosquito-control spending amounted to just $0.64 per resident. By contrast, Monroe County in the Florida Keys spent nearly $208 per capita on mosquito control.

In the summer of 2016, the experts' prediction was realized. Outbreaks of locally acquired Zika virus were discovered in two Miami areas—the upscale Wynwood neighborhood, with its open-air restaurants and shops, and ever-popular Miami Beach. The county soon spent more than $10 million to control the outbreaks, with most of the funding going to independent mosquito-control contractors who were hired to reinforce agency staff. Notably, Florida health and agriculture officials sent fewer than two dozen mosquito traps to aid in the response. (The Florida Department of Agriculture normally handles mosquito control, but responsibility was transferred to the Department of Health once Zika became a public health threat.)

As mosquito-control experts worked to contain the outbreak, civic and health officials at the local and state levels squabbled to attribute blame, with the Miami-Dade County and Miami Beach mayors accusing state health officials of requiring them to keep secret the locations where mosquitoes carrying the Zika virus were captured. By fall 2016, the Florida Department of Health would record more than 100 local mosquito-borne Zika infections.

Discussion and Application Questions

1. In what ways did the preparations for and response to Miami's Zika outbreak demonstrate ineffective public health leadership?
2. How did varying responsibilities for mosquito control between the state health and agriculture departments—as well as between the state and local health departments—contribute to the problematic response to Zika?
3. How could government and public health leaders have responded more effectively?
4. Would the coaching of local public health officials by the Florida Department of Agriculture have been beneficial in controlling the Zika outbreak?

Summary

Mentoring is a personal support process based on concern for the professional success of the individual being mentored. The person who provides guidance is the mentor, and the person who receives guidance is the mentee. An effective mentor should serve as a role model and trusted counselor to the mentee. Mentoring is related to coaching, but the two processes are not the same. Mentoring focuses chiefly on the mentee's career development, whereas coaching is directed toward specific situations. Coaching may be considered part of the larger concept of mentoring. An effective mentoring process benefits the mentee, the mentor, and the organization at large. Mentees can develop their professional abilities, acquire useful information and expertise, and gain a better understanding of the processes by which the organization functions. Mentors often gain self-esteem, respect from peers, and a sense of renewal. As the value of mentoring has become more widely recognized, its use has increased across a variety of fields, including public health.

Establishing an effective mentor–mentee relationship is a complex process. Although some organizations match mentors with mentees in formal programs, the more common approach is for mentees to select their own mentors. In selecting a mentor, the aspiring mentee should set at least one goal for the mentoring process, identify and meet with prospective mentors within the organization, work to implement each prospective mentor's initial suggestions, and determine whether each candidate is a good mentoring fit. Clear communication at the start of the relationship can help build the kind of trusted partnership that is essential for good mentoring.

The Anderson and Shannon mentoring model incorporates mentoring dispositions, relationships, functions, and activities. The three mentoring dispositions—(1) being open to the mentee, (2) leading the mentee incrementally over time, and (3) expressing interest in the mentee's professional and personal needs—are central to the model. In the mentoring relationship, the mentor serves as a role model while also nurturing the mentee and acting as a care giver. According to the model, the five functions of the mentoring process are (1) teaching, (2) sponsoring, (3) encouraging, (4) counseling, and (5) befriending. The mentoring activities coordinate with the lessons of the five functions.

In the application of situational leadership to the mentoring process, individuals' readiness to engage in the process as mentees determines their mentee readiness level (MR1–MR4). Leaders, in turn, use a leadership style (S1–S4) that is appropriate to that readiness level. The mentee readiness levels roughly correspond with other models that specify stages or phases in the mentoring partnership. The four stages identified by Bell are (1) leveling the learning field, (2) fostering acceptance and safety, (3) giving learning gifts, and (4) bolstering self-direction and independence. The four phases identified by Kram are (1) initiation, (2) cultivation, (3) separation, and (4) redefinition.

Coaching, which may be considered part of the mentoring process, has three main components—technical help, personal support, and individual challenge. These components are held together by an emotional bond between the coach and the person being coached. The process of coaching can be broken down into four main steps: (1) preparation, (2) discussion, (3) active coaching, and (4) follow-up. Effective communication and feedback—or even "feedforward," as coined by Goldsmith—are essential to the coaching process.

Discussion Questions

1. What is the difference between mentoring and coaching? How do the two concepts interact?
2. Define the term *mentoring*. What responsibilities exist between the mentor and mentee?
3. What are the benefits of the mentoring process?
4. What are the qualities and roles of an effective public health mentor?
5. Describe how an individual goes about the process of choosing a mentor.
6. Analyze the key features of the Anderson and Shannon mentoring model.
7. How would you employ the situational leadership model of mentoring?
8. What are the myths of mentoring, and how can they be overcome?
9. What are the critical elements of developing a formal mentoring program? Compare and contrast formal and informal mentoring arrangements.
10. For deeper thought: How does effective coaching make public health leaders' jobs easier? How does it enhance their careers?

Web Resources

Chronus. 2017. "How to Start a High-Impact Mentoring Program." Accessed August 15. http://chronus.com/how-to-start-a-mentoring-program.

Management Mentors. 2015. "The Differences Between Coaching and Mentoring." Accessed August 15, 2017. www.management-mentors.com/resources/coaching-mentoring-differences.

Moscinski, P. 2002. "Take Charge of Your Mentoring Experience." American College of Healthcare Executives. Acccssed August 15, 2017. www.ache.org/newclub/career/MentorArticles/Takecharge.cfm.

References

1. Bell, C. R. 2000. "The Mentor as Partner." *Training Development Journal* 54 (2): 52–56.

2. Cobb, M. D., D. L. Fox, J. E. Many, M. W. Matthews, E. McGrail, and G. T. Sachs. 2006. "Mentoring in Literacy Education: A Commentary from Graduate Students, Untenured Professors, and Tenured Professors." *Mentoring and Tutoring* 14 (4): 371–87.

3. Ledlow, G. R., and M. N. Coppola. 2014. *Leadership for Health Professionals: Theory, Skills, and Applications*, 2nd ed. Sudbury, MA: Jones & Bartlett Learning.

4. Levinson, D. J., C. N. Darrow, E. B. Klein, M. H. Levinson, and B. McKee. 1978. *The Seasons of a Man's Life*. New York: Knopf.

5. Kram, K. E. 1988. *Mentoring at Work: Developmental Relationships in Organizational Life*. New York: University Press of America.

6. Crosby, J. n.d. "John Crosby Quotes." FinestQuotes. Accessed February 6, 2017. www.finestquotes.com/author_quotes-author-John%20Crosby-page-0.htm.

7. Harvard Business Essentials. 2004. *Coaching and Mentoring*. Boston: Harvard Business School Press.

8. Biehl, B. 2007. *Mentoring: How to Find a Mentor and How to Become One*. Mt. Dora, FL: Allen.

9. Phillips-Jones, L. 2001. *The New Mentors and Protégés*. Grass Valley, CA: Coalition of Counseling Centers.

10. Rowitz, L. 2014. *Public Health Leadership: Putting Principles into Practice*, 3rd ed. Sudbury, MA: Jones & Bartlett.

11. Alleman, E. 1989. "Two Planned Mentoring Programs That Worked." *Mentoring International* 3 (1): 6–12.

12. Fiedler, F. E., and A. F. Leister. 1977. "Leader Intelligence and Task Performance: A Test of a Multiple Screen Model." *Organizational Behavior and Human Performance* 20 (1): 1–14.

13. Zaleznik, A. 1967. "Management Disappointment." *Harvard Business Review* 45 (6): 59–70.

14. Kram, K. E. 1980. "Mentoring Process at Work: Developmental Relationships in Managerial Careers." Doctoral dissertation, Yale University.

15. Bass, B. M. 2008. *The Bass Handbook of Leadership: Theory, Research, and Managerial Applications*, 4th ed. New York: Free Press.

16. Jennings, E. E. 1967. *Executive Success: Stresses, Problems, and Adjustments*. New York: Appleton-Century-Crofts.

17. Carruthers, J. 1993. "The Principles and Practices of Mentoring." In *The Return of the Mentor: Strategies for Workplace Learning*, edited by B. J. Caldwell and E. M. A. Carter, 9–24. London, UK: Falmer Press.

18. Gray, W. A. 1989. "Situational Mentoring: Custom Designing Planned Mentoring Programs." *International Journal of Mentoring* 3 (1): 19–28.

19. Wickman, F., and T. Sjodin. 1996. *Mentoring*. Chicago: Irwin Professional Publishing.

20. Anderson, E. M., and A. L. Shannon. 1988. "Toward a Conceptualization of Mentoring." *Journal of Teacher Education* 39 (1): 38–42.

21. Churchill, W. n.d. "Winston Churchill Quotes." FinestQuotes. Accessed August 24, 2017. www.finestquotes.com/author_quotes-author-Winston%20Churchill-page-4.htm.

22. Holsinger, J. W., Jr. 2010. *How to Develop Lay Ministry Within a Local Church*. Lewiston, MA: Edwin Mellen Press.

23. Kram, K. E. "Phases of the Mentor Relationship." *Academy of Management Journal* 26 (4): 608–25.

24. Covey, S. R. 1989. *The 7 Habits of Highly Effective People*. New York: Simon & Schuster.

25. Sandler, B. R. 1993. "Women as Mentors: Myths and Commandments." *Chronicle of Higher Education* 39 (27): B3.

26. Noe, R. A., D. B. Greenberger, and S. Wang. 2002. "Mentoring: What We Know and Where We Might Go from Here." In *Research in Personnel and Human Resources Management*, vol. 21, edited by G. R. Ferris and J. J. Martocchio, 129–73. Oxford, UK: Elsevier.

27. Chao, G. T., P. M. Walz, and P. D. Gardner. 1992. "Formal and Informal Mentorships: A Comparison on Mentoring Functions and Contrast with Nonmentored Counterparts." *Personnel Psychology* 45 (3): 619–36.

28. Goldsmith, M. 2006. "Try Feedforward Instead of Feedback." In *Coaching for Leadership*, edited by M. Goldsmith and L. Lyons, 45–49. San Francisco: Pfeiffer.

29. Waldroop, J., and T. Butler. 1996. "The Executive as Coach." *Harvard Business Review* 74 (6): 111–17.

30. Harvard Business School Publishing. 2003. *Harvard ManageMentor on Giving and Receiving Feedback*. Boston: Harvard Business School Publishing.

31. Snopes.com. 2008. "Dragnet 'Just the Facts.'" Updated December 13. www.snopes.com/radiotv/tv/dragnet.asp.

32. Centers for Disease Control and Prevention. 2016. "Zika Virus." Updated September 29. www.cdc.gov/zika/about/index.html.

33. Staletovich, J. 2016. "How Miami-Dade Got Outgunned and Overwhelmed in the War on Zika." *Miami Herald*. Published September 23. www.miamiherald.com/news/local/environment/article103665202.html.

EPILOGUE: EFFECTIVE PUBLIC HEALTH LEADERSHIP

James W. Holsinger Jr. and Erik L. Carlton

I n this book, we have attempted to provide an in-depth overview of effective public health leadership, with attention to both its theoretical bases and its practical applications. We have discussed the various attributes of effective leadership and explored the ways in which those attributes can be applied to leader–follower interactions. We have considered the ways that the situation or context affects leadership within organizations, and we have taken a close look at the relationships that leaders develop with their followers—whether those followers are employees, constituents, or collaborators. Effective public health leaders must be able to engage the organization and its constituents with a sense of collaboration, while at the same time demonstrating a steady commitment to ethical behavior and the mission of public health. We conclude this book with a summary of several key points.

Personal Attributes of Leaders

Effective leaders in public health are not always saints nor sinners; likewise, they are not completely selfless nor selfish. However, they constantly strive to place the needs of their followers and the organization above their own. Effective public health leaders are the chief role models within their organizations. To be effective role models, leaders must control their egos and consistently uphold organizational values.

Leading organizations, groups, and teams is never easy, and it requires a great deal of self-discipline. Since the tone of the organization is set from the top, a leader's failure of self-discipline can plant the seeds for failure throughout the organization. Restraint is an important—though often undervalued—tool of leadership. Leaders cannot allow themselves to "blow off steam" by shouting at followers, employees, constituents, or other collaborators. Effective leaders also embrace innovation and creativity to ensure that the organization produces quality services to meet the needs of the community. High-quality work saves time and money because tasks do not need to be done over; meanwhile, half-finished work is labor lost. Effective leaders build strong trust relationships with followers, employees, constituents, and other collaborators, and these relationships help the organization make a meaningful difference in the lives of the population served.

Leading the Organization

Effective public health leaders must always be aware of the situation or context in which they lead, and they must use a suitable style of leadership for both individuals and groups. A key element of the situation is the mission of the organization or group. Effective leaders must embrace the mission, unite followers in its pursuit, and take appropriate actions to achieve it. By virtue of being assigned to a leadership position, the public health leader obtains both position power and personal power. However, power is in the eye of the beholder, and it depends heavily on the day-to-day perceptions of followers. If followers perceive that the leader is failing to exercise power wisely and effectively, the leader's power—particularly personal power—will be diminished. Even when leaders feel that they are firmly in control, followers are never as submissive as the leaders hope for them to be. Leaders in public health should study the various techniques of leading groups and teams, select a methodology that works for them, and put it into practice on a daily basis.

Relationship to Followers

The key to effective public health leadership lies in the relationship of the leader to the follower, and vice versa. Pursuit of a public health organization's goals requires both good leaders and good followers, and strong relationships between the two are essential for a productive work environment. Both leadership and followership rely on influence and counterinfluence on both sides of the relationship. In maintaining strong relationships, leaders must place the needs of followers ahead of their own needs, building confidence when followers are insecure and supporting all followers in their development. Leaders cannot let themselves become out of touch with their followers, or the followers will perceive that they have no leader. Effective public health leaders recognize that followers are far more important to the leader than leaders are to the followers. Leaders without followers are simply individuals taking a walk—all by themselves!

Collaboration and Systems Leadership

Effective public health leadership in the twenty-first century requires the ability to achieve positive health outcomes through collaboration, both within the public health enterprise and across the interorganizational spectrum. As the practice of public health continues to evolve to meet the demands of emerging health issues, leaders will increasingly activate and empower transdisciplinary public health teams.

More and more, public health activities, and thus public health leadership, are transcending traditional public health functions to incorporate multisector partnerships and policies. The resulting paradigm—sometimes called "Public Health 3.0"[1,2,3]—expands the scope of public health leadership and elevates it to true systems leadership, making coalition building, policy development, interpersonal communication, collective impact, and interorganizational strategic planning increasingly critical.[3,4,5] Public health leaders can no longer simply rely on their own abilities and neglect to collaborate with others. Today's effective leaders engage civic, business, healthcare, education, and other leaders in cross-sector visioning, and they engage the citizens they serve to better inform strategic initiatives. Effective public health leaders are proactive in their collaborative ventures. They do not wait for others to come to the table; rather, they actively strive to align shared human, physical, and financial resources across communities.

Effective public health leaders can and should engage healthcare and other leaders in community health needs assessments and health improvement planning. They can and should work with business and economic development leaders to reinforce the connection between health and economic vitality. They can and should leverage ties to education and faith-based organizations to reach populations they might not otherwise reach. Only in this way can the complex public health problems of the twenty-first century be adequately, effectively, and collectively addressed.

Ethical Leadership

Effective public health leaders understand that everything they seek to accomplish must be performed in a legal, ethical, and moral manner. If they behave unethically, they are failing to provide the leadership expected and demanded by their followers, employees, constituents, and collaborators. Such failure is abject and unconscionable. Effective public health leaders do the right thing, the right way, the first time. They know that power can corrupt, and therefore they commit to using their power responsibly, for the good of their followers and the organization. Effective leaders behave ethically in mentoring and coaching relationships, building trust, maintaining confidentiality, and providing a safe place to foster positive change.

Summary

Our belief is that the vast majority of effective public health leaders are made, not born, and that effective public health leadership is an art that can be developed through education and training. Doing so, however, requires extensive practice. Effective leaders work throughout their careers to constantly develop and perfect their knowledge, skills, and abilities.

A public health practitioner seeking to become an effective public health leader needs to recognize that a variety of leadership theories and models exist, and novice leaders should test-drive a number of these theories to determine which ones fit them best. Once they have made that determination, they must continually practice what they have adopted. Some leaders may focus on a single theory or model, whereas others might incorporate aspects from many. The specific theories and models employed are less important than the leader's continued commitment to the process of effective leadership for the good of the public's health.

References

1. DeSalvo, K. B., P. W. O'Carroll, D. Koo, J. M. Auerbach, and J. A. Monroe. 2016. "Public Health 3.0: Time for an Upgrade." *American Journal of Public Health* 106 (4): 621–22.

2. Fraser, M., B. Castrucci, and E. Harper. 2017. "Public Health Leadership and Management in the Era of Public Health 3.0." *Journal of Public Health Management and Practice* 23 (1): 90–92.

3. United States Department of Health and Human Services. 2016. *Public Health 3.0: A Call to Action to Create a 21st Century Public Health Infrastructure.* Accessed February 9, 2017. www.healthypeople.gov/sites/default/files/Public-Health-3.0-White-Paper.pdf.

4. Kaufman, N. J., B. C. Castrucci, and J. Pearsol. 2014. "Thinking Beyond the Silos." *Journal of Public Health Management and Practice* 20 (6): 557–65.

5. Carlton, E. L. 2014. "Answering the Call for Integrating Population Health: Insights from Health System Executives." *Advances in Health Care Management* 16: 115–38.

APPENDIX

This appendix presents sets of public health leadership competencies developed by the Association of Schools and Programs of Public Health (ASPPH) and the Council on Linkages Between Academia and Public Health Practice.

ASPPH Education Committee—Master's Degree in Public Health Core Competency Development Project (Version 2.3, August 2006)

LEADERSHIP

The ability to create and communicate a shared vision for a changing future; champion solutions to organizational and community challenges; and energize commitment to goals.

Competencies: Upon graduation, it is increasingly important that a student with an MPH be able to...

1. Describe the attributes of leadership in public health.
2. Describe alternative strategies for collaboration and partnership among organizations, focused on public health goals.
3. Articulate an achievable mission, set of core values, and vision.
4. Engage in dialogue and learning from others to advance public health goals.
5. Demonstrate team building, negotiation, and conflict management skills.
6. Demonstrate transparency, integrity, and honesty in all actions.
7. Use collaborative methods for achieving organizational and community health goals.
8. Apply social justice and human rights principles when addressing community needs.

9. Develop strategies to motivate others for collaborative problem solving, decision-making, and evaluation.

Source: Association of Schools of Public Health Education Committee. 2006. *Master's Degree in Public Health Core Competency Model, Version 2.3*. Published August. www.aspph.org/app/uploads/2014/04/Version2.31_FINAL.pdf.

ASPPH Education Committee—Doctor of Public Health (DrPH) Core Competency Model (Version 1.3, November 2009)

LEADERSHIP

The ability to create and communicate a shared vision for a positive future; inspire trust and motivate others; and use evidence-based strategies to enhance essential public health services.

Competencies: Upon graduation a student with a DrPH should be able to…

E1. Communicate an organization's mission, shared vision, and values to stakeholders.

E2. Develop teams for implementing health initiatives.

E3. Collaborate with diverse groups.

E4. Influence others to achieve high standards of performance and accountability.

E5. Guide organizational decision-making and planning based on internal and external environmental research.

E6. Prepare professional plans incorporating lifelong learning, mentoring, and continued career progression strategies.

E7. Create a shared vision.

E8. Develop capacity-building strategies at the individual, organizational, and community level.

E9. Demonstrate a commitment to personal and professional values.

Source: Association of Schools of Public Health Education Committee. 2009. *Doctor of Public Health (DrPH) Core Competency Model, Version 1.3*. Published November. www.aspph.org/app/uploads/2014/04/DrPHVersion1-3.pdf.

Council on Linkages—Core Competencies for Public Health Professionals (June 2014)

Leadership and Systems Thinking Skills (Tier 2)
8B1. Incorporates ethical standards of practice (e.g., Public Health Code of Ethics) into all interactions with individuals, organizations, and communities.
8B2. Describes public health as part of a larger inter-related system of organizations that influence the health of populations at local, national, and global levels.
8B3. Explains the ways public health care and other organizations can work together or individually to impact the health of a community.
8B4. Collaborates with individuals and organizations in developing a vision for a healthy community (e.g., emphasis on prevention, health equity for all, excellence, and innovation).
8B5. Analyzes internal and external facilitators and barriers that may affect the delivery of the 10 Essential Public Health Services (e.g., using root cause analysis and other quality improvement methods and tools, problem solving).
8B6. Provides opportunities for professional development for individuals and teams (e.g., training, mentoring, peer advising, coaching).
8B7. Ensures use of professional development opportunities by individuals and teams.
8B8. Modifies organizational practices in consideration of changes (e.g., social, political, economic, scientific).
8B9. Contributes to continuous improvement of individual program and organizational performance (e.g., mentoring, mentoring progress, adjusting programs to achieve better results).
8B10. Advocates for the role of public health in providing population health services.

Source: Council on Linkages Between Academia and Public Health. 2014. "Core Competencies for Public Health Professionals." Published June. www.phf.org/resourcestools/Pages/Core_Public_ Health_Competencies.aspx.

GLOSSARY

ability: Possession of the manner or skill to do something.

achievement-oriented leadership: A type of leadership behavior that involves setting challenging goals for followers and interactions that are both supporting and demanding.

action mediation: The process by which the leader and the group select an appropriate course of action and create an organizational system for making high-quality decisions.

activist: A follower who engages with the group and acts with considerable passion and energy.

act utilitarianism: A reasoning approach in which every moral decision is made on the basis of a comparative analysis of the particular situation with the aim of maximizing the group good.

adjourning stage: The stage in the team life cycle in which the team dissolves and its members transition to new challenges.

agreeableness: The ability to get along with other people; a key characteristic for resolving conflict and gaining followers.

alienated follower: A follower who thinks independently but has negative energy or passive engagement.

all-inclusive workforce: An approach to organizational diversity that fosters the continuation of subgroup identity within an overarching organizational identity.

altruism: An unselfish concern for the welfare of others.

analogical reasoning: Moral reasoning based on structural comparisons between situations.

Anderson and Shannon mentoring model: A conceptualization of the mentoring process that incorporates mentoring dispositions, relationships, functions, and activities.

assertiveness: The extent to which individuals are aggressive, assertive, or confrontational in relationships.

assessment: Systematically collecting, assembling, analyzing, and making available information about the health of the community.

assigned leadership: Leadership based on a person's assigned position in an organization.

assurance: Ensuring that necessary personal and community health services are provided to every member of the community.

augmentative effect: The idea that transformational leadership augments, or enhances, transactional leadership.

authentic transformational leadership: Transformational leadership motivated by altruism and integrity.

authority: The advantages, duties, rights, and obligations linked to a specific position within an organization.

autonomy: Practitioners' freedom to establish criteria for entry into a profession, to control a body of knowledge and skills, and to oversee professional standards and certification.

bystander: A follower who observes the group but chooses not to participate.

charisma: The ability to connect with followers in a way that produces remarkable performance and attainment.

charismatic authority: A form of authority that is informally granted from below based on an individual's personal characteristics.

coaching: Instructing, training, and directing one or more people to learn specific skills or achieve a goal.

coercive power: Power derived from one's capacity to penalize or punish others.

cognitive style: The way one perceives, processes, interprets, and uses information.

collaboration: A mutually beneficial, well-defined relationship between two or more organizations or individuals that achieves results through working together.

collectivistic values: Cultural views concerning the leader's/follower's relationship to the organization/work, family orientation, and general society.

colorblind approach: An approach to organizational diversity that seeks to develop an overarching identity for all individuals within the organization while ignoring cultural group identities.

commitment: An outcome in which a follower agrees internally with a request or decision made by the leader and works to carry it out.

commutative justice: Fairness in exchange and discourse, including such aspects as confidentiality and truth telling.

compliance: An outcome in which a follower carries out the leader's wishes but is unenthusiastic, making little or no effort to perform effectively.

conceptual skills: Skills that are cognitive in nature and based on concepts and ideas.

Conditions of Trust Inventory (CTI): A validated trust inventory with 11 dimensions: availability, competence, consistency, discreetness, fairness, integrity, loyalty, openness, promise fulfillment, receptivity, and overall trust.

connection power: Power based on the perceived association of the leader with influential people and organizations.

conscientiousness: The ability to remain focused on goals and to pursue them in a purposeful manner.

consequentialism: A type of teleological reasoning in which a desired end can justify the means; includes utilitarianism and hedonism.

contingency: A fact or event that is incidental to or dependent on something else.

contingency theories of leadership: Theories that consider the influence of intervening situational variables on leadership behavior and outcomes; such theories focus on leaders, followers, and the situation.

contingent reward (CR): A transactional leadership approach that sets expectations for followers and offers recognition or rewards when goals are achieved.

core competency model: A framework developed by the Association of Schools and Programs of Public Health that establishes a baseline of knowledge required of candidates for various public health degrees.

core functions of public health: Three central tasks—assessment, policy development, and assurance—to be carried out by all public health agencies at every level of government.

cross-functional team: A type of team in which members from various functional subunits have responsibility for a particular project.

cultural cohesion: The extent of consensus for specific values among an organization's employees and their agreement with the way things are done.

culture: The shared learning of a group or organization, including such elements as values, beliefs, customs, behavior, emotions, and cognition.

culture gap: The difference between the values and behaviors that an organization actually has and those that are appropriate for the context in which the organization functions.

deontological reasoning: Moral reasoning based on categories, which often yield sets of formal rules.

dependency: A source of power based on the leader's control over something that the follower desires or depends on.

determination: The motivation a leader needs to come to a decision, to persevere in the face of obstacles, and to see a job through to completion.

diehard: A follower whose feelings of support or opposition are extremely intense.

diffusion of innovation theory: A model that categorizes individuals based on their receptivity to innovation.

directive leadership: A type of leadership behavior that involves telling followers what is to be accomplished, who is to accomplish it, where and when it should be done, and how the leader wants the task to be performed.

discrimination: Actions that are based on prejudice.

disposition: A person's inclinations or tendencies toward a certain temperament.

distributive justice: The dissemination of goods and costs, both tangible and intangible, in an appropriate or equitable manner throughout society.

diversity: The presence of people from a variety of cultures, backgrounds, or ethnicities.

dyadic framing of leadership: A way of viewing leadership with an emphasis on relational processes between leaders and followers.

dyadic pair: A unit of analysis consisting of a leader (manager) and a follower (subordinate) within the work environment.

dynamic subordinancy: A condition in which individuals assume responsibility for their own behavior and development, as well as for their contributions to the organization, rather than simply relying on directional, autocratic leadership.

ecological power: Power based on the leader's control of the physical work environment, technological systems, and organizational structure in which people work.

emergent leadership: Leadership exercised by an individual who is not assigned to a leadership role.

emotional intelligence: The ability to systematically review the emotions of oneself and other individuals, differentiating between various emotions, appropriately labeling them, and utilizing such information to guide behavior and thought.

emotional stability: The degree to which a person is calm, secure, and well adjusted.

empathy: The capacity to understand the values, motives, and emotions of another person.

enhancer variable: A variable that strengthens relationships between leader behaviors and outcome criteria.

essential values: Fundamental values, proposed in Priester's values framework, that are required for a healthcare system.

ethical leadership: Leadership based on moral reasoning and ethical decision making.

ethics: The analysis of formally expressed and legitimized standards and patterns of behavior.

ethnocentrism: A tendency for individuals to place their own cultural group at the center of their worldview.

expectancy: The perceived probability that a certain behavior will lead to a certain outcome.

expert power: Power based on followers' perceptions of a leader's competence.

external adaptation: The cultural function through which members of an organization understand and adjust to the external environment.

external fit: Alignment of an organization's culture and strategies with the outside environment.

extra-role behavior (ERB): Work-related activities that are not included in the formal description of the employee's role.

extraversion: One's degree of concern and engagement with what is outside the self.

Fiedler's contingency model of leadership effectiveness: A model, developed by Fred Fiedler, based on the idea that effective leadership depends on matching situational demands and leadership style; also known as the *leader-match model.*

five dysfunctions of a team: A model that identifies five forms of dysfunction that arise in team settings: absence of trust, fear of conflict, lack of commitment, avoidance of accountability, and inattention to results.

followership: A follower's efforts to actively help an organization or a cause to succeed while independently exercising critical judgment in completing tasks and solving potential problems.

Followership Continuum: A model in which followers can move (in either direction) across five levels of performance: employee, committed follower, engaged follower, effective follower, and exemplary follower.

forming stage: The stage of team development in which a new group is beginning its orientation and developing awareness.

French-Raven taxonomy of power: A model that, in its expanded form, identifies seven bases of power: legitimate power, reward power, coercive power, information power, ecological power, referent power, and expert power.

full-range leadership: A model that consists of the transformational, transactional, and passive-avoidant leadership styles.

functional work team: A type of team in which members have different responsibilities but work together to perform a common function.

future orientation: The extent to which a culture engages in advance planning and other forward-looking activities.

gender egalitarianism: The degree to which a culture minimizes gender differences in societal roles and encourages gender equality.

great man theory: An approach to leadership study, popular prior to 1950, that focused on the traits of individuals who were thought to be great men.

groupthink: A tendency to think or make decisions as a group, to the point that individual creativity and responsibility are discouraged.

hard power: Power based on the leader's position within the organization and the authority vested in the leader; also called *position power.*

hedonism: A reasoning method that prioritizes self-fulfillment and is contingent upon some significant degree of personal liberty; also known as *rational egoism.*

Hill's team leadership model: A model that focuses on the leader's role in ensuring team effectiveness by diagnosing team problems and taking appropriate steps to correct them.

humane orientation: The degree to which a culture encourages and rewards members' support for community values, sensitivity and caring, altruism, and generosity.

idealized influence attributes and behaviors (IIA and IIB): The collection of ideal qualities and actions that followers look for in leaders.

ideology: A coherent set of beliefs that holds individuals together, based on cause-and-effect relationships.

implementer: A follower who is supportive but unwilling to challenge the leader.

implicit leadership theory: The idea that individuals have certain beliefs and convictions about the traits and behaviors that distinguish leaders from nonleaders and effective leaders from ineffective leaders.

impression management tactics: Behaviors used by individuals to influence the way they are perceived by others.

inclusion: The practice of welcoming diversity and encouraging participation from people representing a wide variety of backgrounds and characteristics.

individual consideration (IC): The way in which a leader acts as a coach or mentor and pays attention to each individual's need for achievement and growth.

individualist: A follower who is not fully supportive but is willing to challenge the leader.

individualized leadership: Use of leadership styles appropriate for each follower, rather than a style that is common for all members of the group.

influence: The way a leader affects a follower, particularly in terms of the impact of requests and decisions.

influence tactics: Behaviors that are used by one individual to change the behaviors, opinions, or attitudes of another.

influential values: A category in Priester's values framework that includes six values that were emphasized in US healthcare during the twentieth century.

information power: Power based on the leader's ability to control the flow of information that followers consider important.

informing stage: The stage at the start of the team development process in which people are notified of their membership in the group and informed about the group's mission.

in-group: A category of vertical dyad linkage in which the follower has a high degree of exchange with the leader and takes on extra roles and responsibilities in the work setting.

in-group collectivism: The degree to which a culture is based on family cohesiveness, devotion, and loyalty.

inspirational motivation (IM): The enthusiasm, encouragement, and optimism that a leader provides to inspire and motivate followers.

institutional collectivism: The degree to which a culture encourages collective activity and is identified with the broader interests of society.

instrumental compliance: An influence process that occurs when a follower completes a task requested by the leader with the understanding that a reward or punishment will result.

instrumental values: Values, proposed in Priester's values framework, that are necessary to support the essential values.

integrity: Consistency between claimed moral values and behavior.

intellectual stimulation (IS): The degree to which a leader provides a stimulating environment through dialogue, innovation, creativity, and collaborative problem solving.

intelligence: The capacity for understanding, reasoning, and perception, including the aptitude for grasping facts and the relationships between them.

internal fit: The degree to which an organization's culture has consensus and consistency in its values and ideologies.

internal integration: The process by which culture establishes unity and collective identity within the group.

internalization: An influence process that occurs when a follower commits to a task requested by the leader because the task is deemed desirable in and of itself and compatible with the follower's beliefs and values.

interpersonal skills: Social skills and skills involving people.

isolate: A follower who is detached and silent, thus often ignored.

job tension: Emotional or mental strain resulting from job stress.

just coercion theory: A theory that combines various moral reasoning methods—including utilitarianism, deontology, and virtue—to explain how governmental power can and should be used; also known as *just war theory*.

justice: The principle of being impartial and fair in resolving situations with competing claims or in assigning deserved rewards and punishments; giving each person his or her due.

laissez-faire (LF) leadership: A passive approach to leadership in which leaders are absent or uninvolved in important issues and decisions; sometimes referred to as *nonleadership*.

leader attribution error: The tendency to overestimate the role of a single leader and underestimate, or altogether ignore, the roles of the many followers.

leader–member exchange (LMX) theory: A leadership model in which the leader develops exchange agreements with each follower and the quality of each exchange relationship influences the follower's performance, decisions, responsibilities, and access to resources; also called *vertical dyad linkage theory*.

leadership: A process in which an individual intentionally acts to influence another individual or group, regardless of the reason, in an effort to achieve a common goal, which may or may not contribute to the success of the organization.

leadership-making model: A model of leader, follower, and organizational development based on the leader's characteristics, the characteristics of the follower, and the level of maturity of the relationship between them.

leadership style: A pattern of behavior that a leader exhibits when dealing with followers.

leadership substitute: A characteristic of a task, organization, or followers that makes relationship- or task-oriented leadership impossible or unnecessary.

Leadership–Teamship–Followership Continuum: A model that describes the way individuals occupy—and move between—various roles of leadership and followership in a team environment.

leadership traits: Personal attributes or characteristics that are commonly associated with the ability to lead.

least-preferred coworker scale (LPC): A scale used in Fiedler's contingency model to measure leadership style and distinguish between task-motivated leaders (low LPC score) and relationship-motivated (high LPC score) leaders.

legitimate power: Power associated with status or formal job authority.

liminality: The absence of clear cultural meaning during periods of challenge or transformation.

locus of control: A concept reflecting the degree to which individuals feel they can control their life situations or are affected by outside forces.

management: Working with and through people in order to complete the work at hand in an effective and efficient manner.

management by exception, active (MBEA): A transactional leadership approach that involves setting clear standards for compliance, specifying what constitutes ineffective performance, closely monitoring for deviances and mistakes, and taking corrective action as quickly as possible when problems occur.

management by exception, passive (MBEP): A passive-avoidant leadership approach in which the leader waits for things to go wrong before taking action.

mediator variable: A variable that represents an intermediate step between independent and dependent variables.

mentee: A person who seeks wisdom and guidance from a mentor.

mentor: A person who provides guidance and shares experiences to help develop the abilities of another person.

mentoring: A support process that is based on concern for the professional success of an individual, is both personal and intimate, and requires face-to-face interaction.

mentoring disposition: A characteristic attributed to a mentor that defines the mentor's actions in a certain situation.

middle axiom: A basic moral principle generally shared by individuals and groups even if they do not agree on the principle's philosophical or theological foundations.

morals: Standards and patterns of behavior that are formally expressed and legitimized.

mores: Standards of good and bad and of right and wrong that are simply assumed without formal expression.

motivation: The internal or external impetus that produces enthusiasm and persistence in followers to carry out a course of action.

motive: A reason for doing something in response to social experiences or stimuli.

multicultural approach: An approach to organizational diversity that considers employees' cultural differences as a benefit and a source of organizational strength.

multiculturalism: The presence of multiple cultures, or subcultures, within a larger system.

Multifactor Leadership Questionnaire (MLQ): A 45-item questionnaire that can be implemented in both self-rated and other-rater formats to measure transformational, transactional, and passive-avoidant leadership.

Myers-Briggs Type Indicator (MBTI): A tool that identifies personality types through the assessment of individual preferences across four dimensions.

need: Something essential or strongly desired, usually physiological in nature.

negative right: A right of a person to be generally free from state interference with regard to speech, religion, assembly, or other matters; also called a *liberty right*.

neutralizer variable: A variable that blocks or weakens leader influence on follower outcomes.

norming stage: The stage of team development in which the team becomes more cohesive and functions according to agreed-upon roles and concepts.

notifiable disease: A disease for which frequent and timely information about individual cases is deemed necessary for public health.

openness: The quality of being intellectually curious and inquisitive, open-minded and learning oriented, and experience based.

organizational citizenship behavior (OCB): Behavior that demonstrates an individual's commitment to the organization and its goals, typically through civic virtue and altruism.

organizational culture: Traditional or customary ways of thinking and acting that are shared by members of an organization and that individuals must acquire, to some extent, to be accepted into the organization.

out-group: A category of vertical dyad linkage in which the follower has a low degree of exchange with the leader and takes on defined roles according to a formal employment arrangement.

participant: A follower who engages with the group and tries to make an impact.

participative leadership: A type of leadership behavior that involves sharing work problems with followers and soliciting their input in the decision-making process.

partner: A follower who both supports and is willing to challenge the leader.

partnership building: A stage in individualized management marked by a positive exchange between the leader and each follower, with a resulting increase in follower performance.

passive-avoidant leadership: A leadership style in which the followers are given the power to make decisions.

path–goal theory: An exchange theory of leadership that explains how contingent rewards function and how such rewards influence subordinates' satisfaction and motivation.

performance orientation: The degree to which a culture encourages and rewards performance excellence and the attainment of goals.

performing stage: The stage of team development in which the team achieves results and develops a sense of pride through interdependence and collaborative work.

personal identification: An influence process that occurs when a follower attempts to imitate the leader's behaviors and thus identifies with the leader's attitudes, goals, and objectives.

personal integrity: Adherence to personal values in day-to-day behavior; the quality of being ethical, trustworthy, and honest.

personality: The combination of qualities and characteristics that form an individual's distinctive character.

personalized leader: A leader who has a significant need for personal power and uses it selfishly and without self-control.

personal power: Power based on a leader's effective use of skills and attributes, as perceived by the followers.

Physician Charter: A document that outlines fundamental professional principles and responsibilities for physicians and other healthcare practitioners.

plastic biological functionality: A person's biological capacity to operate given the social and ecological order.

policy development: Acting in the public interest to establish comprehensive public health policies based on scientific knowledge.

political tactics: Behaviors through which people acquire, develop, and use power, as well as other resources, in an attempt to gain desirable future outcomes.

position power: Power based on a leader's assigned role in the organization.

positive right: A right or entitlement, often to a good or service, that arises out of a society's economic or structural capacity.

power: A leader's ability to influence followers' beliefs, attitudes, and courses of action.

power distance: The degree to which stratification within a culture results in the unequal sharing of power.

practitioner: An individual who practices a profession.

prejudice: A preconceived opinion, attitude, or belief that is based not on actual experience or reason but rather on generalized ideas about certain groups.

Priester's values framework: A model developed by Reinhard Priester in 1992 to show the values that underlie the health system and should be used to guide reform.

principlism: A system of practical ethical decision making that concentrates on the moral principles of autonomy, beneficence, nonmaleficence, and justice.

proactive influence tactics: Behaviors intended to immediately engage the follower in taking on a new task or implementing a change.

profession: A field characterized by specialized knowledge and skills, altruism, self-regulation, and the preservation and expansion of knowledge.

professionalism: The manner of practicing a profession with competence, skill, and a commitment to serving the interests of other people either individually or collectively as a society.

proposed values: A category in Priester's values framework that includes essential values and instrumental values for meeting society's healthcare needs in the future.

protégé: An individual receiving guidance in a long-term leader-development process designed for personal succession.

prudence: Applied wisdom.

pseudotransformational leadership: Use of transformational leadership concepts for self-centered purposes.

public health: A science and art of protecting and improving the health of populations and communities.

public health system: The various governmental and nongovernmental agencies, including advocacy groups, focused on the health of populations and communities.

rational authority: Legal authority associated with a specific role or office and bound by the rules under which it is granted.

reactive influence tactics: Behaviors used by followers to oppose an unwanted influence attempt or to modify the leader's request to improve its acceptability.

referent power: Power based on followers' identification with and liking for a leader.

relationship behavior: Two-way communication in the relationship between leader and follower, including such actions as encouraging, listening, clarifying, and facilitating.

relationship management: The ability to relate to other individuals in a way that makes them feel understood and supported.

relationship-motivated leadership style: The style of leadership most concerned with the development of close interpersonal relationships.

resistance: A outcome in which a follower is opposed to the leader's request or decision and makes a minimal effort to carry it out.

resource: A follower who neither supports nor challenges the leader.

retributive justice: The assignment of a proportionate punishment for criminal behavior.

reward power: Power derived from one's capacity to provide rewards to others.

role finding: The first phase of the leadership-making process, in which the leader and the follower evaluate the other's abilities and motivations; also called *team finding.*

role implementation: The third phase of the leadership-making process, in which the behaviors of the leader and follower become interlocked; also called *team implementation.*

role making: The second phase of the leadership-making process, in which the dyadic relationship develops and both members come to understand how the other will function in specific situations; also called *team making.*

rule utilitarianism: A reasoning approach in which general practices are followed that have strong tendencies toward maximizing the group good.

self-awareness: The ability associated with self-assessment, recognizing and understanding one's own emotions, and knowing one's personal strengths and weaknesses.

self-concept: The identity constructed from the beliefs people have about themselves at the individual, interpersonal, or collective level.

self-confidence: Realistic certainty in one's own judgment, ideas, ability, power, decision making, and skills.

self-managed team: A type of team in which much of the leader's authority and responsibility is turned over to the team members.

self-management: The ability to keep one's emotions in balance; emotional self-control.

self-regulation: Practitioners' control over the practice of a profession under the guidance of a professional organization independent of direct governmental supervision.

sheep or passive follower: A follower who is dependent, does not think critically, and has negative energy or passive engagement.

situational favorability: The degree to which a particular situation provides leaders with control over followers or subordinates.

situational focus: An emphasis on the strong influence that elements of the situation, independent of the individual, have on the emergence and behavior of leaders.

situational leadership: The idea that there is no one best way to influence other people and that the readiness of the people being influenced determines the style that a leader should use.

situational moderator variable: An aspect of a particular situation that might enhance or negate a leader's skills, traits, and behaviors.

skill: The ability to perform activities in an effective manner.

social awareness: The ability to understand the dynamics that occur in individual, group, and community relationships.

social exchange theory: A theory that examines reciprocal influence processes that occur in small groups and determine how power and influence are gained or lost.

social intelligence: The aptitude for understanding the thoughts, feelings, and behaviors of others, and of oneself, in social situations and for acting appropriately based on that understanding.

socialization: The process by which a person learns the deeply held assumptions that make up the heart of a culture.

socialized leader: A leader who uses power to serve higher goals that benefit the organization, other leaders, and followers.

soft power: Power based on the leader's personality characteristics and the personal relationships the leader has with followers; also called *personal power.*

sponsorship: The degree to which the leader supports or backs a follower.

stages of change theory: A model that presents a series of stages representing differing degrees of behavioral change.

star or exemplary follower: A follower who thinks critically with positive energy and active engagement.

stereotyping: Having exaggerated or irrational negative images or beliefs about members of certain groups.

storming stage: The stage of team development in which team members resist one another and advance conflicting ideas.

strategic contingencies theory: A theory that examines how power is gained and lost by various parts of an organization and how such power distribution influences the organization's effectiveness.

Style 1 (S1) leadership: The situational leadership style that involves telling followers what to do, how to do it, when to do it, and where to do it; the "directing" style of leadership.

Style 2 (S2) leadership: The situational leadership style that combines highly directive and highly supportive behaviors; the "coaching" style of leadership.

Style 3 (S3) leadership: The situational leadership style that is high in supportive behavior and low in directing behavior; the "supporting" style of leadership.

Style 4 (S4) leadership: The situational leadership style that is low in both supportive and directive behavior; the "delegating" style of leadership.

supportive leadership: A type of leadership behavior that involves demonstrating concern for the followers' well-being and for each individual's needs.

syndemic: An aggregation of two or more diseases in a population in which some biological interaction exacerbates the negative effects of the diseases.

systems thinking: A leadership practice that emphasizes the system components required to meet an organization's short- and long-term needs.

task behavior: Behavior through which a leader spells out duties and responsibilities to followers; providing direction on what to do, who to do it, when to do it, where to do it, and how to do it.

task-motivated leadership style: The style of leadership most concerned with reaching a goal.

task structure: A situational variable based on the degree to which task requirements are clearly spelled out.

team: A group of interdependent individuals pursuing a common purpose.

team capacity: Shared or distributed team leadership that incorporates the leadership skills of all the team members.

teamship: The act of working together as a team within standards of behavior that each person within the team environment understands.

technical skills: Skills relating to the use of things, such as tools and equipment.

teleological reasoning: Moral thinking directed toward an end.

temperament: A person's nature, particularly with regard to emotionalism or excitability.

top executive team: A team that possesses a high level of autonomy in determining its mission and objectives, as well as in determining how it will function.

traditional authority: Authority based on tradition, established values, and social norms.

trait: A distinguishing characteristic or quality possessed by a person.

transactional leadership: Leadership that emphasizes setting clear objectives and goals for followers and using punishments and rewards to encourage compliance.

transformational leadership: A leadership model that emphasizes efforts to produce positive change in individuals and social systems—particularly, enhancing followers' motivation, morale, and performance.

trust: Belief or faith in another individual; a fundamental and foundational tenet of human relationships.

Tuckman's stages of team development: A sequence of four developmental stages—forming, storming, norming, and performing—through which teams and small groups progress; later versions of the model included additional stages of informing and adjourning.

uncertainty avoidance: The extent to which a culture uses established social norms to minimize uncertainty and increase predictability.

utilitarianism: A reasoning method based on comparing two or more options and choosing the one that does the most overall good for the most people.

valence: The perceived desirability of an outcome associated with a behavior.

value: An attitude or belief dealing with ethics, morals, or what is right and wrong.

values framework: A basic structure of principles and standards of behavior.

vertical dyad linkage (VDL): The pairing of leader (manager) and each follower (subordinate) in an individual relationship.

virtual team: A type of team in which members correspond chiefly through telecommunications technologies and rarely meet face to face.

virtue reasoning: A reasoning method that emphasizes the development of the character of the individual or community as the moral end.

Vroom-Jago model of leadership: A contingency model of leadership that identifies various levels of participative leadership, with each level having an impact on the quality and accountability of the decision being made.

yes-person/conformist follower: A follower who has positive energy and engagement but is dependent and does not think critically.

INDEX

Note: Italicized page locators refer to figures or tables in exhibits.

relationship between followers and, 194; task-oriented, 99–100

Leadership. *See also* Contingency theories of leadership; Followership; Path–goal theory of leadership; Power; Public health leadership; Situational leadership; Transactional leadership; Transformational leadership; Vroom-Jago model of leadership: achievement-oriented, 143, 159; art of, 28; assigned, 25, 39; authentic, 197–98, 287; common goal as prerequisite for, 24; competencies, 28–29, 39; defining, 23–24, 39; describing, 24–26; directive, 143, 145, 159; dyadic framing of, 193; emergent, 25, 39; ethical, 35–37, 40; full-range, 195, 208; global study of, 264–68; influence and, 350–51; integrative model of, 305–6, *306*; interactive, 276; laissez-faire, 203; management and, 40; management *vs.*, 26–28; moral, models of, 224, *224*; participative, 143, 146, 159; passive-avoidant, 195; personal qualities associated with, 28; power and, 25–26, 39; as process, 23–24; research on big five dimensions and, 92; science of, 28; servant, 287; social exchange theory and, 362; supportive, 143, 145, 159; team success and, 317; trait approach to, 84–85; trait research, 82–83; traits commonly associated with, 82; women in, 272–76

Leadership actions: Hill's team leadership model and, 332

Leadership attributes: similarities between followership attributes and, 290, 292

Leadership continuum, *101*, 101–2

Leadership for Physician Executives, 5, 6

Leadership Grid, 100–101, 104

Leadership-making model, 184

Leadership-making process: four key features in, 171; life cycle in, *172, 173*; phases of, 171–72

Leadership outcomes: measuring, 203

Leadership skills, 87–89, 103, 104; conceptual skills, 88–89, *89*, 103, 104; defined, 87; interpersonal or human skills, 87–88, *89*, 103, 104; technical skills, 87, *89*, 103, 104

Leadership styles, 112; autocratic, 100, 101, 104; behavioral approach and, 99–102; defined, 99; democratic, 100, 101, 104; "human relations," 101; integrative model and optimum matching of, 305–6, *306*; laissez-faire, 101; LPC score and, 120–21, 133; mentor, 386–88; path–goal theory and, 145; relationship-motivated, 120, 122; relationship-oriented, 295; research findings on, 101–2; situational leadership and, 124, 127–28; task-motivated, 120, 122; task-oriented, 295; team, 328; transactional, 173; transformational, 173; variation of situational leadership approach and, 329; of women, 275–76

Leadership substitutes: variable criteria for, 114

Leadership–Teamship–Followership Continuum: roles in, 300, 309

Leadership theories: flaws in, 194

Leadership training, 123

Leadership traits, 24–25, 85–87; intelligence, 85–86; personal integrity, 86–87; self-confidence and determination, 86

Leaders participation styles: in Vroom-Jago model of leadership, 150

Least-preferred coworker (LPC) scale: defined, 120

Ledlow, Gerald R., 323

"Left-brain" thinking patterns, 92

ABOUT THE AUTHORS

James W. Holsinger Jr., MD, PhD, has practiced leadership in a variety of organizations both in academia and in federal (civilian and military) and state government. He currently serves as the Charles T. Wethington Jr. Endowed Chair in the Health Sciences at the University of Kentucky. He has faculty appointments in preventive medicine and environmental health and health management and policy in the College of Public Health and in internal medicine, surgery, and anatomy in the College of Medicine.

Dr. Holsinger served for 26 years in the United States Department of Veterans Affairs. During this time, he held appointments as chief of staff and medical center director in various Veterans Affairs medical centers. In 1990, he was nominated by President George H. W. Bush and confirmed by the US Senate as the first presidentially appointed chief medical director of the Veterans Health Administration. In 1992, he became the first undersecretary for health in the Department of Veterans Affairs. From 1994 to 2003, he served as chancellor of the University of Kentucky Medical Center. In 2003, Kentucky Governor Ernie Fletcher appointed Dr. Holsinger as the first secretary of the Cabinet for Health and Family Services of the Commonwealth of Kentucky. After serving in that role for two years, Dr. Holsinger returned to the University of Kentucky faculty in 2005.

Dr. Holsinger served for more than 31 years in the US Army Reserve, serving as the commander of several hospitals, in addition to other appointments. His Army Reserve career culminated in 1989 with his assignment to the Joint Staff as assistant director for Logistics J-4 (Medical Support) and his promotion to major general in 1990. He retired from the US Army Reserve in 1993.

Dr. Holsinger received both his MD (1964) and his PhD (1968) from Duke University. He has been the recipient of numerous awards, including the Gold Medal of the American College of Healthcare Executives, the Exceptional Service Award and Distinguished Career Award of the Department of Veterans Affairs, the Superior Service Award of the Kentucky Cabinet for Health and Family Services, the Distinguished Service Medal and Legion of Merit of the US Army, the Order of Jerusalem of the World Methodist Council, and the Founder's Medal of the Association of Military Surgeons of the United States. Dr. Holsinger holds Mastership in the American College of Physicians.

Erik L. Carlton, DrPH, MS, is assistant professor of health systems management and policy and the director of the Master of Health Administration program at the University of Memphis School of Public Health. He also holds adjunct faculty appointments in preventive medicine and advanced practice and doctoral studies and is an affiliate faculty member with the Center for Health Systems Improvement at the University of Tennessee Health Sciences Center. Dr. Carlton's current research focuses on public health and healthcare leadership, the intersection of public health and primary care systems, and the integration of behavioral health into healthcare and public health systems. He teaches courses in healthcare management leadership, population health management, healthcare quality and outcomes, and health policy and the organization of health systems for the School of Public Health.

Dr. Carlton has nearly two decades of managerial and leadership experience in both private- and public-sector organizations. He has served as a consultant to numerous local health departments, hospital systems, and other healthcare organizations. He is a past chair of the Public Health Academics section of the Tennessee Public Health Association and a past treasurer of the Health Administration section of the American Public Health Association. Dr. Carlton is a behavioral health clinician licensed to practice in marriage and family therapy. He previously operated a private therapy practice, and he continues to consult with public health and healthcare organizations related to behavioral health integration and strategies. Dr. Carlton holds a doctor of public health degree in health services management and a master of science degree in family studies (with an emphasis in marriage and family therapy), both from the University of Kentucky.

ABOUT THE CONTRIBUTORS

Emmanuel D. Jadhav, DrPH, serves as assistant professor in the public health program at the Ferris State University College of Health Professions, where he teaches undergraduate and graduate courses in public health management, leadership, and global health. His research focuses on the application of health services research to organizational theory, leadership, and the role of public health in the care of elder and vulnerable adults. Dr. Jadhav earned graduate degrees in hospital management and zoology, a postgraduate diploma in medical law and ethics, and a doctor of public health degree.

Jennifer Redmond Knight, DrPH, is an assistant professor at the University of Kentucky College of Public Health and a member of the University of Kentucky Markey Cancer Center Cancer Control Program. Dr. Knight earned her BA in communications from Ouachita Baptist University in Arkadelphia, Arkansas; her MPH in epidemiology from the University of Kentucky College of Public Health in Lexington; and her DrPH in health services management from the University of Kentucky College of Public Health. Her work focuses on cancer prevention and control, with current emphases on lung cancer; policy, systems, and environmental changes; and leadership, partnerships, coalitions, and resource planning.

William A. Mase, DrPH, is an assistant professor at the Georgia Southern University Jiann-Ping Hsu College of Public Health. His primary line of research focuses on public health and associated healthcare professionals workforce development. His current active research is in the area of rural and critical access hospital operations, finance, and sustainability. He teaches master's and doctoral-level courses in health policy, regulation, and ethics.

Donna J. Schmutzler, DrPH, graduated from the University of Kentucky College of Public Health with a doctor of public health degree focused in the core area of health service management. Since graduation, she has traveled in developing countries, teaching and studying their healthcare systems. Professionally, she has served as a certified nurse-midwife, providing healthcare services to women and their unborn infants, and has taught students from various healthcare specialties in the clinical setting.

James R. Thobaben, PhD, is a professor of ethics and dean of the School of Theology and Formation at Asbury Theological Seminary. Prior to assuming his current position, he was vice president of a physical rehabilitation facility centered on the treatment of people with traumatic brain injuries and spinal cord injuries. His academic fields are bioethics, social ethics, and sociology of religion, and he has academic degrees from Oberlin College (BA), Yale University (MDiv and MPH), and Emory University (PhD). Dr. Thobaben served as visiting ethics scholar in molecular biology at the University of Missouri. In the past, he has been an occasional part-time professor at the University of Kentucky College of Public Health. He is the author of *Healthcare Ethics: A Comprehensive Christian Resource*, in addition to numerous articles.